Case-Based Interventional Neuroradiology

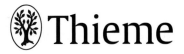

Your *Case-Based* book includes free bonus access to RadCases online!

RadCases is an extensive online database of key cases for your rounds, rotations and exams.

Simply visit http://RadCases.thieme.com **and, when prompted during the registration process, enter the scratch-off code below to get started today.**

This book cannot be returned once this panel has been scratched off.

Expand on your *Case-Based* book with access to 250 core cases online.

The scratch-off code above provides 12 months of access to an additional 250 neuro imaging cases via **RadCases.thieme.com**, our searchable online database of must-know cases.

You can also purchase e-subscriptions to key cases in other subspecialties by visiting **RadCases.thieme.com**.

Features of RadCases online include:

- A **user-friendly layout** that is ideal for self-study or quick reference
- Stress-free way to **study and review the most common and most critical cases**
- Clearly labeled, **high-quality radiographs** allow you to absorb key findings at-a-glance
- A **flexible search function** that lets you locate specific cases by age, differential diagnosis, modality, and more
- The ability to **bookmark cases** you want to revisit or '**hide' cases** you've already learned

System requirements for optimal use of RadCases online

	WINDOWS	**MAC**
Recommended Browser(s) **	Microsoft Internet Explorer 7.0 or later, Firefox 2.x, Firefox 3.x ** all browsers should have JavaScript enabled	Firefox 2.x, Firefox 3.x, Safari 3.x, Safari 4.x
Flash Player Plug-in	Flash Player 8 or Higher * * Mac users: ATI Rage 128 GPU does not support full-screen mode with hardware scaling	
Minimum Hardware Configurations	Intel® Pentium® II 450 MHz, AMD Athlon™ 600 MHz or faster processor (or equivalent) 128 MB of RAM	PowerPC® G3 500 MHz or faster processor Intel Core™ Duo 1.33 GHz or faster processor 128 MB of RAM
Recommended for optimal usage experience	Monitor resolutions: • Normal (4:3) 1024×768 or Higher • Widescreen (16:9) 1280×720 or Higher • Widescreen (16:10) 1440×900 or Higher DSL/Cable internet connection at a minimum speed of 384.0 Kbps or faster	

Case-Based Interventional Neuroradiology

Timo Krings, MD, PhD, FRCP (C)
Professor, Department of Medical Imaging, University of Toronto
Division of Neuroradiology, Toronto Western Hospital
Toronto, Canada
Professor, Department for Neuroradiology
University Hospital of the Technical University RWTH
Aachen, Germany
Practicien Attaché, Service de Neuroradiologie Diagnostique et Thérapeutique
CHU Le-Kremlin-Bicetre
Paris, France

Sasikhan Geibprasert, MD
Staff Neurointerventionalist, Department of Radiology
Ramathibodi Hospital
Mahidol University
Bangkok, Thailand
Fellow, Department of Diagnostic Imaging
Hospital for Sick Children
University of Toronto
Toronto, Canada

Karel G. ter Brugge, MD, FRCP (C)
The David Braley and Nancy Gordon Chair in Interventional Neuroradiology,
University of Toronto
Professor, Department of Medical Imaging and Surgery, University of Toronto
Head, Division of Neuroradiology, Toronto Western Hospital
Toronto, Canada

Thieme
New York • Stuttgart

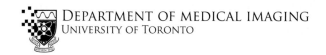
DEPARTMENT OF MEDICAL IMAGING
UNIVERSITY OF TORONTO

Thieme Medical Publishers, Inc.
333 Seventh Avenue
New York, NY 10001

Executive Editor: Timothy Y. Hiscock
Managing Editor: J. Owen Zurhellen IV
Editorial Assistant: Elizabeth D'Ambrosio
Editorial Director: Michael Wachinger
Production Editor: Marcy Ross, MPS Content Services
International Production Director: Andreas Schabert
Compositor: MPS Content Services, A Macmillan Company

Library of Congress Cataloging-in-Publication Data

Krings, Timo.
    Case-based interventional neuroradiology / Timo Krings, Sasikhan Geibprasert, Karel G. ter Brugge.
        p. ; cm.
    Includes bibliographical references and index.
    ISBN 978-1-60406-373-8 (alk. paper)
    1. Nervous system—Interventional radiology—Case studies. I. Geibprasert, Sasikhan. II. Brugge, K. G. ter (Karel G. ter) III. Title.
    [DNLM: 1. Cerebrovascular Disorders—radiotherapy—Case Reports. 2. Central Nervous System—blood supply—Case Reports. 3. Radiology, Interventional—methods—Case Reports. WL 355]
    RD594.15.K75 2011
    616.8'04754—dc22

                                                                    2010029281

Important note: Medical knowledge is ever-changing. As new research and clinical experience broaden our knowledge, changes in treatment and drug therapy may be required. The authors and editors of the material herein have consulted sources believed to be reliable in their efforts to provide information that is complete and in accord with the standards accepted at the time of publication. However, in view of the possibility of human error by the authors, editors, or publisher of the work herein or changes in medical knowledge, neither the authors, editors, nor publisher, nor any other party who has been involved in the preparation of this work, warrants that the information contained herein is in every respect accurate or complete, and they are not responsible for any errors or omissions or for the results obtained from use of such information. Readers are encouraged to confirm the information contained herein with other sources. For example, readers are advised to check the product information sheet included in the package of each drug they plan to administer to be certain that the information contained in this publication is accurate and that changes have not been made in the recommended dose or in the contraindications for administration. This recommendation is of particular importance in connection with new or infrequently used drugs.

Some of the product names, patents, and registered designs referred to in this book are in fact registered trademarks or proprietary names even though specific reference to this fact is not always made in the text. Therefore, the appearance of a name without designation as proprietary is not to be construed as a representation by the publisher that it is in the public domain.

Printed and bound in India by Replika Press Pvt. Ltd.

5 4 3 2

ISBN 978-1-60406-373-8

To our teachers

CONTENTS

PART III

Cranial Dural Arteriovenous Shunts

PART IV

Head and Neck Vascular Lesions

PART V

Tumors

PART VI

Trauma

PART VII

Stroke

FOREWORD

Writing a book at the beginning of the twenty-first century about interventional neuroradiology, still widely known as "endovascular neurosurgery," is an extraordinarily risky bet. It is therefore worth trying to determine whether the authors of this book, under the direction of Karel ter Brugge, have successfully met the challenge that they have set for themselves. Those wishing to disseminate specialized personal knowledge should not only be highly skilled in their specific field, but also, and especially, have the maturity that comes only with wide experience. Timo Krings, Sasikhan Geibprasert, and Karel ter Brugge are core members of Pierre Lasjaunias' famous school, and benefit from the vast experience they have obtained by working under his direction. The expertise of this team is thus innately based on exceptional radioanatomical and clinical foundations as well as on very human qualities that combine scientific rigor, honesty, and ethics.

Given the irreproachable quality of the information conveyed by such an elite team, globally esteemed and respected as they are, we may yet consider the technique that they have utilized in its presentation. Indeed, in this Internet era, with its capacity for the extraordinarily rapid, even "instant," transmission of information, the continuing relevance of the traditional printed book may be brought into question. Compared to scientific journals and especially information rendered on a website, the lag inherent in the printed book can contribute to the rapid obsolescence of the information being presented. This is especially true since the continuing evolution of interventional neuroradiology is itself extraordinarily rapid. Closely dependent on technological progress, interventional neuroradiology takes a quantum leap forward with each technological innovation.

The techniques of endovascular interventional neuroradiology have evolved steadily towards ever-smaller applications and the emergence of the third dimension has radically transformed their precision and thus the safety of our interventions. The miniaturization of our surgical instruments has greatly contributed to our progress, and the ongoing development of nanotechnology will very likely enable further innovations that are even harder to visualize today.

It is in this particularly difficult context that the brilliance of this book's design stands out. Its major importance lies in the fact that it is actually not a traditional textbook, because the authors have clearly taken the gamble of trying to stimulate personal reflection on the reader's part. The chapters are in fact a succession of carefully described and analyzed observations that consequently require a direct and thoughtful participation. On examining these various observations, which range over virtually the entire field of vascular pathology, readers are challenged to methodically ask themselves the key questions that absolutely must be answered before choosing a therapeutic approach. Selecting the optimum strategy, that is, the one most effective and least hazardous to the patient, is unquestionably the core of the therapeutic process. Confronted with daily reality, readers are thus constantly forced to practice selecting the best indication as well as the most appropriate therapeutic technique.

Technical knowledge is indeed indispensible, but alone it is insufficient for successful implementation without an exacting intellectual process. Given that there are frequently multiple therapeutic possibilities, the approaches advocated by the authors are not didactically imposed but are carefully argued and thus manifestly well justified, admirably demonstrating the authors' excellent instructional abilities. This orientation of the book's content is crucial, because at the present time the poor quality of therapeutic indications chosen by many surgical teams around the world is certainly the Achilles' heel of early twenty-first-century interventional neuroradiology.

This overarching concern for the proper choice of therapeutic indications is highlighted by the authors' honesty and courage in describing the complications that can arise even within the best teams. These observations, carefully selected, analyzed, and described will enable readers to become aware of the actual risks to which patients are exposed, as they learn at the same time to make a timely diagnosis and take appropriate measures to best mitigate any adverse consequences.

In the same vein, this book is remarkable for its rational approach in the deepest sense of the word. Indeed, ongoing development is so rapid due to the continual introduction of new surgical instruments that the top teams lack sufficient time to properly assess the actual clinical outcomes of their interventions. This is why many procedures are being performed to "experiment" with new, and apparently improved, surgical instruments, whereas we know very well that the outcomes of clinical developments in the medium and long term can be mediocre or frankly even poor despite "satisfactory radioanatomic controls."

It is noteworthy that the authors have also taken on the challenge of covering virtually the entire spectrum of pathological conditions accessible to treatment by interventional neuroradiology. Their discriminating choice of observations has enabled them to cover practically all the situations encountered, even the most difficult ones. The systematic nature of the book's organization enables the reader to find information quickly on any given observation. Of course, this leads to some repetition, but we know that repetition of important elements is the basis of a well-organized course of instruction. The sections entitled "Pearls and Pitfalls" are highly relevant. For example, when the authors write that skin disinfection is an essential step for infiltration or intraspinal injections, it should not be taken lightly, because it is absolutely true. The repetition of "minor" steps in a protocol can lead to over-familiarity and make us forget the need for their rigorous application. Many readers will also appreciate the bibliographical sources, available for each clinical case, which provide immediate references relevant to the case being considered.

This book thus perfectly reflects the immense clinical, radioanatomical, technical. and human qualities of the team of Timo Krings, Sasikhan Geibprasert, and Karel ter Brugge. It is therefore not only useful but, in my opinion, really essential that all those wishing to train in interventional neuroradiology should read and reread this book, taking time for contemplation as needed, to gradually reach the level of maturity indispensable to the practice of this exciting but extremely difficult specialization. When making a difficult decision, many practitioners will benefit from reading the chapter that corresponds to the case at hand, and they will certainly find it helpful in reaching their decision. This book will most certainly contribute to the improvement of outcomes in interventional neuroradiology.

I would therefore like to congratulate the authors and to thank them warmly for making this resource for training and development available to all those with an interest in brain and spinal pathology. It will enable them to make real progress in providing the patients in their care with the greatest possible benefit.

Luc Picard, Prof. Dr. Dr. h.c.
Professor Emeritus of Neuroradiology
Honorary President of the World Federation of Interventional and Therapeutic Neuroradiology
President of the World Federation of Neuroradiological Societies

PREFACE

Interventional neuroradiology has become an integral component of the multidisciplinary management of patients with disorders of the head, neck, and spine. Patient acceptance and clinical outcome have proved better with minimally invasive procedures than with traditional open surgical approaches. Yet, we need to be vigilant to ensure that the new treatment techniques are indeed enhancing patient care and are carried out with the full realization that other treatment options may exist.

The authors of this book have a long experience with interventional neuroradiologic techniques in Asia, Europe, and North America, which will benefit our readers. Contributions by other experts in the field have further enhanced the comprehensive coverage of all aspects of interventional neuroradiology.

The unique strength of this book is that it also provides the background information on which the principles of treatment are based. In each case report, the clinical and imaging findings are interpreted so that the reader can fully understand and formulate the reasons for the treatment and the specific goals to be achieved.

The authors have made a deliberate attempt to be unbiased in their choice of materials used, to provide background information regarding their choices under each circumstance, and to outline the risks and benefits of their choices versus those of other options. Safety is paramount in this field, and proper training and continued education are the pillars on which the best possible patient care rests. This is particularly relevant in our field, as more and more asymptomatic patients are referred whose disorders are incidentally discovered. Several case reports describe in detail how to manage such situations, highlighting once again the importance of knowing the natural history of the diseases we are asked to treat so that clinicians will offer the best choice for their patients in their overall risk management strategy.

We did not select exotic, bizarre, or exceptional cases, nor did we include "heroic" procedures (being well aware that the "hero" in those procedures is never the doctor but rather the patient). Instead, we chose to describe those cases that the interventionalist will see in his or her daily practice. Periprocedural complications do occur, even in the best hands, the difference being that experienced practitioners will recognize them early and know how to best manage them. This is why we added examples of "classic" periprocedural complications.

We believe that this book fills a unique void in the field of interventional neuroradiology in that it provides extensive information about the pathologic mechanisms involved in the diseases that we are asked to treat and describes in detail the latest treatment options available. We hope that you and your patients will derive the full benefit of our experience as described herein.

CONTRIBUTORS

Ronit Agid, MD
Staff Neuroradiologist, Division of Neuroradiology
Toronto Western Hospital
University of Toronto
Toronto, Canada

Florian Elgeti, MD
Staff Radiologist, Department of Radiology
Charité Universitätsmedizin Berlin
Berlin, Germany

Richard I. Farb, MD
Staff Neuroradiologist, Division of Neuroradiology
Toronto Western Hospital
University of Toronto
Toronto, Canada

Sasikhan Geibprasert, MD
Staff Neurointerventionalist, Department of
    Radiology
Ramathibodi Hospital
Mahidol University
Bangkok, Thailand
Fellow, Department of Diagnostic Radiology
Hospital for Sick Children
University of Toronto
Toronto, Canada

Pakorn Jiarakongmun, MD
Staff Neurointerventionalist, Department of
    Radiology
Ramathibodi Hospital
Mahidol University
Bangkok, Thailand

Timo Krings, MD, PhD
Staff Neuroradiologist, Division of Neuroradiology
Toronto Western Hospital
University of Toronto
Toronto, Canada

Pierre L. Lasjaunias, MD, PhD [Deceased]
Head of Neuroradiology
CHU Le-Kremlin-Bicetre
Paris, France

Vitor Mendes Pereira, MD, MSc
Head of Interventional Neuroradiology
University Hospital
Geneva, Switzerland

Sirintara Pongpech, MD
Head, Department of Radiology
Chief, Interventional Radiology Section
Ramathibodi Hospital
Mahidol University
Bangkok, Thailand

Roger M. L. Smith, MD
Staff Neuroradiologist, Division of Neuroradiology
Toronto Western Hospital
University of Toronto
Toronto, Canada

Karel G. ter Brugge, MD
The David Braley and Nancy Gordon Chair in
    Interventional Neuroradiology
Head, Division of Neuroradiology
Toronto Western Hospital
University of Toronto
Toronto, Canada

Jan E. Vandevenne, MD, PhD
Interventional Radiologist
Ziekenhuizen-Oost-Limburg, Genk
University of Hasselt
Diepenbeek, Belgium

Linda Vanormelingen, MD, PhD
Department of Morphology
University of Hasselt
Diepenbeek, Belgium

Robert A. Willinsky, MD
Staff Neuroradiologist, Division of Neuroradiology
Toronto Western Hospital
University of Toronto
Toronto, Canada

CASE 1

Case Description

Clinical Presentation

A 54-year-old man presents with the sudden acute onset of headache, nausea, and vomiting. When he arrives in the emergency department, he has a decreased level of consciousness and is not fully oriented. Emergency CT is performed.

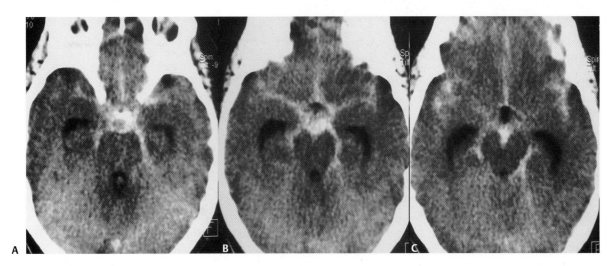

Fig. 1.1 (A–C) Unenhanced axial CT reveals nearly symmetric hyperdensity within the basal cisterns, corresponding to diffuse SAH. Prominent size of the temporal horns of the lateral ventricles is noted. Note the small round hypodense area within the hyperdense clot at the level of the prepontine cistern, suspicious for a basilar tip aneurysm.

Radiologic Studies

CT

CT demonstrated a basal subarachnoid hemorrhage (SAH) with a nearly symmetric distribution, a small blood clot in the fourth ventricle, and no evidence of intraparenchymal hemorrhage. Enlargement of the ventricles (especially the temporal horns) was noted. Within the prepontine cistern, a focal round area without subarachnoid blood was seen (**Fig. 1.1**). CTA confirmed the suspicion of a single basilar tip aneurysm, and angiography with the intention to treat was performed during the same session.

DSA

Injection of the left vertebral artery demonstrated a basilar tip aneurysm. 3D rotational angiography revealed an irregular shape with a cranial daughter aneurysm (or bleb), which was regarded as the probable point of rupture. The aneurysm size was 12 × 10 × 9 mm. The neck of the aneurysm was considered to be moderately wide (5 mm). A cranial fusion–type of basilar apex was present, and the most proximal portions of both P1 segments were incorporated in the neck. No focal vasospasm was seen (**Fig. 1.2**).

1

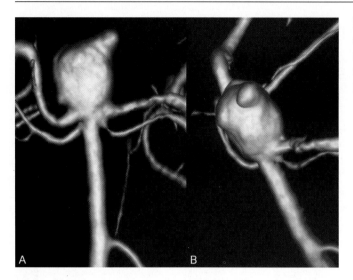

Fig. 1.2 DSA of the vertebral artery. 3D reconstruction in **(A)** AP and **(B)** oblique lateral views shows a basilar tip aneurysm with a rather wide neck. A daughter bleb is noted at the left posterior aspect of the aneurysm dome.

Diagnosis

Ruptured aneurysm of the basilar tip

Treatment

EQUIPMENT

- Standard 6F access (puncture needle, 6F vascular sheath)
- A 6F multipurpose catheter (Guider Soft Tip; Boston Scientific, Natick, MA) with continuous flush and a 0.035-in hydrophilic guidewire (Terumo, Somerset, NJ)
- A 45-degree angled microcatheter with a 1.7F tip and a 0.0165-in inner lumen (Excelsior SL 10; Boston Scientific) with a 0.014-in guidewire (Synchro 14; Boston Scientific)
- Coil selection: for framing, GDC 10 soft 360-degree coils 1 mm × 20 cm, 10 mm × 20 cm, and 9 mm × 20 cm; for subsequent filling and finishing, GDC 10 soft 2D SR coils 7 mm × 10 cm, 5 mm × 8 cm and two coils 4 mm × 8 cm (Boston Scientific)
- Contrast material
- Heparin

DESCRIPTION

The 6F multipurpose catheter was placed in the distal vertebral artery. Control injections demonstrated good flow and no vasospasm surrounding the guiding catheter. Following a roadmap in the working projection, the microcatheter was advanced via the micro-guidewire and carefully placed in the lower one-third of the aneurysm. Here, the first coils were deployed, with care taken not to advance the coils into the cranial daughter aneurysm. With the first three complex-shaped coils, a stable frame for subsequent filling of the aneurysm could be established. Control runs demonstrated no protrusion of coils into the parent vessels and good framing of the aneurysm neck. Subsequently, the microcatheter was advanced as far distally into the aneurysm as possible to continue coiling from the dome to the neck with 2D coils, which allowed dense packing of the aneurysm with only two coil loops (of smaller, soft coils) protruding into the daughter aneurysm. If protrusion beyond the frame was noted caudally, the coils were repositioned. A control run demonstrated complete exclusion from the aneurysm and a dense coil mesh (**Fig. 1.3**). No thromboembolic complications were noted, and all distal vessels were well preserved. The procedure was carried out with the patient on heparin (5000 IE), which was not reversed following the procedure.

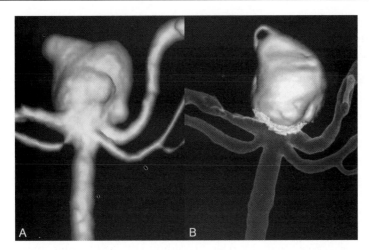

Fig. 1.3 3D rotational angiography in PA view **(A)** before and **(B)** following coil embolization demonstrates the dense coil mesh. No contrast material is noted entering the aneurysm. Only a few loops are seen in the daughter bleb.

Discussion

Background

Saccular aneurysms are the most frequently encountered form of aneurysm. They arise at arterial bifurcations and resemble berry-like outpouchings of the vessel wall. Their etiology and pathophysiology are complex and poorly understood. Although genetic factors likely contribute to their development, other factors, such as aging, elevated blood pressure, blood shear stresses, and cigarette smoking, are also thought to contribute to the formation and/or rupture of aneurysms.

The average annual risk for SAH is 10 to 21 per 100,000 people, with higher incidence rates encountered in Finland and Japan. Risk factors for hemorrhage include female gender, increasing age, previous symptomatic aneurysm, larger size, and location in the posterior circulation.

The prognosis following untreated aneurysmal SAH is poor; in a community-based study, the mortality rates were 12% before patients reached the hospital, 43% within the first week, and 56% at day 30 if the aneurysm was left untreated. In a meta-analysis of untreated ruptured aneurysms performed by Heros in 1990, significant morbidity and mortality after the first hemorrhage were estimated to be 50%, with a further mortality of 35% after the second bleed. The risk for rebleeding without treatment is ~1% per day for the first 9 days, increases to 4% at day 10, then fluctuates at ~ 2 to 3% per day during days 11 through 15. The cumulative risk for rebleeding is ~20% in the first 2 weeks and 30 to 50% in 6 months.

Aneurysms typically arise at branch points on the parent artery. The branch point may be formed by the origin of a side branch from the parent artery (e.g., posterior communicating artery) or by subdivision of a main arterial trunk into two trunks (e.g., middle cerebral artery or terminal internal carotid artery bifurcation, tip of the basilar trunk). Sidewall aneurysms are rare and if present usually arise at a turn or curve in the artery and point in the direction that the blood would have flowed if the curve were not present. At both the branch points and the curves, local alterations in intravascular hemodynamics are present that exert high shear stress forces on those regions that receive the greatest force of the pulse wave. Therefore, the aneurysm dome typically points in the direction of the maximal hemodynamic thrust in the pre-aneurysmal segment of the parent artery. Aneurysms that are encountered on a straight, nonbranching segment of an intracranial artery should raise the suspicion of a dissecting process because saccular aneurysms are infrequently encountered at these sites. More than 90% of all saccular intracranial aneurysms are located at one of the following five sites: (1) internal carotid artery at the origin of the posterior communicating artery; (2) junction of the anterior cerebral and anterior communicating arteries; (3) proximal bifurcation of the middle cerebral artery; (4) terminal bifurcation of the basilar artery into the posterior cerebral arteries; and (5) terminal bifurcation of the carotid artery into the anterior cerebral and middle cerebral arteries. In the anterior circulation, other common sites of aneurysms are the origins of the ophthalmic, superior hypophyseal, and anterior choroidal arteries. In the posterior circulation, the origin of the posterior inferior cerebellar, anterior inferior cerebellar, and superior cerebellar arteries and the junction of the basilar and vertebral arteries are likely sites of aneurysm formation.

Noninvasive Imaging Workup

PHYSICAL EXAMINATION

- Patients typically report the abrupt onset of the "worst headache of their life." Loss of consciousness, meningismus, focal neurologic deficits, and nausea may be present.
- Many patients report earlier, milder headaches over the days preceding the acute event, most likely representing small "sentinel bleeds" from an unstable aneurysm.
- On physical examination, patients are photophobic and demonstrate nuchal rigidity.
- Cerebrospinal fluid (CSF) analysis is necessary in patients whose CT is negative but in whom an SAH is strongly suspected.
- The rate of rebleeding is significantly higher in patients with poor overall clinical status than in those with good clinical status.

CT/CTA

- In the acute setting of patients with the "worst headache of their life," CT is the first method of choice to detect SAH and the aneurysm, following CTA.
- The presence of additional intraparenchymal hemorrhage (with or without mass effect) and/or acute hydrocephalus will prompt emergency neurosurgical treatment in the appropriate clinical setting.
- In patients with large aneurysms, the aneurysm "ghost" can be seen within the subarachnoid blood as a focal area of SAH sparing.
- CTA has a high sensitivity and specificity, and in most instances, the treatment decision can be based on the 3D reconstruction of CTA; however, if CTA is negative in the presence of a classic SAH, DSA is still necessary.

MRI/MRA

- In the acute setting, MRI or MRA is rarely needed. FLAIR-weighted sequences will demonstrate the subarachnoid blood with a slightly higher accuracy than that of CT as a high signal (unsuppressed CSF) within the subarachnoid spaces. In later stages following an SAH, pial hemosiderosis can be seen that is best detected by susceptibility or T2*-weighted sequences.

Invasive Imaging Workup

- Diagnostic cerebral angiography combined with 3D rotational angiography remains the gold standard for evaluating patients presenting with SAH and suspected intracranial aneurysms. DSA and 3D DSA have the highest temporal and spatial resolution and provide the most precise depiction of intracranial vessel morphology and hemodynamic analysis. It is therefore still needed in CTA-negative cases of SAH. If the quality of the noninvasive images is suboptimal, treatment decisions can be obtained after careful analysis of the angiography. For aneurysmal detection and pre-therapeutic planning, 3D rotational angiography is considered the gold standard. If not available, additional oblique views with magnification should be obtained for aneurysm detection and detailed pre-therapeutic morphologic analysis. Analysis must include location of the aneurysm, incorporation of vessels in the aneurysm neck, width of the neck, size of the aneurysm, presence and location of associated daughter aneurysms, vasospasm, and additional aneurysms. Should the studies prove negative for aneurysm, they must then address vasculitis, cranial dural arteriovenous fistulae, and sinus thrombosis as possible alternate etiologies for SAH.

Differential Diagnosis

- Although more than 80% of SAHs are caused by aneurysmal rupture, other sources of SAH include trauma (typically more peripheral and local and associated with other sequelae of trauma), arteriovenous malformation hemorrhage (classically associated with intraparenchymal bleed), dural arteriovenous fistula with cortical venous reflux (especially a dural arteriovenous fistula within the posterior fossa, which can present with SAH).
- Perimesencephalic SAH: Patients are classically neurologically intact, with only slight nuchal rigidity and a small amount of subarachnoid blood layered within and adjacent to the perimesencephalic cistern.

Treatment Options

CONSERVATIVE OR MEDICAL MANAGEMENT

- Given the high rate of rebleeding, conservative management of an acutely ruptured aneurysm is not recommended unless the patient's clinical condition precludes active intervention. Aneurysms should in principle be treated as soon as possible.
- In the time interval between arrival in the hospital and treatment, principles of general care include management of headache (paracetamol with or without codeine). Hypertension should not be treated aggressively because it may act as a compensatory mechanism for the increased intracranial pressure.

SURGICAL TREATMENT

- Whether to clip or to coil is extensively discussed in Case 2. In the present case of a patient with a large basilar tip aneurysm, the endovascular option is undoubtedly in most centers the therapy of choice.
- Treatment of hydrocephalus may be necessary in the acute setting together with extraventricular drainage.
- An indication for emergency surgical intervention is an aneurysm associated with a space-occupying hematoma in a patient with a decreased level of consciousness.

ENDOVASCULAR TREATMENT

- Endovascular options are considered the method of first choice in ruptured aneurysms of the posterior circulation.
- The general principle of treating these aneurysms is endosaccular deployment of platinum spirals (coils), either with or without the assistance of devices such as balloons or stents (see Cases 5 and 6).
- In many cases, the bleb (daughter aneurysm) indicates the point of rupture and therefore a segment of the aneurysm sac that is weaker than the remainder. Coiling of this bleb has to be done either very carefully or not at all. In the present case, we allowed only one loop of a single coil to enter the presumed point of rupture to avoid periprocedural repeated rupture. In cases in which the bleb is located proximal to or very close to the neck, surgery may be indicated rather than coil embolization.

Possible Complications

- Periprocedural hemorrhage
- Thromboembolic complications
- Recanalization of the aneurysm

Published Literature on Treatment Options

Given the high risk for rebleeding with its associated mortality, there is no question that acutely ruptured aneurysms should be treated. Concerning the timing of treatment, in most centers an acute treatment is advocated. Even with an early and successful intervention, SAH is a devastating disease, and the risk for a poor outcome is high. Factors associated with a poor outcome are poor clinical status on admission, a large SAH, increasing age, posterior circulation location of the aneurysm, and preexisting medical conditions. Neurologic complications due to hydrocephalus and vasospasm and systemic complications with infections, cardiac problems (arryhthmia, myocardial infarction), or pulmonary edema may all lead to a poor outcome.

Basilar apex aneurysms arise where the posterior cerebral arteries branch off from the tip of the basilar artery. At the aneurysm site, the blood flow changes from vertical to nearly horizontal, so these aneurysms project upward in the direction of the long axis of the basilar artery. The majority of patients with basilar tip aneurysms display a relatively short basilar artery (caudal fusion disposition), with the tip of the basilar artery near the caudal end of the interpeduncular fossa. The neck of the basilar aneurysm is preferentially located at the caudal part of the fusion. The largest and most important perforators to arise from the basilar tip are the posterior thalamoperforating arteries (retromammillary arteries). These originate from the basilar tip and P1 segment, enter the brain through the posterior perforated substance in the interpeduncular fossa medial to the cerebral peduncles, and ascend through the midbrain to the thalamus. On occasion, a single P1 perforator may supply both thalami. Typically, the caudal portions of P1 supply their own sides, whereas the cranial segments of P1 may supply bilateral territories. In patients with caudal fusions of the basilar artery, the posterior communicating artery flows caudally and is likely to supply diencephalic-mesencephalic territories. In patients with cranial fusion of the basilar artery, there is likely to be a basilar contribution to the supply of this area. The risks from occlusion of these vital perforating vessels include visual loss, weakness, memory deficits, autonomic and endocrine imbalance, abnormal movements, diplopia, and depression of consciousness. Given the risk for surgical perforator occlusion, especially in larger aneurysms, endovascular approaches have been widely adopted to treat basilar apex aneurysms.

The aim of endovascular treatment with platinum coils is to permanently occlude the aneurysm lumen based on the following assumptions: Immediately after the coils are deployed in the aneurysm, thrombocytes adhere to the coil loops because of changes in hemodynamics and flow velocity followed by fibrous organization of the primary thrombus over the course of the following days. According to the theory, mechanical stability is further increased over the next weeks by collagenous extracellular matrix and granulation tissue between the coil loops that may then create a foundation for neoendothelial sprouting from healthy vessel walls. Although these theoretical considerations seem appealing, experimental results are not always accordant; the newly developed thrombus, which mainly consists of erythrocytes captured within thin fibrin strings, may not be able to withstand the arterial blood pressure and the presence of fibrinolytic agents in the circulating blood. Moreover, physiologic thrombus retraction, the physical effects of the so-called water hammer effect on the coil material, and the possible presence of old thrombus within the aneurysm dome into which coil loops may be shifted, can lead to a delayed aneurysm regrowth. Despite the potential of delayed recanalization of the aneurysm, the rebleeding rates of sufficiently coiled aneurysms are low, and endovascular treatment of cerebral aneurysms is an established option in the management of ruptured aneurysms.

PEARLS AND PITFALLS

- The average annual risk for SAH is 10 to 21 per 100,000 people per year.
- Untreated ruptured aneurysms have a poor prognosis. Rebleeding is associated with a high mortality rate and occurs more frequently in patients with poor clinical grades and within the first 48 hours following the acute SAH. Early treatment is therefore recommended.
- Aneurysms are classically found at branching points of the large basal intradural arteries.
- "Thunderclap" headaches are the most common presenting symptom and should lead to prompt CT and (if negative) CSF analysis.
- DSA should be employed if CTA is negative in the setting of a classic SAH.
- Coiling of basilar tip aneurysms is safe and effective in preventing recurrent hemorrhage. Follow-up controls are mandatory to detect reopening, especially in large aneurysms.

Further Reading

Bederson JB, Connolly ES Jr, Batjer HH, et al; American Heart Association. Guidelines for the management of aneurysmal subarachnoid hemorrhage: a statement for healthcare professionals from a special writing group of the Stroke Council, American Heart Association. Stroke 2009;40(3):994–1025

Brisman JL, Song JK, Newell DW. Cerebral aneurysms. N Engl J Med 2006;355(9):928–939

Guglielmi G, Viñuela F, Dion J, Duckwiler G. Electrothrombosis of saccular aneurysms via endovascular approach. Part 2: Preliminary clinical experience. J Neurosurg 1991;75(1):8–14

Guglielmi G, Viñuela F, Sepetka I, Macellari V. Electrothrombosis of saccular aneurysms via endovascular approach. Part 1: Electrochemical basis, technique, and experimental results. J Neurosurg 1991;75(1):1–7

Heros RC. Intracranial aneurysms. A review. Minn Med 1990;73(10):27–32

Pakarinen S. Incidence, aetiology, and prognosis of primary subarachnoid haemorrhage. A study based on 589 cases diagnosed in a defined urban population during a defined period. Acta Neurol Scand 1967;43(Suppl 29):29, 1–28

Peluso JP, van Rooij WJ, Sluzewski M, Beute GN. Coiling of basilar tip aneurysms: results in 154 consecutive patients with emphasis on recurrent haemorrhage and re-treatment during mid- and long-term follow-up. J Neurol Neurosurg Psychiatry 2008;79(6):706–711

Sellar R, Molyneux A. ISAT: The International Subarachnoid Aneurysm Trial. Lessons and update. Interventional Neuroradiology 2008;14:50–51

van Gijn J, Kerr RS, Rinkel GJ. Subarachnoid haemorrhage. Lancet 2007;369(9558):306–318

CASE 2

Case Description

Clinical Presentation

A 51-year-old man has an acute onset of headache without loss of consciousness and without focal neurologic deficits. On arrival in the emergency department, he exhibits photophobia and nuchal rigidity. Emergency CT demonstrates a diffuse symmetric subarachnoid hemorrhage (SAH) and no evidence of hydrocephalus. CTA reveals a multilobulated anterior communicating artery aneurysm. Angiography is performed.

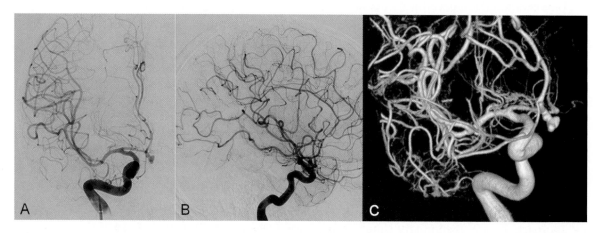

Fig. 2.1 DSA. Right ICA angiogram in **(A)** AP and **(B)** lateral views and **(C)** 3D reconstruction reveals a lobulated outpouching at the anterior communicating artery pointing anteroinferiorly, representing a ruptured aneurysm.

Radiologic Studies

DSA

After injection into the right internal carotid artery (ICA), the anterior communicating artery aneurysm was identified pointing anteriorly and inferiorly with at least three lobules, each measuring ~4 mm. The neck of the aneurysm measured 3.8 mm. A rather acute angle between the ICA termination and A1 was present (**Fig. 2.1**).

Diagnosis

Ruptured aneurysm of the anterior communicating artery

Treatment

EQUIPMENT

- Standard 6F access (puncture needle, 6F vascular sheath)
- A 6F multipurpose catheter (Envoy; Cordis, Warren, NJ) with continuous flush and a 0.035-in hydrophilic guidewire (Terumo, Somerset, NJ)
- A 45-degree angled microcatheter with a 1.7F tip and a 0.0165-in inner lumen (Excelsior SL 10; Boston Scientific, Natick, MA) with a 0.014-in guidewire (Synchro 14; Boston Scientific)

- Coil selection: for framing of the distal (bilobed) portion, GDC 360-degree soft coil 5 mm × 9 cm (Boston Scientific) and subsequent filling with DeltaPaq coil 3 × 8 (Micrus, San Jose, CA); for the proximal portion, MicruSphere 3 mm × 5.4 cm (Micrus) and subsequent filling with DeltaPaq coil 2 mm × 2 cm (Micrus)
- Contrast material
- Heparin

DESCRIPTION

The 6F multipurpose catheter was advanced into the right distal ICA. Over a J-shaped micro-guidewire, the acutely angulated A1 segment was catheterized by retracting the J-shaped guidewire from the M1 segment to hook up into the A1 segment and then slowly advancing both the microcatheter and the guidewire. To navigate the microcatheter around the acute curve, the guidewire was subsequently placed into the right distal A2 segment. Once the microcatheter was within the A1 segment, the guidewire was retracted and navigated into the aneurysm. The slack was removed from the system, and the catheter was slowly navigated into the distal lobulated part of the aneurysm. The first two coils were aimed at framing the distal part of the aneurysm. This part was then filled with DeltaPaq coils, which allowed good filling of the distal part of the aneurysm. The catheter was then gently retracted, and the second part of the aneurysm was coiled. Given its rounder shape, a MicruSphere coil was chosen for framing, followed by DeltaPaq coils for subsequent filling. The final result demonstrated complete occlusion of the aneurysm and no missing branches (**Fig. 2.2**). The patient had an uneventful recovery.

Discussion

Background

For ruptured aneurysms, two major treatment options are available: neurosurgical clip ligation and endovascular coil treatment. Following its first clinical use in 1990, coil embolization was primarily reserved for those aneurysms that were difficult to access surgically and for patients with poor clinical grades. Since publication of the results of the International Subarachnoid Aneurysm Trial (ISAT), however, the endovascular treatment of cerebral aneurysms has gained more acceptance and is now regarded in most centers as the technique of choice for the treatment of ruptured aneurysms. The ISAT demonstrated that patients with aneurysms rated by both the neurosurgeon and the interventional neuroradiologist as possible candidates for their respective therapies had a better outcome

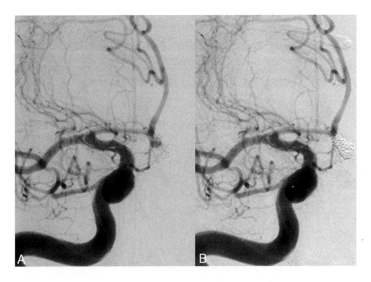

Fig. 2.2 Right ICA angiogram in the working projection following embolization of **(A)** the distal and **(B)** the proximal compartments. No filling of the aneurysm sac with contrast is seen after the coiling.

concerning morbidity, dependency, and mortality when they underwent endovascular treatment. Approximately 10,000 patients with acute SAH were screened; of those, slightly more than 20% (*n* = 2143) were included in the study as eligible for both treatment options and were randomized to either surgery or coiling. The rate of death or dependency was 23.7% in the endovascular group and 30.6% in the surgical group at 1 year, resulting in relative and absolute risk reductions for death or dependency after endovascular treatment of 22.6% (95% CI [confidence interval], 8.9–34.2%) and 6.9% (95% CI, 2.5–11.3%), respectively. The study concluded that outcome in terms of survival free of disability at 1 year was better with endovascular options. The recently published long-term results (mean follow-up, 9 years; range, 6–14 years) confirm the positive trend for endovascular treatment options, with a significantly decreased risk for death at 5 years in the endovascular group (relative risk, 0.77; 95% CI, 0.61–0.98; *p* = 0.03). However, the proportions of survivors at 5 years who were independent did not differ between the two groups: endovascular 83% (626 of 755) and neurosurgical 82% (584 of 713). The risk for rebleeding was higher in the endovascular group (11 rebleeds vs. 2); however, it was still very low, with a cumulative risk for rebleeding after 6 years of ~1%.

Noninvasive and Invasive Imaging Workup

- Imaging workup (CT, CTA, or DSA) must detail imaging features that are important in deciding whether to treat by neurosurgical or endovascular approaches and, if an endovascular approach is chosen, what kinds of devices and techniques to employ for the procedure.
- Brain
  - Hydrocephalus
  - Intraparenchymal blood, mass effect, midline shift
  - Fisher grade of SAH and blood distribution
  - Edema/swelling
- Arterial access
  - Tortuosity of vessels at the neck
  - Calcifications or stenoses of major arteries supplying brain
  - Arterial variations
- Aneurysm morphology
  - Size, configuration, and direction of the aneurysm dome; presence or absence and location of aneurysm blebs (daughter aneurysms)
  - Neck morphology, including width of the aneurysm neck, incorporation of parent vessel, perforator or branching vessel into the neck of the aneurysm
  - Calcifications of the aneurysm neck or its dome
  - Location of adjacent perforating arteries, presence of local or global vasospasm
  - Other aneurysms

Treatment Options

SURGICAL TREATMENT

- Microsurgical clip ligation is considered a durable treatment for ruptured intracranial aneurysms; its success is based on surgical accessibility.
- Surgical access to the middle cerebral artery, the ICA termination, and the posterior communicating artery is relatively easily obtained. Access to the anterior communicating artery allows, in addition to clip ligation, fenestration of the lamina terminalis, which may reduce the number of cases of shunt-dependent hydrocephalus. Access to the posterior circulation, or the supra-ophthalmic ICA, is considered more challenging.

- Anterior communicating artery aneurysms that are pointing caudally and anteriorly are considered to be more readily accessible than those pointing cranially and posteriorly.
- Surgery during the acute phase of SAH in a patient with an edematous brain may require more brain retraction, especially if the aneurysm has a deep location.

ENDOVASCULAR TREATMENT

- Endovascular coil embolization is an established alternative to surgical treatment options.
- Its success is mainly based on aneurysm morphology (size of the aneurysm, neck-to-dome ratio, perforators at the neck) and arterial access (tortuosity of vessels).

Possible Complications

See also Cases 6, 8, 9, and 10.

- Thromboembolic complications
- Periprocedural rupture
- Unproven long-term stability

Published Literature on Treatment Options

The percentage of patients harboring a residual neck or body remnant of the aneurysm after coil treatment ranges between 5 and 20%, and 15 to 35% of patients will in time demonstrate recanalization of the aneurysm. Consequently, the risk for rebleeding is higher after coiling than after clipping. As late rebleeding occurs more often in patients treated by coil embolization (0.152%/y in ISAT, up to 0.3%/y in the literature vs. 0.03% for surgery), the question arises whether in younger patients with a longer life expectancy the superiority of the initial post-interventional results may be offset by the rate of late rebleeding. In addition, the ISAT subgroup analysis of patients younger than 40 years demonstrated that the difference between poor outcome rates of coiled versus clipped aneurysms was very small in this age group. This led to the conclusion in a recently published study by Mitchell et al that in the younger age group, clip ligation may be favored over coil placement. This notion is further supported by experimental results that demonstrated stable aneurysm occlusion, with neoendothelium covering the former aneurysm neck in clipped aneurysms, whereas in coiled aneurysms no stable occlusion was visualized. However, over the past years, endovascular methods have improved considerably, with new coils and device-assisted coiling, whereas there has been very little change in neurosurgical techniques. It is therefore likely that the rate of recurrent SAH will decrease while the safety of the endovascular treatments will increase. This was confirmed by Schaafsma et al in a study of recurrent SAH within the first 8 years after treatment in 283 coiled patients with a total follow-up of 1778 patient-years; the cumulative incidence was 0.4% (95% CI, –0.4 to 1.2) after coiling versus 2.6% (95% CI, 1.2–4.0) after clipping. The rates of rebleeding after adequate coiling of aneurysms are therefore equal to those after clipping.

The results of ISAT, including the long-term results, indicate the superiority of endovascular treatment options for those aneurysms deemed suitable for both surgery and endovascular approaches. The results can therefore not be generalized to all ruptured aneurysms and all neurosurgical/endovascular teams. Instead, the results of ISAT must be extrapolated to individual patients after all the different factors that may play a role in the treatment decision have been considered, including the etiology of the aneurysm, the age and clinical status of the patient, the respective neurosurgical and endovascular experience and skills available, the anatomy and location of the aneurysm with regard to feasibility of the endovascular or surgical approach, and the equipment and material available and the comfort with which the treating team may use them. Finally, factors such as the health care environment and the patient's or family's wishes may play a role in the treatment decision.

PEARLS AND PITFALLS

- Endovascular treatment should be favored over surgical treatment if both the neurosurgeon and the interventionalist agree that the aneurysm is suitable for treatment with both methods.
- The imaging workup must provide the details needed for the treatment decision.
- An anterior communicating artery aneurysm may not be visualized on angiography because of flow competition phenomenon from the contralateral A1 segment. In these instances, compression of the contralateral ICA during contrast injection or bilateral ICA injections may be helpful.

Further Reading

Holmin S, Krings T, Ozanne A, et al. Intradural saccular aneurysms treated by Guglielmi detachable bare coils at a single institution between 1993 and 2005: clinical long-term follow-up for a total of 1810 patient-years in relation to morphological treatment results. Stroke 2008;39(8):2288–2297

Komotar RJ, Hahn DK, Kim GH, et al. Efficacy of lamina terminalis fenestration in reducing shunt-dependent hydrocephalus following aneurysmal subarachnoid hemorrhage: a systematic review. Clinical article. J Neurosurg 2009;111(1):147–154

Krings T, Busch C, Sellhaus B, et al. Long-term histological and scanning electron microscopy results of endovascular and operative treatments of experimentally induced aneurysms in the rabbit. Neurosurgery 2006;59(4):911–923, discussion 923–924

Mitchell P, Kerr R, Mendelow AD, Molyneux A. Could late rebleeding overturn the superiority of cranial aneurysm coil embolization over clip ligation seen in the International Subarachnoid Aneurysm Trial? J Neurosurg 2008;108(3):437–442

Molyneux AJ, Kerr RS, Birks J, et al; ISAT Collaborators. Risk of recurrent subarachnoid haemorrhage, death, or dependence and standardised mortality ratios after clipping or coiling of an intracranial aneurysm in the International Subarachnoid Aneurysm Trial (ISAT): long-term follow-up. Lancet Neurol 2009;8(5):427–433

Molyneux A, Kerr R, Stratton I, et al; International Subarachnoid Aneurysm Trial (ISAT) Collaborative Group. International Subarachnoid Aneurysm Trial (ISAT) of neurosurgical clipping versus endovascular coiling in 2143 patients with ruptured intracranial aneurysms: a randomised trial. Lancet 2002;360(9342):1267–1274

Schaafsma JD, Sprengers ME, van Rooij WJ, et al. Long-term recurrent subarachnoid hemorrhage after adequate coiling versus clipping of ruptured intracranial aneurysms. Stroke 2009;40(5):1758–1763

van der Schaaf I, Algra A, Wermer M, et al. Endovascular coiling versus neurosurgical clipping for patients with aneurysmal subarachnoid haemorrhage. Cochrane Database Syst Rev 2005;(4):CD003085

Wermer MJ, Greebe P, Algra A, Rinkel GJ. Incidence of recurrent subarachnoid hemorrhage after clipping for ruptured intracranial aneurysms. Stroke 2005;36(11):2394–2399

Willinsky RA, Peltz J, da Costa L, Agid R, Farb RI, terBrugge KG. Clinical and angiographic follow-up of ruptured intracranial aneurysms treated with endovascular embolization. AJNR Am J Neuroradiol 2009;30(5):1035–1040

CASE 3

Case Description

Clinical Presentation

A 44-year-old woman with a long-standing history of migraines has what she describes as atypically severe headaches 4 days before admission. Because the headaches do not vanish and have increased slightly over time, she seeks the advice of her family physician, who orders CT.

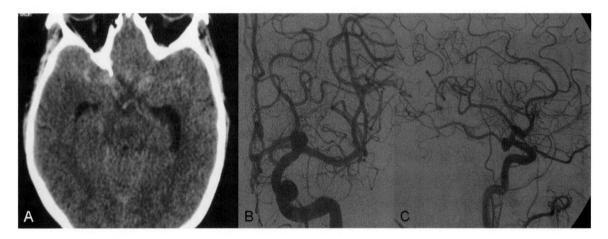

Fig. 3.1 **(A)** Unenhanced axial CT shows minimal symmetric hyperdensity along the suprasellar and MCA cisterns bilaterally. **(B)** Left ICA angiogram in AP view and **(C)** right ICA angiogram in lateral view reveal aneurysms at the left carotid termination and right posterior communicating artery origin.

Radiologic Studies

CT

Unenhanced CT demonstrated a small amount of subarachnoidal blood with a symmetric distribution (**Fig. 3.1A**). There was mild enlargement of the ventricles.

DSA

After injection into the left internal carotid artery (ICA), a round carotid termination aneurysm was found, and injection into the right ICA demonstrated a posterior communicating artery aneurysm (**Fig. 3.1 B,C**).

Diagnosis

Multiple aneurysms

13

Treatment

EQUIPMENT

- Standard 6F access (puncture needle, 6F vascular sheath)
- A 6F multipurpose catheter (Guider Soft Tip; Boston Scientific, Natick, MA) with continuous flush and a 0.035-in hydrophilic guidewire (Terumo, Somerset, NJ)
- A 45-degree angled microcatheter with a 1.7F tip and a 0.0165-ininner lumen (Excelsior SL 10; Boston Scientific) with a 0.014-in guidewire (Synchro 14; Boston Scientific)
- Coil selection: left ICA termination, GDC 10 360-degree soft SR coils 6 mm × 11 cm; right posterior communicating artery, GDC 10 360-degree soft SR coils 5 mm × 9 cm); subsequent filling with GDC 10 2D soft SR coils and GDC 10 Ultrasoft (all, Boston Scientific)
- Contrast material
- Heparin

DESCRIPTION

Because it could not be decided which aneurysm was ruptured and because both aneurysms were not deemed accessible via the same craniotomy, embolization with occlusion of both aneurysms was performed in the same setting. The 6F multipurpose catheter was placed in the left ICA, and 3D angiography was performed to obtain the working projection. Catheterization and subsequent coiling of the left ICA termination aneurysm was performed under roadmap conditions in the working projection after framing with a complex (GDC 10 360-degree) coil and subsequent filling with soft helical coils. Subsequently, the same procedure was repeated for the right side with uneventful coiling of the right posterior communicating artery aneurysm (**Fig. 3.2**). The procedure was performed under heparin. The patient awoke from anesthesia without neurologic deficits and had an uneventful recovery. She will be followed with noninvasive imaging to evaluate the stability of the coiled aneurysms and to screen for possible de novo aneurysms.

Discussion

Background

The incidence of multiple intracranial aneurysms appears to be extremely variable, depending in part on the patient population (whether the series included surgical, radiologic, or autopsy findings and whether the aneurysms were ruptured or unruptured). The prevalence of multiple intracranial aneurysms varies between 25 and 31% in autopsy series and between 12 and 26% in larger clinical series. Female patients account for 60 to 81% of those with multiple aneurysms. The ICA and middle cerebral artery (MCA) are most prone to the formation of multiple aneurysms. A special subgroup of multiple aneurysms are the "mirror-like" or "twin" aneurysms at symmetric sites on each side. Twin aneurysms occur in ~5 to 10% of all patients with aneurysms, but in as many as 36% of all patients with multiple aneurysms. They are found in all intracranial vessels but are most common in the MCA.

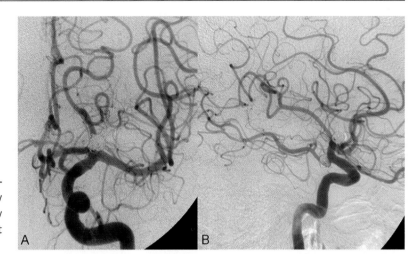

Fig. 3.2 DSA. Post-coiling angiograms of **(A)** the left ICA in AP view and **(B)** the right ICA in lateral view demonstrate no residual contrast filling of both aneurysms.

They exhibit a familial association, and they tend to rupture earlier in life than "classic" aneurysms. If multiple aneurysms are found in a patient presenting with a subarachnoid hemorrhage (SAH), the question of which one of the aneurysms has ruptured must be raised. Imaging can in most instances help to define the culprit aneurysm, which can then be targeted for priority treatment.

Noninvasive Imaging Workup

CT/MRI

- If intraparenchymal blood is present, the ruptured aneurysm will be easy to identify because it will point toward the blood clot. Classic sites of intraparenchymal bleeding are the orbitofrontal gyri or the gyrus rectus in anterior communicating artery aneurysms and the frontal operculum in MCA aneurysms.
- The subarachnoidal blood distribution can also help to determine the culprit aneurysm (**Fig. 3.3**). Focal clot surrounding the ruptured aneurysm may be present. Lateralized aneurysms (MCA, ICA termination, or posterior communicating artery) will classically have a lateralized blood distribution, and the more lateral their location, the more pronounced the lateralization of blood. Midline aneurysms (basilar tip, anterior communicating artery) will have a more symmetric blood distribution. In the craniocaudal direction, a more prominent blood distribution in the posterior fossa, surrounding the brainstem, in the quadrigeminal, cistern, or along the tentorium speaks in favor of posterior communicating artery, vertebral artery, or basilar artery tip aneurysms, whereas ruptured MCA and anterior communicating artery aneurysms tend to have more blood in the supratentorial compartments (interhemispheric fissure and sylvian fissure, respectively).
- As demonstrated in the present case, the pattern of blood distribution is valid only in the acute stages of an SAH.

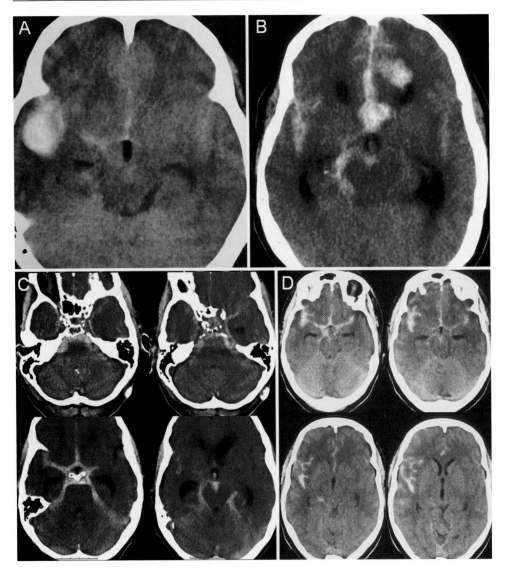

Fig. 3.3 (A–D) Unenhanced CT scans from different patients demonstrating blood distribution patterns that can predict the location of a ruptured aneurysm. **(A)** Intraparenchymal hemorrhage close to the MCA cistern from a ruptured MCA aneurysm. **(B)** Hemorrhage in the orbitofrontal and cingulate gyri from a ruptured anterior communicating artery aneurysm. **(C)** Symmetric blood distribution (−> midline location) that is more pronounced infratentorially from a ruptured basilar artery tip aneurysm. **(D)** Asymmetric supratentorial blood distribution from a ruptured MCA aneurysm.

CTA/MRA OR DSA

- Angiography can also reveal information about the culprit aneurysm, which is classically larger than the unruptured aneurysm and more irregular in shape (**Fig. 3.4**).
- Aneurysms blebs, or "daughter aneurysms," are classic indicators of rupture.
- Contrast stagnation within a bleb on the late venous phases of DSA speaks clearly in favor of the rupture point.
- Extravasation of contrast at the time of angiography very rarely occurs but will identify the bleeding aneurysm.
- An aspect ratio (i.e., the ratio of the depth of the aneurysm to the width of the aneurysm neck) of more than 1.6 is present in the vast majority of ruptured aneurysms (80%), whereas an aspect ratio of less than 1.6 is present in 90% of unruptured aneurysms.
- Focal localized vasospasm is classically present at the ruptured aneurysm site.

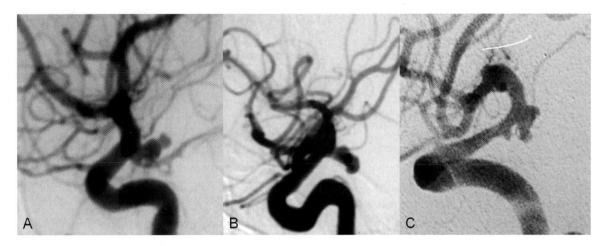

Fig. 3.4 (A–C) The classic morphologic identifiers of a ruptured aneurysm are presented here in three different ruptured posterior communicating artery aneurysms, all of which have an irregular shape with **(A)** an additional "bleb," **(B)** a high aspect ratio, and **(C)** focal vasospasm localized to the parent vessel (ICA).

Treatment Options

- If a patient with multiple aneurysms presents with SAH and it is uncertain which one is responsible for the bleed, then all aneurysms must be treated and secured.
- Surgical and endovascular treatments are available, as discussed in Cases 1 and 2. In the case of multiplicity, surgery has been advocated for those aneurysms that can be reached via the same craniotomy, whereas, in our opinion, endovascular options should be favored if multiple craniotomies are necessary to occlude all aneurysms.

Possible Complications

- All the complications detailed in Cases 8, 9, and 10 may occur.

Published Literature on Treatment Options

Surgery has been recommended for patients with multiple aneurysms because of the ability to treat the different aneurysms via the same surgical exposure and in the same surgical session. It has been estimated that between 50 and 70% of patients with multiple aneurysms can have all their aneurysms treated via a single craniotomy. Because multifocality may indicate an underlying vessel wall weakness with a subsequently higher risk for aneurysm regrowth over time, a more definitive treatment, such as clipping, may also speak in favor of surgery. However, for patients in whom multiple craniotomies would be necessary to treat all the aneurysms, the benefits of surgery are less obvious, and one may instead argue that an endovascular approach is much less invasive as long as the multiple aneurysms can be treated within a single endovascular setting, as was done in our case.

In our practice, we first determine which is the ruptured aneurysm by means of imaging data, as outlined above. The treatment decision is then based on neurosurgical versus endovascular accessibility and predicted outcome, with the International Subarachnoid Aneurysm Trial (ISAT) data taken into account. It is only secondarily that the argument with respect to multiplicity is taken into account based on the considerations described in the first paragraph of this section. If we are unsure about which aneurysm has ruptured, all aneurysms are treated at the same time.

Previous aneurysmal SAH is considered a major risk factor for subsequent hemorrhage from another, yet unruptured aneurysm. Therefore, treatment of these aneurysms is recommended. In

ISAT, of 24 observed rebleeds, 11 occurred from another aneurysm, four of which had been present at the initial angiogram and the remainder of which presented as de novo aneurysms. In a cohort of more than 600 patients treated with clipping, 129 aneurysms were detected after a mean interval of 8 years; 20% of these were at the site of previous rupture, 80% were remote from it. Thirty percent of them were truly de novo aneurysms, the others having already been there at presentation. Growth was noted in 25% of the followed aneurysms. This underlines in our opinion the need and benefit of continuous screening of patients with SAH to detect the development of additional aneurysms.

In patients with multiple aneurysms, the physician should actively seek an underlying disease such as polycystic kidney disease, connective tissue diseases (fibromuscular dysplasia, Marfan syndrome, Ehlers-Danlos type 4 syndrome), neurofibromatosis, and familial occurrence with potential genetic influences, and also rarer diseases such as cardiac myxoma. Patients must be discouraged from smoking because smoking is a major risk factor for rebleeding from a secondary aneurysm.

PEARLS AND PITFALLS

- Multiple aneurysms occur in 20% of cases, and a detailed angiographic workup (either by four-vessel angiography or high-quality noninvasive imaging) is therefore necessary in all patients with SAH.
- Blood distribution on CT and aneurysm morphology can determine the culprit aneurysm in most instances. If the culprit aneurysm cannot be identified, all aneurysms must be treated.
- Patients with a previous SAH have a substantial risk for new aneurysm formation and the enlargement of untreated aneurysms. Screening these patients may be beneficial, especially those with multiple aneurysms, hypertension, and a history of smoking.
- Surgery has been advocated for those aneurysms that can be treated via the same craniotomy.

Further Reading

Baccin CE, Krings T, Alvarez H, Ozanne A, Lasjaunias P. Multiple mirror-like intracranial aneurysms. Report of a case and review of the literature. Acta Neurochir (Wien) 2006;148(10):1091–1095, discussion 1095

Imhof HG, Yonekawa Y. Management of ruptured aneurysms combined with coexisting aneurysms. Acta Neurochir Suppl (Wien) 2005;94:93–96

Porter PJ, Mazighi M, Rodesch G, et al. Endovascular and surgical management of multiple intradural aneurysms: review of 122 patients managed between 1993 and 1999. Interventional Neuroradiology 2001;7(4):291–302

Ujiie H, Tamano Y, Sasaki K, Hori T. Is the aspect ratio a reliable index for predicting the rupture of a saccular aneurysm? Neurosurgery 2001;48(3):495–502, discussion 502–503

Wermer MJ, van der Schaaf IC, Velthuis BK, Algra A, Buskens E, Rinkel GJ; ASTRA Study Group. Follow-up screening after subarachnoid haemorrhage: frequency and determinants of new aneurysms and enlargement of existing aneurysms. Brain 2005;128(Pt 10):2421–2429

CASE 4

Case Description

Clinical Presentation

A 20-year-old woman with a positive family history of subarachnoid hemorrhage (SAH) is screened for aneurysms. (The patient's mother and the mother's sister both had aneurysmal SAH.) MRA shows an internal carotid artery (ICA) termination aneurysm, and the patient is referred to us for further management. The patient is a heavy smoker.

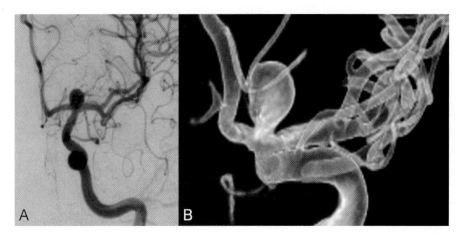

Fig. 4.1 DSA. Left ICA angiogram in **(A)** AP view and **(B)** 3D transparent volume rendering shows a left carotid termination aneurysm.

Radiologic Studies

DSA

After injection into the left ICA, a carotid termination aneurysm was seen with a maximum diameter of 6 mm, a small neck, and no daughter aneurysms (**Fig. 4.1**). The remainder of the examination was unremarkable.

Diagnosis

Unruptured aneurysm of the ICA termination

Treatment

EQUIPMENT

- Standard 6F access (puncture needle, 6F vascular sheath)
- A 6F multipurpose catheter (Envoy; Cordis, Warren, NJ) with continuous flush and a 0.035-in hydrophilic guidewire (Terumo, Somerset, NJ)
- A 45-degree angled microcatheter with a 2 tip and a 0.019-in inner lumen (Excelsior 10–18; Boston Scientific, Natick, MA) with a 0.014-in guidewire (Synchro 14; Boston Scientific)
- Coil selection: for framing, GDC 18 360-degree coils 6 mm × 20 cm; for subsequent filling and finishing, GDC 10 regular and soft coils (stretch-resistant) with progressive downsizing (Boston Scientific)
- Contrast material
- Heparin

DESCRIPTION

Although the International Study on Unruptured Aneurysms (ISUIA) reported a 5-year risk for the rupture of anterior circulation aneurysms less than 7 mm in size to be close to 0 and the treatment-related risk to be ~10%, treatment was decided upon in this case, given the expected lower risk of treatment in a young patient with a medium-size aneurysm having a small neck and the expected higher natural history risk in a patient with (1) a positive family history, (2) female gender, (3) a long life expectancy, and (4) a history of smoking. A 6F multipurpose catheter was introduced into the left ICA, and 3000 units of heparin were given. Following a roadmap in the working projection, the microcatheter was advanced over the micro-guidewire and placed close to the entrance of the aneurysm, from which deployment of the first coil was started. Once this coil was deployed, the catheter was slightly advanced into the aneurysm, and subsequent coiling with smaller and softer coils was performed until a dense coil mesh was obtained. Control series via the guiding catheter demonstrated complete occlusion of the aneurysm (**Fig. 4.2**). The micro-guidewire was advanced, straightening the catheter, and the microcatheter was slowly withdrawn from the aneurysm, with care taken to prevent any coil loops from exiting the aneurysm. The patient awoke without any neurologic deficits. Follow-up control after 1 year demonstrated stable results and no de novo formation of aneurysms.

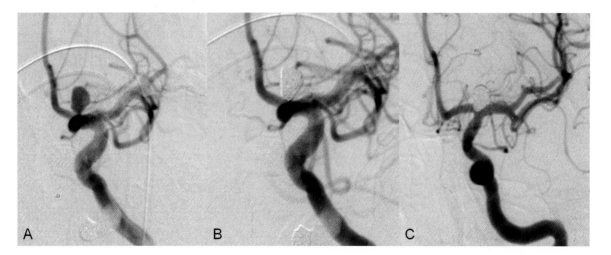

Fig. 4.2 DSA. Left ICA angiograms in the working projection **(A)** before and **(B)** after coiling. **(C)** Final control angiogram of the left ICA in AP view shows no residual filling of the aneurysm sac.

Discussion

Background

Depending on the study cited, the prevalence of arterial aneurysms is between 2 and 5% of the general population, approximately 10 times higher than the frequency of arteriovenous malformations in the same group. In a recent meta-analysis, a prevalence of intracranial aneurysms in adults of 2.3% was found, with an increasing prevalence in elderly patients and a slight predominance in females. A positive family history and the presence of polycystic kidney disease were associated with a higher rate of intracranial aneurysms. Given the high morbidity and mortality rates associated with aneurysms, the treatment of incidental aneurysms has to be based on a comparison of the risks of their natural history versus the risks of treatment. The risk for rupture of intracranial aneurysms was evaluated in a recent meta-analysis by Wermer et al. They found that the risk for rupture was increased in female patients, in those with a history of smoking, in elderly patients, and in patients of Japanese or Finnish descent. Larger aneurysms, posterior circulation aneurysms, and aneurysms in patients who had other, previously ruptured aneurysms were also associated with a higher risk for hemorrhage. This meta-analysis found the overall annual risk for hemorrhage of an unruptured aneurysm to be 0.7%. In the WHO MONICA study of stroke by Ingall et al, a total of 3368 SAH events recorded during 35.9 million person-years of observation in 11 populations in Europe and China comprising 25- to 64-year-old men and women resulted in SAH rates of 7 to 21 per 100,000 persons per year. Given the rate of aneurysm occurrence of ~2%, a risk for rupture of unruptured aneurysms of 0.3 to 1% per year can therefore be expected. These values (derived from a meta-analysis of 19 studies including ISUIA and a validated prospective population-based study) are in striking contradiction to those of ISUIA 2 and ISUIA 3. ISUIA prospectively investigated the natural history of unruptured aneurysms and evaluated the risks of surgical and endovascular treatment in 4060 patients, 1692 of whom received no treatment.

Table 4.1 demonstrates the cumulative risks for bleeding in 5 years stratified according to aneurysm location (anterior circulation [excluding the posterior communicating artery] versus posterior circulation), aneurysm size, and history of previously bled aneurysm (group 2) versus no previously ruptured aneurysm (group 1). The discrepancy between these findings and our clinical experience in daily practice (i.e., most ruptured aneurysms are anterior circulation aneurysms < 7 mm in size) has been the subject of considerable discussion. Likewise, the procedural risks reported in this study (a surgical therapeutic risk of slightly > 10% and an endovascular risk of ~9%) are in striking contrast to those reported in other, larger studies on treatment-related risks, which are in the range of 4%. Although it is beyond the scope of this book, which is a case-based compilation of endovascular

Table 4.1 From ISUIA 2: 5-Year Cumulative Rupture Rates According to Size and Location of Unruptured Aneurysm

	< 7 mm, %	7–12 mm, %	13–24 mm, %	≥ 25 mm, %
Cavernous carotid artery	0*	0[†]	0	3.0	6.4
Anterior circulation (excluding PcomA)	0*	1.5[†]	2.6	14.5	40
Posterior circulation (including PcomA)	2.5*	3.4[†]	14.5	18.4	50

*Patients without previous SAH from other aneurysm

[†]Patients with previous SAH from other aneurysm

Abbreviations: ISUIA, International Study on Unruptured Aneurysms; PcomA, posterior communicating artery

Source: Wiebers DO, Whisnant JP, Huston J 3rd, et al. Unruptured intracranial aneurysms: natural history, clinical outcome, and risks of surgical and endovascular treatment. Lancet 2003; 362(9378):103–110. Reprinted with permission.

procedures, to discuss in detail the potential shortcomings of ISUIA, the following comments can be made: The hemorrhagic risk in the anterior circulation, despite being low, is implausibly low at 0; likewise, the procedural risk of 10% is implausibly high. The study does not take into consideration individual features of the aneurysm (e.g., aneurysm morphology [aspect ratio, blebs, irregular shape], aneurysm growth over time, intra-aneurysmal flow dynamics or associated vessel wall disease, aneurysm etiology, associated calcifications, multiplicity of aneurysms, associated arterial variations), nor does it account for individual patient characteristics (female vs. male gender, family history of aneurysms or SAH, history of smoking or hypertension, ethnic descent). Finally, it does not take into account the experience of the local treatment team that the neurointerventionalists and neurosurgeons must quote to the patient during the process of informed consent. Therefore, a strict adherence to the numbers in this study without a consideration of the individual patient, the individual aneurysm, and the experience of the local treating team is in our opinion not correct.

Noninvasive Imaging Workup

PHYSICAL EXAMINATION

- Unruptured aneurysms are usually clinically silent.
- Posterior communicating artery and superior cerebellar aneurysms may become symptomatic with oculomotor nerve palsy due to pulsations, and the sudden occurrence of a cranial nerve III palsy is in our opinion a warning sign of the acute growth of an aneurysm. These patients are treated urgently, even if they do not present with SAH.
- Giant aneurysms may become symptomatic because of mass effect. The treatment of these lesions is detailed in Case 11.
- In patients with the sudden onset of severe headache without evidence of SAH on cerebrospinal fluid analysis or CT, a warning leak must be taken into consideration, and treatment of these aneurysms may be expedited.

CT/CTA

- Although unenhanced CT plays a role in detecting calcifications and demonstrating mass effect, CTA will demonstrate the aneurysm, its size, the neck, the potential for endovascular access, and other, associated aneurysms and thereby will risk-stratify the individual unruptured aneurysm.
- CTA can be used to follow untreated patients to evaluate potential lesion growth; however, radiation issues may make time-of-flight (TOF) MRA preferable.

MRI/MRA

- MRI and MRA are used to screen patients with familial aneurysms because no radiation is necessary and no contrast has to be given. We employ TOF MRA, preferably at 3 tesla (T), to screen and, if a conservative management is adopted, to follow the patient.
- With current treatment-associated morbidities taken into consideration, screening of the first-degree relatives of patients with sporadic aneurysmal SAH is not indicated; to prevent one SAH, 149 relatives must be screened.
- However, screening of relatives is indicated in the case of familial aneurysms because the relative risk for aneurysms in first-degree relatives is 4.2 (compared with 1.8 in families in which only one member has had an aneurysm). In addition, in the subgroup of patients with familial aneurysms, the risk for an SAH resulting from an aneurysm is four times greater than the risk in the general population.
- Screening is also necessary in the identical twin of a patient with an aneurysm.
- Repeat screening is recommended approximately every 5 years.

Invasive Imaging Workup

- With better image quality and image reconstruction algorithms, angiography is rarely needed for the diagnostic workup of patients with unruptured aneurysms because the data needed to decide on treatment or conservative management as well as the treatment modality are readily obtainable by noninvasive imaging modalities. If endovascular options are contemplated, we perform a 3D rotational angiography as well as standard AP and lateral views of the vessel of interest, followed by an injection in the working projection.

Treatment Options

CONSERVATIVE OR MEDICAL MANAGEMENT

- As detailed above, conservative treatment must be considered, especially in the case of small aneurysms in the anterior circulation in elderly patients and in patients with a shorter life expectancy.

SURGICAL TREATMENT

- Surgical management consists of clip ligation of the aneurysm following craniotomy.

ENDOVASCULAR TREATMENT

- Endovascular treatment options for small unruptured aneurysms are coil embolization (with or without device assistance; e.g., stent, balloon). In small-necked aneurysms, like the one in this case, unassisted endovascular coiling is in most instances possible. For unruptured aneurysms, we tend to use the slightly stiffer 18 coils.

Possible Complications

- Thromboembolic complications
- Periprocedural aneurysm rupture
- Aneurysm recanalization

Published Literature on Treatment Options

Based on the above-mentioned considerations regarding the shortcomings of ISUIA and based on other studies of the natural history risk of unruptured aneurysms, we recommend the treatment of posterior circulation unruptured intracranial aneurysms (including those of the posterior communicating artery) larger than 3 mm and the treatment of anterior circulation aneurysms larger than 7 mm. The treatment of anterior circulation unruptured aneurysms smaller than 7 mm should be individualized based on the age and family history of the patient, previous hemorrhage, and the aneurysm shape and growth. If conservative management is adopted, follow-up noninvasive imaging is performed in our center (preferably with unenhanced TOF MRA at 3 T) to rule out aneurysm growth over time. If invasive management is proposed, then as the next step the treatment modality has to be determined. Again, this has to be individualized based on the age of the patient, the location and shape of the aneurysm, the treatment team's capability (including its morbidity and mortality record), and the patient's preference. In ISUIA, there was a slightly better outcome in patients treated by endovascular means. However, this has to be weighed against (1) the higher risk for residual aneurysms after coiling (5–20% in the literature following coiling, 0–3% after clipping), (2) the higher risk for aneurysm recanalization after coiling (15–35% vs. 0–5%), and consequently the higher re-treatment rates following coiling (5–13%). In addition to these considerations, decisions about what therapy to choose depend on the location of the aneurysm (with posterior circulation aneurysms more likely candidates for endovascular treatments), its morphology (incorporation of vessels at the aneurysm neck favors surgical techniques, whereas perforators surrounding the neck are more easily treated by endovascular options), and its size (very small and very large aneurysms are more likely to be treated surgically). If calcifications are present at the aneurysm neck, surgery may be more dangerous. On the other hand, in patients with kidney disease, the contrast material and the necessity of follow-up studies will likely favor surgical therapy. In patients with significant atherosclerosis and significant tortuosity and ectasia of the vasculature, endovascular access may be difficult and dangerous.

PEARLS AND PITFALLS

- The risk for future rupture of an unruptured aneurysm increases when the patient is female; has a history of previous SAH from a different aneurysm; an aneurysm larger than 7 mm; an aneurysm of the posterior circulation, or a family history of aneurysm; and lives in certain geographic locations.
- Screening in familial forms of SAH is recommended.
- Treatment recommendations should take into account the individual history, the aneurysm morphology, and the experience of the treating team and should not be based only on ISUIA.

Further Reading

Clarke M. Systematic review of reviews of risk factors for intracranial aneurysms. Neuroradiology 2008;50(8):653–664

Ingall T, Asplund K, Mähönen M, Bonita R. A multinational comparison of subarachnoid hemorrhage epidemiology in the WHO MONICA stroke study. Stroke 2000;31(5):1054–1061

Pierot L, Spelle L, Vitry F; ATENA Investigators. Immediate clinical outcome of patients harboring unruptured intracranial aneurysms treated by endovascular approach: results of the ATENA study. Stroke 2008;39(9):2497–2504

Magnetic Resonance Angiography in Relatives of Patients with Subarachnoid Hemorrhage Study Group. Risks and benefits of screening for intracranial aneurysms in first-degree relatives of patients with sporadic subarachnoid hemorrhage. N Engl J Med 1999;341(18):1344–1350

Rinkel GJ, Djibuti M, Algra A, van Gijn J. Prevalence and risk of rupture of intracranial aneurysms: a systematic review. Stroke 1998;29(1):251–256

Schievink WI, Schaid DJ, Michels VV, Piepgras DG. Familial aneurysmal subarachnoid hemorrhage: a community-based study. J Neurosurg 1995;83(3):426–429

Standhardt H, Boecher-Schwarz H, Gruber A, Benesch T, Knosp E, Bavinzski G. Endovascular treatment of unruptured intracranial aneurysms with Guglielmi detachable coils: short- and long-term results of a single-centre series. Stroke 2008;39(3):899–904

van Rooij WJ, Sluzewski M. Procedural morbidity and mortality of elective coil treatment of unruptured intracranial aneurysms. AJNR Am J Neuroradiol 2006;27(8):1678–1680

Wermer MJ, Rinkel GJ, van Gijn J. Repeated screening for intracranial aneurysms in familial subarachnoid hemorrhage. Stroke 2003;34(12):2788–2791

Wermer MJ, van der Schaaf IC, Algra A, Rinkel GJ. Risk of rupture of unruptured intracranial aneurysms in relation to patient and aneurysm characteristics: an updated meta-analysis. Stroke 2007;38(4):1404–1410

Wiebers DO, Whisnant JP, Huston J III, et al; International Study of Unruptured Intracranial Aneurysms Investigators. Unruptured intracranial aneurysms: natural history, clinical outcome, and risks of surgical and endovascular treatment. Lancet 2003;362(9378):103–110

CASE 5

Case Description

Clinical Presentation

A 57-year-old woman is found unconscious by her daughter. On arrival in the emergency department, she has a Glasgow Coma Scale score of 5. Emergency CT demonstrates subarachnoid hemorrhage with a significant amount of intraventricular blood. Following bilateral external ventricular drainages, the patient localizes to pain stimulation and treatment is contemplated.

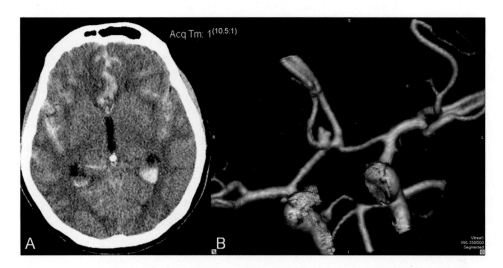

Fig. 5.1 (A) Unenhanced axial CT shows diffuse subarachnoid hemorrhage bilaterally and focal clot within the interhemispheric fissure. Intraventricular hemorrhage in the lateral ventricles is also observed bilaterally. **(B)** 3D CTA reveals a large lobulated aneurysm of the anterior communicating artery.

Radiologic Studies

CT/CTA

CT demonstrated bilateral symmetric blood, intraventricular hemorrhage, and blood in the interhemispheric fissure. CTA demonstrated as the source of bleeding a lobulated 4 × 3-mm anterior communicating artery aneurysm with a 3.5-mm broad neck (**Fig. 5.1**).

Diagnosis

Wide-necked ruptured aneurysm of the anterior communicating artery

Treatment

EQUIPMENT

- Bifemoral standard 6F access (puncture needle, 6F vascular sheath)
- A 2 × 6F multipurpose catheter (Envoy; Cordis, Warren, NJ) with continuous flush and a 0.035-in hydrophilic guidewire (Terumo, Somerset, NJ)

25

- A straight microcatheter with a 1.7F tip and a 0.0165-in inner lumen (Excelsior SL 10; Boston Scientific, Natick, MA) with a 0.014-in guidewire (Transend 10 Platinum Tip, Boston Scientific)
- A 4 × 7-mm HyperForm balloon (ev3, Plymouth, MN)
- Coil selection: for framing, 3.5 × 5 TruFill DCS orbit (Cordis); for subsequent filling and finishing, MicroPlex 10 HyperSoft helical coils 2 mm × 3 cm, 2 mm × 1 cm, 2 mm × 1 cm (MicroVention, Tustin, CA)
- Contrast material
- Heparin

DESCRIPTION

The 6F multipurpose catheter was placed in the left internal carotid artery (ICA). An attempt was made to navigate the balloon from the left ICA across the anterior communicating artery and the aneurysm neck into the right A2 segment; however, the guidewire could not be positioned into the

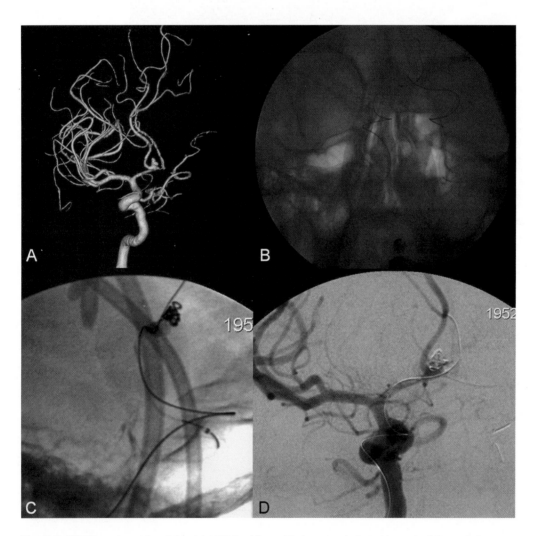

Fig. 5.2 (A) 3D angiography of the right ICA in oblique AP view reveals the wide neck of the anterior communicating artery aneurysm. **(B)** Unsubtracted image before deployment of the first coil shows the balloon crossing from the right ICA into the left A2 segment, bridging the aneurysm neck, and the microcatheter being placed from the left ICA into the aneurysm. **(C)** Unsubtracted image demonstrates the "down-the-barrel" view of the coil with the balloon inflated. **(D)** Right ICA angiogram in the working projection shows subsequent remodeling of the parent vessel and the result of the first framing coil.

A2 segment. Subsequently, the guiding catheter was navigated into the right ICA, from which balloon placement over the neck into the left A2 segment proved possible. Given the caliber of the A1 segment, we decided to introduce the microcatheter from the left side, and a second guiding catheter was introduced. The microcatheter could be introduced into the aneurysm, where the first coil was subsequently deployed with the balloon inflated to prevent coil protrusion into the parent artery. Deflation of the balloon verified stability of the coil, which was then detached (**Fig. 5.2**). The same procedure was repeated for the other coils, resulting in complete occlusion of the aneurysm with no evidence of thromboembolic complications (**Fig. 5.3**). At the end of the procedure, given the rather broad neck of the aneurysm, heparin was not reversed.

Discussion

Background

One of the main factors limiting the endovascular treatment of intracranial aneurysms is the shape of the aneurysmal sac, particularly the width of the neck. Wide-necked aneurysms were therefore treated with surgery rather than with endovascular options. The balloon-remodeling technique that was first described by Moret et al in 1997 helped to overcome this problem and expanded the number of aneurysms treatable by endovascular means.

Noninvasive Imaging Workup

CTA/DSA

- In cases in which the imaging workup demonstrates a wide-necked aneurysm, accessibility for the potential use of a balloon system must be evaluated.
- Because balloon deployment may include crossover techniques, the size of the anterior and posterior communicating arteries must be determined if they are to be a potential route by which to advance the balloon over the aneurysm neck.

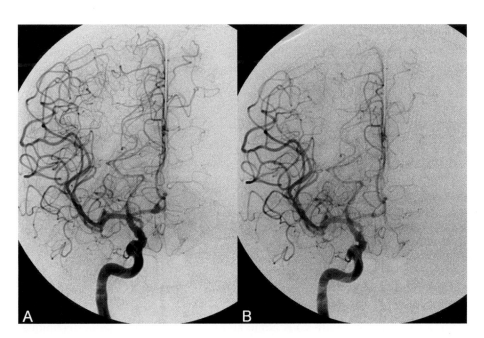

Fig. 5.3 DSA. Right ICA angiogram in AP view **(A)** before and **(B)** after coiling demonstrating complete exclusion of the aneurysm and no thromboembolic complications.

- Choosing the working projection is extremely important when balloon remodeling is used. We try to position the image intensifier to produce a "down-the-barrel" view of the parent artery; the second view should demonstrate the neck of the aneurysm in its widest plane (which is classically perpendicular to the plane in the aforementioned "down-the-barrel" view).

Treatment Options

SURGICAL TREATMENT

- In wide-necked ruptured aneurysms, surgery has to be considered a viable option because even after balloon remodeling, long-term stability is less than that in small-necked aneurysms.
- In our opinion, surgery has to be contemplated in those wide-necked aneurysms in which the point of rupture (defined by a bleb, or daughter aneurysm) is close to the neck because inflation of the balloon may cause repeated rupture, and protection of the aneurysm by endovascular techniques may be more difficult.

ENDOVASCULAR TREATMENT

- In wide-necked aneurysms, GDC 3D coils (Boston Scientific) and MicruSphere and Presidio coils (Micrus) are considered in our practice to lead to a good remodeling of the neck, even without the use of balloons.
- In addition to balloons, stents may be employed to treat wide-necked aneurysms and are discussed in greater detail in Case 6.
- Different guide-dependent balloon types are available: oval balloons for side wall aneurysms, round balloons for terminal or bifurcation aneurysms, and compliant balloons that remodel the neck of any type of aneurysm in a slightly less aggressive way; compliant balloons are used mostly in distal vessels.
- Navigation of the balloons may be difficult with the guidewires currently available for most balloons. Therefore, crossover techniques may sometimes be necessary, as in this case.

Possible Complications

- In addition to the complications of coil embolization, balloon-assisted embolization may increase the rate of thromboembolic events and is feared to lead to a higher rate of periprocedural ruptures.
- In blister-like aneurysms and dissections, with their extremely fragile walls, balloons are in our opinion not indicated because of a higher estimated risk for rupture of the aneurysm.

Published Literature on Treatment Options

The goal of balloon remodeling is threefold: (1) to protect coil loops from protruding into the parent artery, (2) to increase packing density in the aneurysm, and (3) to stop bleeding once a rupture has occurred during the coil embolization procedure. However, there is controversy about the safety and efficacy of balloon remodeling in the current literature.

In a study of more than 500 patients with unruptured aneurysms, Pierot et al note similar rates of adverse events with coiling alone and with the balloon-remodeling technique. The overall rates of adverse events related to the treatment, regardless of whether the adverse events led to clinical consequences, were ~11% for treatment with coils alone and 12% for the remodeling technique.

Morbidity and mortality rates did not differ significantly between the groups (~3% for each). These authors concluded that the remodeling technique is as safe as the standard treatment with coils. Their results are in striking contrast to those of a study by Sluzewski et al of more than 750 patients (~10% of whom were treated with balloon remodeling). Procedure-related complications leading to death or dependency were significantly higher with balloon remodeling (14.1%) than with unassisted coil embolization (3%). In addition, packing densities and the results of 6-month follow-up angiography studies did not differ significantly between the two types of treatments. These authors concluded that balloon remodeling should be used only if conventional coiling of aneurysms is impossible and if the anticipated surgical risks are too high. However, the most recent meta-analysis, by Shapiro et al (which did not include some of the publications that reported a rather high procedural complication rate, such as the aforementioned study by Sluzewski et al), suggested that balloon remodeling is not associated with higher rates of thrombotic complication than those of traditional, unassisted coiling.

The aim of balloon remodeling is not only to prevent coil loops from entering the parent artery but also to allow a higher packing density; it has been argued that a higher packing density may lead to more stable results. However, this assumption has also been challenged in a recent study by Piotin et al, who demonstrated in a retrospective assessment of 225 patients that both recurring and stable aneurysms had the same mean packing density (27%). However, one cannot use this study to argue in favor of the reverse (i.e., that incomplete packing of an aneurysm is sufficient). As the authors themselves stated, they performed embolization "until aneurysmal circulatory exclusion was achieved or until no more coils could be delivered." Therefore, the study simply states that even if complete occlusion is achieved, recurrence is possible. Incomplete occlusion is, however, more likely to result in compaction, aneurysm recurrence, or even early rebleed.

In our experience, balloon assistance is necessary in ~10% of aneurysms, and undoubtedly the use of this technique has increased the number of patients who can be treated with endovascular techniques. As with all endovascular treatments, experience with a device is directly related to peri-procedural safety. This implies that general guidelines on whether or not to use these devices cannot be established. Instead, the individual interventionalist has to balance the risks of the proposed procedure against those of the experience of the surgical team in the sometimes challenging treatment of wide-necked aneurysms.

PEARLS AND PITFALLS _____

- Balloon remodeling of the parent artery allows embolization of wide-necked aneurysms.
- A "down-the-barrel" view is helpful to determine successful remodeling of the parent vessel.
- There is no consensus as to whether balloon assistance increases the complications rates of endovascular therapies, but most studies do not report an increased rate of thromboembolic or hemorrhagic complications.
- Recanalization may occur despite high packing densities, and surgery may therefore still play a role in the management of some wide-necked aneurysms.

Further Reading
Moret J, Cognard C, Weill A, Castaings L, Rey A. Reconstruction technic in the treatment of wide-neck intracranial aneurysms. Long-term angiographic and clinical results. Apropos of 56 cases [in French]. J Neuroradiol 1997;24(1):30–44

Pierot L, Spelle L, Leclerc X, Cognard C, Bonafé A, Moret J. Endovascular treatment of unruptured intracranial aneurysms: comparison of safety of remodeling technique and standard treatment with coils. Radiology 2009;251(3):846–855

Piotin M, Spelle L, Mounayer C, et al. Intracranial aneurysms: treatment with bare platinum coils—aneurysm packing, complex coils, and angiographic recurrence. Radiology 2007;243(2):500–508

Shapiro M, Babb J, Becske T, Nelson PK. Safety and efficacy of adjunctive balloon remodeling during endovascular treatment of intracranial aneurysms: a literature review. AJNR Am J Neuroradiol 2008;29(9):1777–1781

Sluzewski M, van Rooij WJ, Beute GN, Nijssen PC. Balloon-assisted coil embolization of intracranial aneurysms: incidence, complications, and angiography results. J Neurosurg 2006;105(3):396–399

Sluzewski M, van Rooij WJ, Slob MJ, Bescós JO, Slump CH, Wijnalda D. Relation between aneurysm volume, packing, and compaction in 145 cerebral aneurysms treated with coils. Radiology 2004;231(3):653–658

Spelle L, Piotin M, Mounayer C, Moret J. Saccular intracranial aneurysms: endovascular treatment—devices, techniques and strategies, management of complications, results. Neuroimaging Clin N Am 2006;16(3):413–451, viii

CASE 6

Case Description

Clinical Presentation

In 2001, a 40-year-old woman had a subarachnoid hemorrhage (SAH) resulting from a right posterior communicating artery aneurysm that was subsequently clipped. In January 2008, she experienced a second SAH, and DSA demonstrated again a sizeable right posterior communicating artery aneurysm that was subsequently coiled (**Fig. 6.1 A,B**).

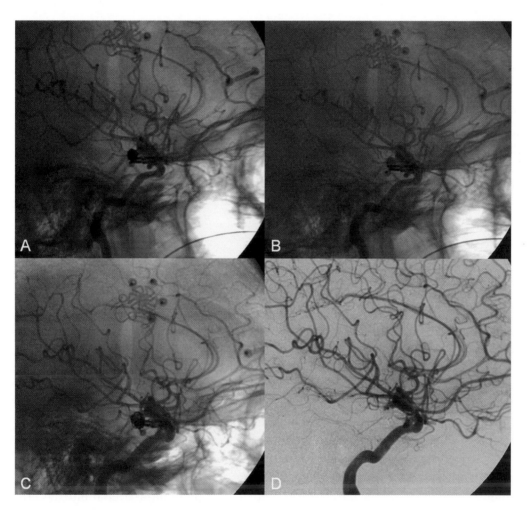

Fig. 6.1 Unsubtracted right ICA angiogram after the patient's second SAH due to aneurysm regrowth of a previously clipped aneurysm **(A)** before coiling and **(B)** after coiling. Follow-up right ICA angiograms in lateral view. **(C)** Unsubtracted and **(D)** DSA images after 1 year demonstrating displacement of the coil mesh and significant recanalization of the aneurysm.

31

Radiologic Studies

DSA

Despite initial good occlusion, follow-up after 1 year demonstrated the recurrence of perfusion in the cranial aspects of the coiled aneurysm and a broad communication with the internal carotid artery (ICA; **Fig. 6.1 C,D**). The patient was put on clopidogrel and aspirin and was scheduled for possible stent-assisted treatment of the aneurysm recurrence.

Diagnosis

Recurrent broad-based posterior communicating artery aneurysm

Treatment

EQUIPMENT

- Standard 6F access (puncture needle, 6F vascular sheath)
- A 6F multipurpose catheter (Envoy; Cordis, Warren, NJ) with continuous flush and a 0.035-in hydrophilic guidewire (Terumo, Somerset, NJ)
- A 45-degree angled microcatheter with a 1.7F tip and a 0.065-in inner lumen (Excelsior SL 10; Boston Scientific, Natick, MA) with a 0.014-in guidewire (Transend Soft Tip; Boston Scientific)
- Prowler Select Plus Microcatheter (Cordis)
- Coil selection: MicroPlex 3 mm × 7 cm complex coil (MicroVention, Tustin, CA)
- Enterprise stent 4.5 mm × 28 mm (Cordis)
- Contrast material
- Heparin

DESCRIPTION

Under roadmap guidance, an Excelsior SL 10 microcatheter was introduced over a Transend Soft Tip wire into the aneurysm. A MicroVention 3 mm × 7 cm complex coil was introduced. A control run showed satisfactory positioning of the coil, and the coil was detached. However, the control run also demonstrated mechanical vasospasm of the cervical ICA around the tip of the guiding catheter with stasis of contrast in the ICA. Although the guiding catheter was carefully pulled back into the common carotid artery, the microcatheter was displaced from the aneurysm, and one of the coil loops protruded with the catheter into the parent vessel lumen, given the broad neck of the aneurysm. The pulsatile motion of this loop suggested its unstable position in the ICA lumen. We therefore decided to place an Enterprise 4.5 mm × 28 mm stent to jail this loop. In addition, stent placement was considered to possibly strengthen the vessel wall (because the aneurysm had regrown after both clipping and coiling) and to ensure dense packing in a subsequent session, given the unfavorable dome-to-neck ratio. Administration of cutaneous nitroglycerin paste and 25 µg of intra-arterial nitroglycerin was necessary to resolve the spasm and allow subsequent stent positioning. The guiding catheter was again introduced into the distal ICA, and a Prowler Select Plus Microcatheter was introduced over the micro-guidewire into the middle cerebral artery. The stent was then introduced and deployed from the ICA terminus to the ICA siphon. During deployment, the coil loop was "jacked" back into the aneurysm. A control run showed delayed filling of the residual aneurysmal lumen and stasis of contrast within the aneurysm (**Fig. 6.2**). Because of the recurrence of ICA vasospasm and the fact that flow into the aneurysm had been significantly altered, we decided to stop the procedure at this point and bring the patient back after 3 months for further coil embolization. The control angiogram after 3 months, however, demonstrated complete obliteration of the aneurysm from the circulation with no evidence of in-stent stenosis.

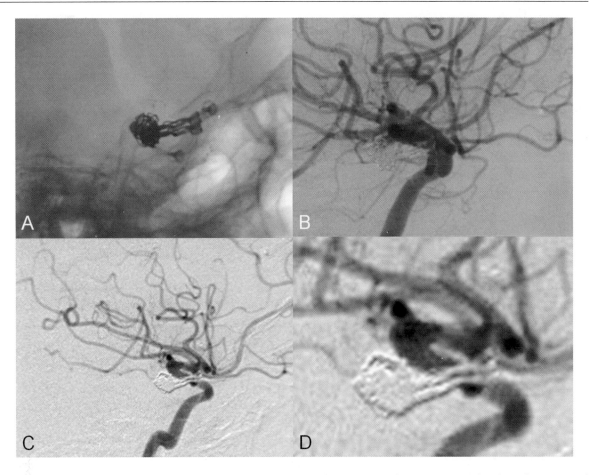

Fig. 6.2 **(A)** Plain radiograph and **(B)** right ICA angiogram in lateral view after stent-assisted coiling show minimal delayed filling of the residual aneurysmal lumen with stasis of the contrast. Follow-up right ICA angiograms in **(C)** lateral and **(D)** magnified views 3 months after the last embolization demonstrate complete obliteration of the aneurysm.

Discussion

Background

At follow-up, ~20% of all coiled intracranial aneurysms show reopening, compared with ~3% of clipped aneurysms. According to the literature, re-treatment is considered mandatory in approximately half of these cases. Risk factors for aneurysm reopening following coiling are location in the posterior circulation, size larger than 10 mm, wide neck, and previous rupture. Because wide-necked aneurysms tend to recur more often, unassisted coiling may not be sufficient to treat these challenging lesions. Balloon-assisted coiling or stenting should be considered for the treatment of these recurrent lesions. In theory, there is a threefold beneficial effect of the stent: (1) The stent may change the hemodynamics within the aneurysm, leading to diversion of the blood flow into the parent artery and away from the aneurysm; (2) the stent will prevent coil loops from protruding into the parent artery, thereby enabling dense packing of the aneurysm; and (3) the stent may provide a scaffold for future neointimal growth from the proximal and distal portions of the (healthy) vessel distant from the aneurysm orifice, thereby excluding the aneurysm from the circulation. If the jailing technique is performed (i.e., entry into the aneurysm with the coil-deploying microcatheter, followed by stent deployment), a fourth desired effect is to stabilize the coil-deploying microcatheter in the aneurysm and prevent it from being displaced into the parent artery during subsequent coiling.

Noninvasive Imaging Workup

CT/CTA

- In our opinion, CT and CTA do not play a role in determining aneurysm recanalization following coiling. CTA may, however, be used to evaluate post-surgical aneurysm remnants.

MR/MRA

- Contrast-enhanced MRA is the best method to evaluate the long-term stability of coiled aneurysms because no other method can demonstrate contrast filling within the coil mass.
- Follow-up must detail the remainder of the intradural vessels because de novo aneurysm formation may occur.

Invasive Imaging Workup

- The role of invasive angiography to detect aneurysm recanalization is in our opinion limited; coil artifacts in 3D rotational angiography may be present, and because of the "helmet effect," recanalization invaginating the coil mass may remain unnoticed on angiography.
- Invasive imaging poses a risk for the patient and is associated with considerably higher costs.

Treatment Options

CONSERVATIVE OR MEDICAL MANAGEMENT

- Selection of those patients who may benefit from re-treatment after aneurysm recurrence may be difficult. The low risk for bleeding from partially filled aneurysms must be balanced against the procedure-related risks of re-treatment.

SURGICAL TREATMENT

- The microsurgical treatment of previously coiled aneurysms is an option in aneurysm recurrence and may consist of direct clipping or of bypasses in coiled aneurysms that cannot be clipped.

ENDOVASCULAR TREATMENT

- In wide-necked aneurysm remnants, balloon-assisted coiling, stenting (alone, in combination with coil placement, or in a staged approach with stent placement first and subsequent coiling in a second session), or flow diversion with densely woven stents may be performed.
- Because this treatment is planned in most instances, patients are pre-treated with aspirin and clopidogrel 3 days before the procedure to prevent thromboembolic complications.
- Stents may be employed either alone or in conjunction with coils that may be implanted in the same session or in a second session. If additional coiling is contemplated, a jailing technique or subsequent catheterization through the stent mesh can be done. Benefits of jailing are additional stability of the coil-deploying catheter.
- Because the newly deployed stent may not be fully implanted in the parent vessel, coil loops may be pushed between the wall of the vessel and the stent. Some authors therefore prefer subsequent coiling in a second session.
- Stent jacking is a technique in which the stent is used as a "jack" to push coils back into the aneurysm.
- Stents may be used to jail migrated coil loops against the vessel wall if they cannot be retrieved with a snare.

Possible Complications

- With the patient on double antiplatelet medication, thromboembolic complications are rare.
- The newly deployed stent can still move, and caution must be taken when the stent is reentered with a microcatheter because the stent may dislodge or the catheter may enter the space between the stent struts and vessel wall.

Published Literature on Treatment Options

The risk that aneurysm remnants or recurrent aneurysms will rebleed is low and has to be balanced against treatment-related risks. Technical difficulties during surgery are the lesser degree of aneurysm sac mobility in previously coiled aneurysms and a higher risk for neck rupture during clip placement because of the intra-aneurysmal coil mass. These challenges are reflected in a combined surgical morbidity and mortality rate of ~10%. The values are considerably worse than those of endovascular re-treatment, with a combined morbidity and mortality rate for re-treatment close to 2%. Because multiple re-treatments may, however, be necessary, endovascular options with stents may prove a viable alternative in the attempt to achieve stable results.

In a recent long-term study of Sedat et al, the technical success rate of stents was 97%, with a procedural morbidity rate of 2% and no mortality. Aneurysm regrowth was seen in 10% of cases at the first follow-up, and after the first control angiogram, no delayed recanalization or regrowth was observed, testifying to the long-term durability of stents. These positive results, confirmed by other groups, have to be balanced against stent-related problems such as delayed in-stent stenosis, which occurs in 6 to 22% of patients. Occlusion of the treated artery and neurologic complications have been reported and may occur as early as 3 months following the procedure. On the other hand, mid- and long-term follow-up of patients with in-stent stenosis has shown no significant associated clinical symptoms and reversal of the stenosis in some patients.

PEARLS AND PITFALLS

- Contrast-enhanced MRA is the method of choice to follow coiled aneurysms.
- In wide-necked aneurysms, stent-assisted coiling may be beneficial and lead to long-term stability.
- In-stent stenosis may occur in up to 22% of patients

Further Reading

Agid R, Willinsky RA, Lee SK, Terbrugge KG, Farb RI. Characterization of aneurysm remnants after endovascular treatment: contrast-enhanced MR angiography versus catheter digital subtraction angiography. AJNR Am J Neuroradiol 2008;29(8):1570–1574

Ferns SP, Sprengers ME, van Rooij WJ, et al. Coiling of intracranial aneurysms: a systematic review on initial occlusion and reopening and retreatment rates. Stroke 2009;40(8):e523–e529

Fiorella D, Albuquerque FC, Woo H, Rasmussen PA, Masaryk TJ, McDougall CG. Neuroform in-stent stenosis: incidence, natural history, and treatment strategies. Neurosurgery 2006;59(1):34–42, discussion 34–42

Henkes H, Fischer S, Liebig T, et al. Repeated endovascular coil occlusion in 350 of 2759 intracranial aneurysms: safety and effectiveness aspects. Neurosurgery 2006;58(2):224–232, discussion 224–232

Mocco J, Snyder KV, Albuquerque FC, et al. Treatment of intracranial aneurysms with the Enterprise stent: a multicenter registry. J Neurosurg 2009;110(1):35–39

Sedat J, Chau Y, Mondot L, Vargas J, Szapiro J, Lonjon M. Endovascular occlusion of intracranial wide-necked aneurysms with stenting (Neuroform) and coiling: mid-term and long-term results. Neuroradiology 2009;51(6):401–409

Tähtinen OI, Vanninen RL, Manninen HI, et al. Wide-necked intracranial aneurysms: treatment with stent-assisted coil embolization during acute (<72 hours) subarachnoid hemorrhage—experience in 61 consecutive patients. Radiology 2009;253(1):199–208

Waldron JS, Halbach VV, Lawton MT. Microsurgical management of incompletely coiled and recurrent aneurysms: trends, techniques, and observations on coil extrusion. Neurosurgery 2009; 64(5, Suppl 2)301–315, discussion 315–317

CASE 7

Case Description

Clinical Presentation

A 41-year-old man with a positive family history of aneurysms (mother and sister both died of subarachnoid hemorrhage [SAH]) is found to have a wide-necked carotid side wall aneurysm opposite the ophthalmic artery. The aneurysm has an intradural location on high-resolution coronal T2-weighted MRI. The patient is pre-treated with clopidogrel and acetylsalicylic acid 3 days before treatment in preparation for stent-assisted coiling.

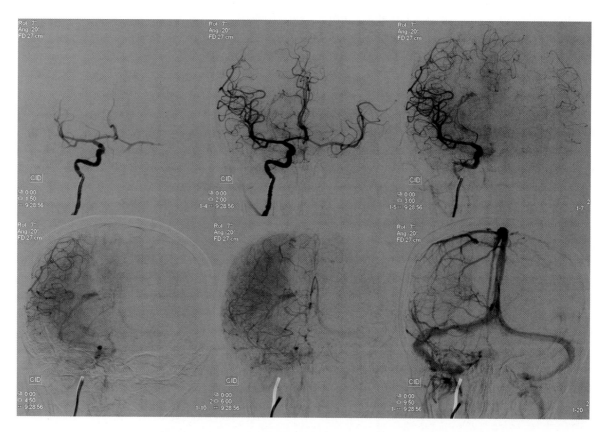

Fig. 7.1 DSA. Right ICA angiogram in AP view demonstrates vasospasm of the right ICA with stagnation of contrast **(upper row)**. Immediate withdrawal of the guiding catheter results in washout of the contrast **(lower row)**.

Radiologic Studies

DSA

Injection into the right internal carotid artery (ICA) demonstrated significant vasospasm surrounding the tip of the catheter with contrast stagnation in the supraclinoid ICA and delayed washout. The vasospasm was noted during the injection, and the catheter was immediately withdrawn, resulting in a good outflow of the contrast material (**Fig. 7.1**). However, subsequent test injections demonstrated persistent and progressive vasospasm in the proximal ICA.

Diagnosis

Mechanically induced vasospasm before stent-assisted coiling

Treatment

EQUIPMENT

- Standard 6F access (puncture needle, 6F vascular sheath)
- A 6F multipurpose catheter (Envoy; Cordis, Warren, NJ) with continuous flush and a 0.035-in hydrophilic guidewire (Terumo, Somerset, NJ)
- A straight microcatheter with a 1.7F tip and a 0.065-in inner lumen (Excelsior SL 10; Boston Scientific, Natick, MA) with a 0.014-in guidewire (Synchro 14, Boston Scientific)
- Coil selection: for framing, MicruSphere 4 × 7.5 (Micrus, San Jose, CA); for subsequent filling and finishing, Ultipaq 3 mm × 4 cm and 2 mm × 4 cm (Micrus)
- Neuroform stent 4.5 mm × 20 mm (Boston Scientific)
- Contrast material
- Heparin
- Nimodipine 2 mg diluted with 0.9% saline to 50% concentration

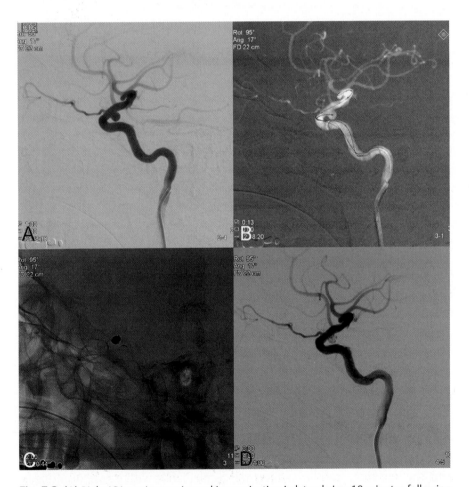

Fig. 7.2 (A) Right ICA angiogram in working projection in lateral view 10 minutes following infusion of nimodipine demonstrating no residual vasospasm. **(B)** Roadmap image demonstrates the position of the stent delivery microcatheter, which will jail the coil delivery microcatheter within the aneurysm. **(C)** Plain radiograph shows the dense coil mesh and stent at the end of the procedure. **(D)** Control right ICA angiogram in the working projection reveals nearly complete occlusion of the aneurysm sac.

DESCRIPTION

The 6F multipurpose catheter was advanced into the right ICA. At angiography, spasm at the tip of the guiding catheter was noted, and the catheter was immediately pulled back. Because the spasm did not resolve, a solution of 2 mg of nimodipine diluted with saline to a 50% concentration was slowly infused through the guiding catheter over 10 minutes, during which time the arterial pressure was carefully monitored. After control angiography demonstrated resolution of the spasm, the Neuroform stent was navigated into the intracranial ICA but not yet deployed. Subsequently, the aneurysm was catheterized with the microcatheter and the stent was deployed, jailing the microcatheter in the aneurysm (**Fig. 7.2**). The aneurysm was then embolized with a total of six coils. The final control run demonstrated no residual vasospasm (**Fig. 7.3**), and the patient awoke without neurologic deficits.

Discussion

Background

Vasospasm, or the contraction of smooth-muscle fibers in the wall of a vessel, is a well-known adverse event that may complicate an endovascular procedure by limiting distal blood flow. Vasospastic complications can occur during both diagnostic and therapeutic angiography and can be induced by the guiding catheter. They can also be caused by other inserted devices, such as protection devices used during carotid artery stenting, balloons, and microcatheters, especially if the anatomy is tortuous and the catheterization prolonged. The larger the lumen of the inserted device, the higher its radial shear stress against the wall, and the more prolonged the duration of the impact of the device against the vessel wall, the higher the likelihood of vasospasm. Young patients are more prone to vasospasm, and it seems

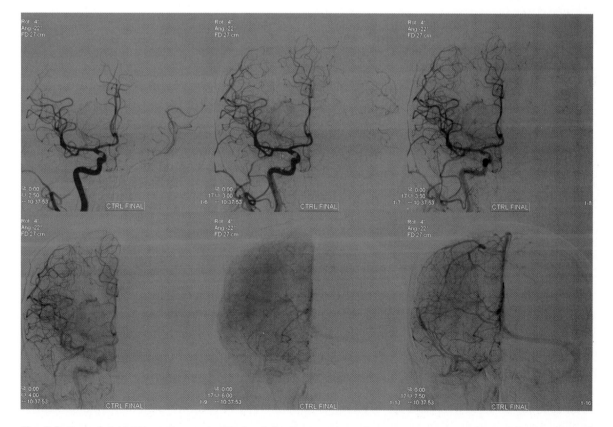

Fig. 7.3 Control right ICA angiogram in AP view following treatment demonstrates no vasospasm with normal cranial circulation time.

to occur more often in female than in male patients. Mechanically induced vasospasm in medium and large vessels, unlike SAH-induced vasospasm, is not the result of inflammation or a functional nitric oxide deficiency (see Case 11), but rather of direct physical irritation of the endothelium. With the increasing endovascular armamentarium, larger-bore catheters for deploying new tools, longer interventional treatment times, and the potentially devastating sequelae of limited distal blood flow, the recognition and treatment of mechanically induced vasospasm are of increasing importance.

Invasive Imaging Workup

- Angiography will demonstrate the extent of the vasospasm and its impact on the cerebral circulation. The classic imaging finding of proximal mechanically induced vasospasm is a "string-of-beads" sign.

Differential Diagnosis

- An acute dissection of the vessel has to be ruled out. In dissections, an intimal flap is commonly seen, and the narrowed segment classically does not demonstrate a string-of-beads sign.

Treatment Options

CONSERVATIVE OR MEDICAL MANAGEMENT

- Different drugs can be used to alleviate vasospasm: intravenous or cutaneous nitrates (depending on the body weight of the patient), intra-arterial papaverine, and intra-arterial or intravenous calcium channel antagonists.

ENDOVASCULAR TREATMENT

- Withdrawing the offending device, removing slack from the system, or pointing the tip of the guiding catheter away from the vessel wall may be helpful.

Possible Complications

- Hypotension and bradycardia may occur as a result of calcium channel antagonists, and nitrates can cause an increase in intracranial pressure (ICP).

Published Literature on Treatment Options

The best way to avoid this complication is to prevent it by gentle catheterization with the aid of a guidewire and careful control to ensure that the tip of the catheter is not directed against the vessel wall. If vasospasm occurs despite these precautions, the easiest way to treat mechanical spasm is to simply withdraw the offending device. However, such a passive treatment may be undesirable in certain conditions when the device (e.g., the catheter system or a protection device) needs to remain in position. In some instances, although vasospasm is present, blood flow is not significantly altered, and just gentle repositioning of the catheter and waiting will be sufficient to restore good flow.

Intravenous nitrates can be used to prevent vasospasm during endovascular procedures; however, their cardiovascular and ICP effects may limit their acute use because they can cause an increase in ICP and a decrease in intracranial compliance. The intra-arterial administration of papaverine has been used for SAH-induced vasospasm, either as monotherapy or together with balloon angioplasty, to alleviate spasm in distal intracranial vessels (see Case 11). However, papaverine therapy is short-acting and may elevate the ICP, and its efficacy in larger-vessel spasm and mechanically induced vasospasm is not proven.

Therefore, calcium channel antagonists, such as verapamil, nifedipine, nimodipine, and amlodipine, have been suggested because they reduce the tone of a muscular artery by inhibiting calcium influx into smooth-muscle cells. In some countries, however, nimodipine is available only as an oral medication and may therefore take too long to produce an effect. The intra-arterial administration of verapamil has been used for the prevention of mechanical vasospasm during endovascular procedures and for the reversal of spasm in coronary grafts, and it has also been reported to be safe and effective in the treatment of cerebral SAH-induced vasospasm. It is well tolerated systemically, although hypotension may occur. In our experience, it is the treatment of choice if vasospasm cannot be relieved by withdrawal of the offending device; our dose is 1 to 2 mg of verapamil given intra-arterially as a bolus with close supervision of the blood pressure and heart rate.

PEARLS AND PITFALLS _____

- In acute mechanically induced vasospasm, the first strategy should be to remove the offending device; however, if this is not possible, calcium antagonists or nitrates can be used to alleviate vasospasm.

Further Reading

Coon AL, Colby GP, Mack WJ, Feng L, Meyers P, Sander Connolly E Jr. Treatment of mechanically-induced vasospasm of the carotid artery in a primate using intra-arterial verapamil: a technical case report. BMC Cardiovasc Disord 2004;4:11

Feng L, Fitzsimmons BF, Young WL, et al. Intraarterially administered verapamil as adjunct therapy for cerebral vasospasm: safety and 2-year experience. AJNR Am J Neuroradiol 2002;23(8):1284–1290

Qureshi AI, Luft AR, Sharma M, Guterman LR, Hopkins LN. Prevention and treatment of thromboembolic and ischemic complications associated with endovascular procedures: Part II—Clinical aspects and recommendations. Neurosurgery 2000;46(6):1360–1375, discussion 1375–1376

Schirmer CM, Hoit DA, Malek AM. Iatrogenic vasospasm in carotid artery stent angioplasty with distal protection devices. Neurosurg Focus 2008;24(2):E12

CASE 8

Case Description

Clinical Presentation

A 46-year-old woman is referred to our aneurysm clinic after having had a severe headache 2 months earlier. At that time, she went to the emergency department but did not receive a CT or lumbar puncture. MRI 6 weeks after the event demonstrated a left-sided, irregularly shaped posterior communicating artery aneurysm. Because of a strong suggestion of a previous subarachnoid hemorrhage, the patient is scheduled to undergo endovascular aneurysm treatment.

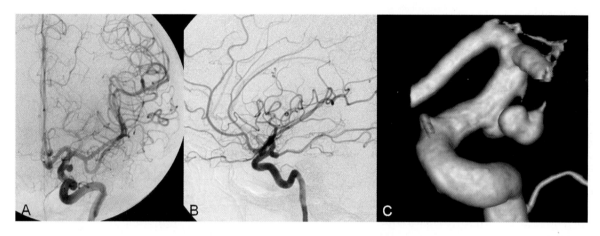

Fig. 8.1 DSA. Left ICA angiogram in **(A)** AP and **(B)** lateral views and **(C)** 3D reconstruction image demonstrates a multilobulated aneurysm at the origin of the left fetal-type posterior communicating artery.

Radiologic Studies

DSA

Diagnostic angiograms with biplane and rotational views confirmed the presence of a multilobulated aneurysm at the origin of the left fetal-type posterior communicating artery measuring ~5.7 × 4.0 mm in its largest diameters (**Fig. 8.1**).

Diagnosis

Aneurysm of the posterior communicating artery

Treatment

EQUIPMENT

- Standard 6F access (puncture needle, 6F vascular sheath)

- A 6F multipurpose catheter (Envoy; Cordis, Warren, NJ) with continuous flush and a 0.035-in hydrophilic guidewire (Terumo, Somerset, NJ)
- A 45-degree angled microcatheter with a 1.7F tip and a 0.065-in inner lumen (Excelsior SL 10; Boston Scientific, Natick, MA) with a 0.014-in guidewire (Synchro 14; Boston Scientific)
- Coil selection: TruFill 5 mm × 15 cm, 5 mm × 10 cm, 4 mm × 7 cm (Cordis)
- HyperForm balloon 4 mm × 7 cm (ev3, Plymouth, MN)
- Contrast material
- Heparin, protamine

DESCRIPTION

Following catheterization of the aneurysm with the microcatheter, the first coil was deployed, which framed the aneurysm satisfactorily (**Fig. 8.2A**). During placement of the final loops of the second coil, one loop prolapsed outside the aneurysmal sac, close to the dome (**Fig. 8.2B**). A control run confirmed the intraprocedural rupture (**Fig. 8.2 C–F**). The coil was deployed, the heparin was reversed with protamine, and a balloon was prepared and placed over the aneurysm neck to tampon the aneurysm and stop the bleeding. The balloon was left in place and inflated for 10 minutes (**Fig. 8.3**) while a third coil was prepared. However, this coil could not be deployed, and the microcatheter was pushed out of the aneurysm. Control runs demonstrated that the bleeding had stopped. Further control runs

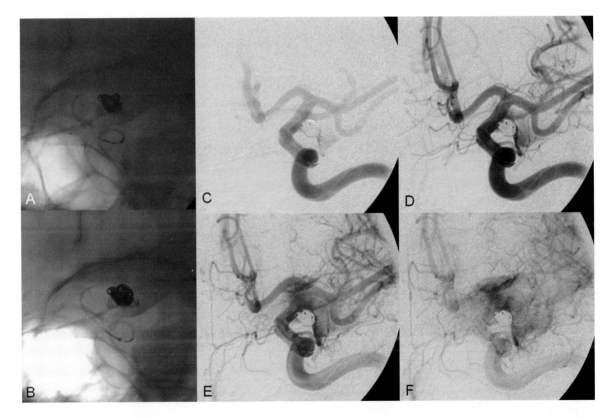

Fig. 8.2 Unsubtracted images during deployment of the **(A)** first and **(B)** second coils. During deployment of the second coil, one prolapsed loop outside the aneurysmal sac near the dome is noted. **(C–F)** Left ICA angiogram in the working projection confirms intraprocedural rupture with extravasation of contrast.

performed at 5 and 30 minutes confirmed these results (**Fig. 8.4**). The patient was extubated and had no neurologic deficits. Follow-up MRI demonstrated no ischemia and complete occlusion of the aneurysm.

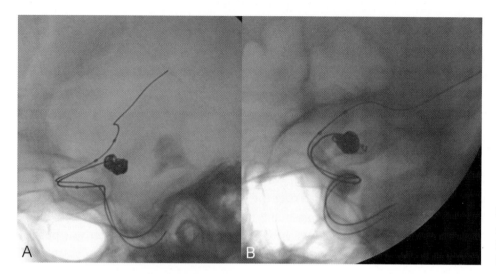

Fig. 8.3 (A,B) Plain radiographs show the position of the balloon in the aneurysm neck to tamponade the bleeding.

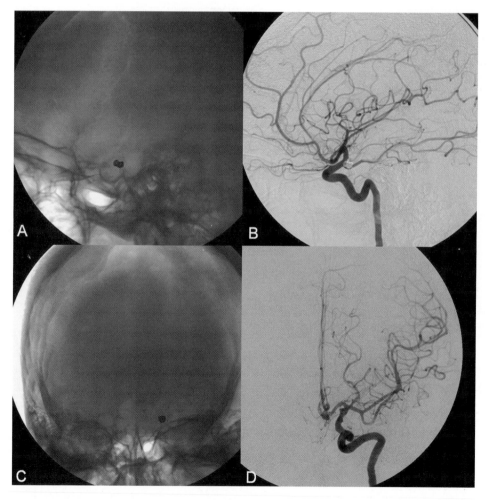

Fig. 8.4 (A,C) Plain radiographs and **(B,D)** left ICA angiograms in lateral and AP views after 30 minutes demonstrating occlusion of the aneurysm and no further extravasation of contrast.

Discussion

Background

Rupture of an intracranial aneurysm during embolization is a feared event that occurs in ~1 to 5% of aneurysm embolization procedures. Although in rare cases it may occur spontaneously as part of the natural course of the disease, other potential causes of a rupture during the diagnostic part of the angiography may be overdrainage via an extraventricular drain and excessive injection of contrast. However, in most instances rupture is caused by a guidewire, microcatheter, or coil perforation. Of these, uncontrolled forward migration of the microcatheter is probably the most common cause of aneurysm rupture. Risk factors for periprocedural rupture are small aneurysm size and previous rupture. A meta-analysis of periprocedural rupture events showed that for patients with ruptured aneurysms, intraprocedural aneurysm perforation was associated with a 33% risk for death and a 5% risk for disability, whereas for those with unruptured aneurysms, the risks for death and disability were 14% each. Worse prognoses are associated with iatrogenic rupture during the coiling of posterior circulation lesions and rupture caused by the coil or the catheter (as opposed to perforation related to the micro-guidewire).

Noninvasive Imaging Workup

PHYSICAL EXAMINATION

- During the acute perforation, patients classically demonstrate a typical or atypical Cushing hemo-dynamic response (acute hypertension and bradycardia or tachycardia) to the sudden increase in intracranial pressure (ICP).

CT/CTA

- CT after the procedure will demonstrate a combination of contrast material and blood within the subarachnoid space; therefore, a follow-up control image obtained after 1 day is more likely to demonstrate the extent of subarachnoid blood following periprocedural rupture.

Invasive Imaging Workup

- Angiography will demonstrate the exact point of rupture; however, once aneurysmal rupture is confirmed, repeated angiographies should be avoided to save time and limit extravasation of contrast into the subarachnoid space.

Differential Diagnosis

- Stagnation of contrast in a focal, not coiled, outpouching of the aneurysm or within a daughter aneurysm must be differentiated from focal extravasation.
- If the coils extend beyond the visible lumen of the aneurysm, they may be extending into a thrombosed part of the aneurysm rather than perforating its wall.

Treatment Options

CONSERVATIVE OR MEDICAL MANAGEMENT

- Immediate reversal of heparin with protamine is recommended once a periprocedural hemor-rhage has occurred (intravenous injection of 10 mg of protamine for 1000 IU of heparin given; if > 30 minutes after heparin administration, 5 mg of protamine for 1000 IU of heparin given).

SURGICAL TREATMENT

- If the clinical signs or CT findings are indicative of progressively increased ICP, placement of a ventricular drain is warranted.
- Surgical inspection may be discussed, depending on the location of the rupture; rupture close to the aneurysm neck may be difficult to control with endovascular means and may cause repeated rupture

ENDOVASCULAR TREATMENT

- To prevent the most common mechanism of perforation (forward jumping of the microcatheter), positioning of the microcatheter must be monitored; the forward progress of the catheter tip must be commensurate with the forward progress of the catheter shaft proximally, not only during catheterization of the aneurysm but also during coil deployment. After coil detachment, forward thrust that has built up may be released, which is why the "slack" in the system must be observed and eventually released before detachment.
- Friction accumulates (and may suddenly be released) in long, tortuous, and narrow vessel segments. Tri-axial approaches may be helpful in controlling microcatheter advancement by releasing friction on the microcatheter.
- It can be debated whether the perforating device should be pulled out or not. The device may be partially occluding the perforation, and pulling it out may result in further injury to the aneurysm wall. Placing a second microcatheter in the aneurysm to complete the embolization before pulling out the first may therefore be an alternative approach.

Possible Complications

- Reversal of heparin may increase the risk for subsequent thromboembolic complications.
- If a rupture occurs at the aneurysm neck, the risk for delayed rebleeding (after the ICP or the vasospasm has decreased) is high.

Published Literature on Treatment Options

Periprocedural rupture of aneurysms is not uncommon; in a subgroup analysis of the Cerebral Aneurysm Rerupture After Treatment (CARAT) study, periprocedural rupture occurred in 14.6% of 1010 patients (299 of whom were treated with coiling and 711 with clipping). Periprocedural rupture occurred significantly more often during clipping than during coiling (19% vs. 5%). However, the impact of the periprocedural rupture was more pronounced in patients undergoing endovascular treatment. Among patients whose aneurysms were clipped, death or disability occurred in 31% of those with periprocedural rupture and in 18% of those without periprocedural rupture; among patients whose aneurysms were treated with coils, death or disability occurred in 63% of those with periprocedural rupture and in 15% of those without intraprocedural rupture. Coronary artery disease and an initially lower Hunt and Hess grade were independent predictors of periprocedural rupture.

When perforation is recognized, treatment consists of immediate reversal of anticoagulation in addition to fast and dense completion of the coil embolization. One may consider leaving the perforated device in place and catheterizing the aneurysm with a second microcatheter to prevent further hemorrhage. Careful retraction with a "salvage" coil at the tip of the catheter (and a new roadmap) and subsequent fast coiling may also be performed. Repeated angiographies are in our opinion not necessary. In our clinical practice, we do not use liquid embolic agents or coils across the perforation site. Placement of such a coil risks exerting tension on the wall and may even impede further hemostasis. Immediate neurosurgical intervention is seldom necessary unless rupture has occurred close to the aneurysm neck. In these cases, balloon occlusion to induce hemostasis followed by surgical inspection may be warranted. Following the rupture, neurosurgical intervention may be necessary to decrease the ICP via emergency ventriculostomy or extraventricular drainage.

PEARLS AND PITFALLS

- Aneurysm rupture occurs more often in small and previously ruptured aneurysms.
- Perforations occur in ~5% of patients undergoing endovascular treatment and in 20% of patients undergoing treatment with surgical clipping.
- Reversal of heparin, fast and dense coiling, and management of an eventually increased ICP with extraventricular drainage are the three major strategies for treatment. They require good teamwork on the part of anesthesia, neurologic intervention, and neurosurgery.
- Not all cases of migration of coils, guidewires, or microcatheters beyond the confines of the aneurysm lumen represent perforation because some aneurysms may be partially thrombosed.

Further Reading

Brisman JL, Niimi Y, Song JK, Berenstein A. Aneurysmal rupture during coiling: low incidence and good outcomes at a single large volume center. Neurosurgery 2005;57(6):1103–1109, discussion 1103–1109

Cloft HJ, Kallmes DF. Cerebral aneurysm perforations complicating therapy with Guglielmi detachable coils: a meta-analysis. AJNR Am J Neuroradiol 2002;23(10):1706–1709

Elijovich L, Higashida RT, Lawton MT, Duckwiler G, Giannotta S, Johnston SC. Cerebral Aneurysm Rerupture After Treatment (CARAT) Investigators. Predictors and outcomes of intraprocedural rupture in patients treated for ruptured intracranial aneurysms: the CARAT study. Stroke 2008;39(5):1501–1506

Sluzewski M, Bosch JA, van Rooij WJ, Nijssen PC, Wijnalda D. Rupture of intracranial aneurysms during treatment with Guglielmi detachable coils: incidence, outcome, and risk factors. J Neurosurg 2001;94(2):238–240

Tummala RP, Chu RM, Madison MT, Myers M, Tubman D, Nussbaum ES. Outcomes after aneurysm rupture during endovascular coil embolization. Neurosurgery 2001;49(5):1059–1066, discussion 1066–1067

Willinsky R, terBrugge KG. Use of a second microcatheter in the management of a perforation during endovascular treatment of a cerebral aneurysm. AJNR Am J Neuroradiol 2000;21(8):1537–1539 (AJNR)

CASE 9

Case Description

Clinical Presentation

A 57-year-old woman has mild headaches 10 days before admission. CT and CTA performed at an outside institution demonstrate a left superior cerebellar artery aneurysm. Cerebrospinal fluid analysis is unremarkable, and she is scheduled for elective coiling. On the weekend before admission, she presents with the acute onset of severe headaches. CT and CTA demonstrate an acute subarachnoid hemorrhage (SAH). Subsequent deterioration of her condition due to hydrocephalus necessitates extraventricular drainage.

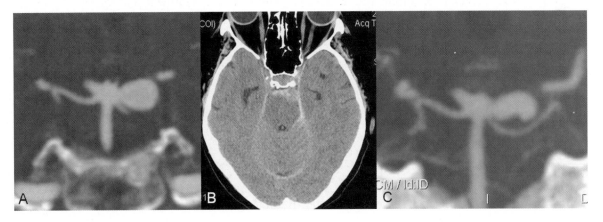

Fig. 9.1 (A) Initial CTA, (B) plain axial CT, and (C) CTA after the SAH. Note the change in the aneurysm shape.

Radiologic Studies

CT/CTA/MRI

Initial CT demonstrated a left superior cerebellar artery aneurysm with a round shape. Ten days later, before her scheduled elective coiling, she presented with an acute SAH. CTA demonstrated a marked change in the shape of the aneurysm (**Fig. 9.1**). The patient proceeded to angiography with coiling.

Diagnosis

Aneurysm of the superior cerebellar artery

Treatment

EQUIPMENT

- Standard 6F access (puncture needle, 6F vascular sheath)

- A 6F multipurpose catheter (Guider Soft Tip; Boston Scientific, Natick, MA) with continuous flush and a 0.035-in hydrophilic guidewire (Terumo, Somerset, NJ)
- A 45-degree angled microcatheter with a 1.7F tip and a 0.065-in inner lumen (Excelsior SL 10; Boston Scientific) with a 0.014-in guidewire (Synchro 14; Boston Scientific)
- Coil selection: for framing, GDC 360-degree coils 7 mm × 15 cm; for subsequent filling and finishing, two GDC 360-degree coils 5 mm × 9 cm (Boston Scientific) and DeltaPaq coils 5 mm × 10 cm, 4 mm × 8 cm, 2.5 mm × 6 cm (Micrus, San Jose, CA)
- Contrast material
- Heparin
- Abciximab (ReoPro; Eli Lilly, Indianapolis, IN) adapted to body weight
- AngioSeal VIP 6F (St. Jude Medical, St. Paul, MN)

DESCRIPTION

The 6F multipurpose catheter was placed in the right vertebral artery at the C5-C6 level. Angiography revealed the superior cerebellar artery (SCA) aneurysm and clot in the entrance of the aneurysm. The aneurysm measured 9 × 5 mm, with a 3-mm neck. The aneurysm neck partially incorporated the origin of the left SCA. The left P1 segment was hypoplastic. Note was also made of a tiny incidental basilar apex aneurysm measuring 1 to 2 mm. An Excelsior SL 10 microcatheter was navigated over a Synchro 14 guidewire into the aneurysm, and placement of a GDC 360-degree 7 mm × 15 cm coil led to satisfactory occlusion of the distal part of the aneurysm body. Following further embolization with two GDC 360-degree 5 mm × 9 cm coils and DeltaPaq 5 mm × 10 cm and 4 mm × 8 cm coils, control angiography demonstrated thrombus surrounding the proximal coil loops and the microcatheter extending into the distal basilar artery (**Fig. 9.2**). Abciximab was administered according to the patient's body weight as an intravenous bolus and a subsequent drip. Subsequently, the aneurysm coiling was finished with additional coils. Control angiography demonstrated resolution of the clot and no evidence of distal emboli. There was good flow into the SCA and complete exclusion of the aneurysm from the circulation. An AngioSeal closure device was used in the right groin. The patient awoke from anesthesia without neurologic deficits, and follow-up MRI after the treatment demonstrated no acute ischemia or infarctions (**Fig. 9.3**).

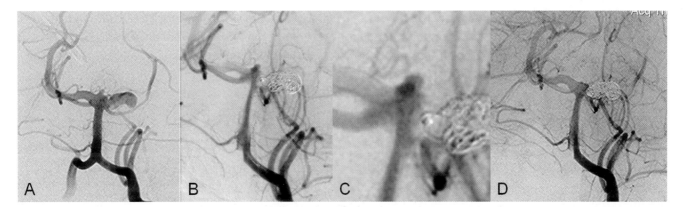

Fig. 9.2 DSA. Left vertebral artery angiograms in AP view **(A)** before the treatment and **(B,C)** during the treatment show progression of the filling defect, representing clot around the aneurysm neck. **(D)** Final control left vertebral artery angiogram following intravenous administration of abciximab and coiling demonstrates complete resolution of the clot.

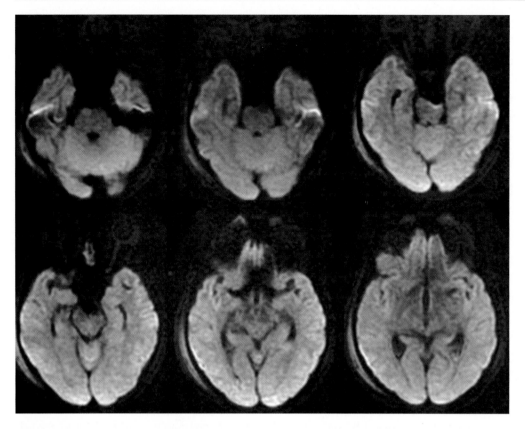

Fig. 9.3 MRI with diffusion-weighted scans after treatment shows no evidence of sequelae of the transient thromboembolic complication.

Discussion

Background

The two most commonly observed and potentially grave complications during aneurysm embolization are thromboembolism and hemorrhage, the former more common than the latter. These complications are more likely to occur during the treatment of ruptured than of unruptured aneurysms, and they are also likely to be linked to the experience of the physicians involved. In larger series, procedural thromboembolic complications leading to morbidity or mortality are present in ~6% of patients with ruptured aneurysms and in 3% of patients with unruptured aneurysms. However, the total rate of occurrence of thromboembolic events (without and with sequelae) is higher and ranges between 3 and 30%. When diffusion-weighted MRI is used, microemboli can be detected in up to 60% of cases. Risk factors for thromboembolic complications that have been discussed are large aneurysm size, previous rupture, long catheterization time, elderly patients, and difficult arterial access. Controversy exists about an increased complication rate when device-assisted embolization strategies are used (see Case 5).

Thrombosis is due to alterations of blood flow and the thrombogenicity of both the endothelial surface and circulating activated hemostatic factors. During SAH, activation of the coagulation system increases the thrombogenicity of circulating hemostatic factors. Thrombogenicity of the endothelial surface will be increased in cases requiring prolonged catheterization or multiple repositioning of coils, with subsequent intimal denudation within the aneurysm or at the aneurysm neck and the potential for endothelial damage. Finally, the blood flow is altered depending on the inserted material, including guiding catheters, coils, and stents. During electrolytic detachment, negatively charged platelets may be attracted by the positive charge induced. All these events will lead to platelet aggregation with subsequent "white thrombus" formation (i.e., a thrombus composed of densely packed platelets and fibrin). Platelet aggregation is mediated via glycoprotein (GP) IIb/IIIa receptors expressed on the platelet surface that bind to fibrinogen and via adhesive proteins that make platelets cross-link.

Given the high rate of thromboembolic events and their potentially devastating consequences, the neurointerventionalist must know how to prevent and manage these situations.

Noninvasive Imaging Workup

PHYSICAL EXAMINATION

- A new neurologic deficit following endovascular coil obliteration is in most instances related to a thromboembolic event and warrants further investigation with MRI or CT.

CT/CTA

- CT may demonstrate a focal area of hypoattenuation in an arterial territory. Given the significant number of metal artifacts, the immediate vicinity of the aneurysm cannot be evaluated, though. CTA can demonstrate distal thrombotic occlusions only in larger vessels; however, it cannot demonstrate thrombus close to the coil mesh.

MR/MRA

- MRI will demonstrate diffusion-weighted abnormalities as a sign of cytotoxic edema. These may be punctate or encompass a wedge-shaped distal arterial territory.

Invasive Imaging Workup

- Because the vast majority of thromboembolic complications occur during a procedure, angiography is the most important means to detect them and treat them rapidly.
- Missing distal branches, contrast stagnation, and an abrupt termination of a vessel as well as a missing capillary blush in the affected territory are the typical signs of distal vessel thrombus.
- Before these findings appear, however, a gradual buildup of thrombus in and around the coil mesh can be seen as a focal absence of contrast in the immediate vicinity of the coil mesh. The challenge for the interventionalist is to recognize this finding before distal migration of the thrombus takes place.

Differential Diagnosis

- The clinical differential diagnosis of a new neurologic deficit after coiling includes mass effect of the coils, perifocal edema surrounding the coiled aneurysm, and focal intraparenchymal hemorrhage.
- The angiographic differential diagnosis of a focal absence of contrast material includes inflow artifacts from other vessels (via the anterior or posterior communicating artery or the contralateral vertebral artery).

Treatment Options

CONSERVATIVE OR MEDICAL MANAGEMENT

- Heparin is a glycosaminoglycan that binds to and activates the enzyme inhibitor antithrombin, thereby inactivating thrombin and other proteases involved in blood clotting. It acts as an anticoagulant, preventing the formation and extension of thrombi within the blood, but it does not break down clots that have already formed. Heparin reverses the effects of excessive thrombin formation. The dosage is guided by bedside measurements of the activating clotting time (for endovascular therapies, the activated clotting time should be approximately between 200 and 350 seconds.

- Acetylsalicylic acid (ASA) acts by irreversibly inhibiting the formation of thromboxane. Thromboxane participates in a platelet receptor–mediated positive feedback loop, further amplifying regional platelet activation, and in the recruitment of additional platelets to the site of thrombus formation.

- Clopidogrel is a prodrug whose active metabolite inhibits adenosine diphosphate from binding to its platelet surface receptor. This binding leads to regional platelet activation and conversion of the GP IIb/IIIa receptor to a high-affinity state. Therapeutic levels (even after a loading dose is given) are not reached until after 6 hours.

- Abciximab is an irreversible GP IIb/IIIa receptor antagonist that binds to and eliminates this receptor and thereby blocks the final common pathway for platelet aggregation. It has a short plasma half-life; however, inhibition of platelet function persists for 4 to 6 hours after termination of the intravenous infusion. The dosage is typically an intravenous bolus of 0.25 mg/kg followed by a continuous infusion of 0.125 µg/kg per minute (maximum of 10 µg/min) for 12 hours.

- Tirofiban (Aggrastat; Medicure, Winnipeg, Manitoba) and eptifibatide (Integrilin; Schering-Plough, Kenilworth, NJ) are reversible GP IIb/IIIa receptor antagonists with a lower affinity for the receptor. Their plasma half-life is 1.5 hours. After discontinuation of the drug infusion, bleeding times return toward normal within ~15 minutes (eptifibatide) and ~4 hours (tirofiban). The currently recommended dosage is two boluses of eptifibatide administered 10 minutes apart, followed by a continuous infusion of 2.0 µg/kg of body weight per minute. Tirofiban is administered as a bolus of 10 µg/kg of body weight, followed by an infusion of 0.15 µg/kg of body weight per minute for 12 hours. Reversal of the effect of these drugs requires platelet transfusion. When GP IIb/IIIa inhibitors are used in conjunction with heparin, the dose of heparin should be decreased slightly.

- Tissue plasminogen activator (tPA) is a thrombolytic enzyme that catalyzes the conversion of plasminogen to plasmin, thereby degrading fibrin. Thrombus that is already established (rather than thrombus that is about to form) is therefore the target of this drug.

- Increasing the blood pressure slightly may help to increase the perfusion pressure.

ENDOVASCULAR TREATMENT

- In our opinion and supported by Ries et al, medical treatment is the first choice when thromboembolic complications are encountered. Mechanical thrombolysis (as discussed in Cases 48 and 49) for acute stroke treatment is usually not necessary, given the physiology of thrombus.

- Because most agents work well intravenously, we do not think that treatment with intra-arterial thrombolysis is necessary, although this remains an issue of debate.

Possible Complications

- Rebleeding from the aneurysm may occur if the aneurysm is not completely coiled. This risk is higher with tPA than with GP IIb/IIIa antagonists.

- Each drug has specific side effects, including thrombocytopenia after the administration of heparin or GP IIb/IIIa antagonists and systemic hemorrhagic complications after the administration of tTPA, ASA, and clopidogrel, especially in combination.

- Nonresponders to ASA (5–40%) and clopidogrel (5–25%) are not uncommon.

Published Literature on Treatment Options

Given the physiology of the blood clotting system and the different mechanisms of action of the drugs described above, their use in the prevention and management of thromboembolic events differs. There are no established guidelines for anticoagulant and antiplatelet management, and therefore practice varies widely.

It is generally agreed that heparin should be used during aneurysm coiling. Heparin reverses the effects of excessive thrombin formation that may be induced by the foreign material inserted or implanted. Because heparin does not break down clots that have already formed, it is believed to be safe even in the context of acutely ruptured and not yet coiled aneurysms, and it is therefore given in most centers once the sheath is inserted. In a recent meta-analysis regarding aneurysm perforation (also cited in Case 9) Cloft reported no increase in morbidity and mortality after intraprocedural perforation in patients given heparin versus patients not given heparin.

ASA and clopidogrel can be used as prophylactic drugs in unruptured aneurysm coiling. In cases in which stent implantation is being considered, both drugs are strongly suggested before treatment. At a minimum, the patient will take 100 mg of ASA and 75 mg of clopidogrel on 3 consecutive days before the intervention. Whether the use of one or both of these drugs in "uncomplicated" (i.e., small neck) unruptured aneurysms is necessary remains at the discretion of the interventionalist, but it has been recommended in a recent review article by Fiehler and Ries. In the same article, it is proposed that ASA be given intravenously after the first coil is deployed in a ruptured aneurysm or, because the intravenous form of ASA is not available in all countries, via a gastric tube. With this strategy, the rate of thromboembolic events could be reduced from ~18% without intraprocedural ASA to 9% with intraprocedural ASA. In the experience of these authors, the outcome after iatrogenic aneurysmal perforation did not differ between patients given ASA and those not given ASA.

While heparin, ASA, and clopidogrel are used to *prevent* thromboembolic complications, the acute management of thrombus formation requires other drugs, including tPA or GP IIb/IIIa antagonists. Given the mechanism of action described above, tPA will act better on established ("red") thrombi, which are rich in fibrin with trapped erythrocytes and classically occur in low-flow situations (e.g., because of an incompletely flushed guiding catheter). "White" thrombi, due to platelet aggregation related to coil or microcatheter manipulations or due to the activated blood clotting system in acute SAH, respond much better to GP IIb/IIIa antagonists, and treatment with tPA is not recommended, given the potentially disastrous complications of tPA. In the International Subarachnoid Aneurysm Trial (ISAT), all five patients who received thrombolytic therapy with tPA rebled and died, presumably because the protective slow-flow thrombus within the aneurysm that was induced by the coils resolved. Platelet inhibition with the GP IIb/IIIa antagonists dissolves hyperacute thrombus; however, it does not seem to cause resolution of the slow-flow red thrombus needed to protect the aneurysm and is therefore considered the method of choice in acute thromboembolic complications. Because after discontinuation of the drug infusion bleeding times return toward normal within a short period (15 minutes), eptifibatide may be considered safer than tirofiban (4 hours) or abciximab (up to 6 hours).The latter drugs should be considered if acute stenting is to be performed in an acutely ruptured aneurysm in the absence of premedication with clopidogrel or aspirin.

PEARLS AND PITFALLS

- The prophylaxis of thromboembolic complications is best managed with heparin, ASA, and clopidogrel.

- Intraprocedural acute thromboembolic events are best managed with GP IIb/IIIa antagonists because in most instances platelet aggregation thrombus is present.
- Thromboembolic complications occur more often in ruptured aneurysms.
- Bleeding into preexisting infarctions may occur.

Further Reading

Brilstra EH, Rinkel GJ, van der Graaf Y, van Rooij WJ, Algra A. Treatment of intracranial aneurysms by embolization with coils: a systematic review. Stroke 1999;30(2):470–476

Fiehler J, Ries T. Prevention and treatment of thromboembolism during endovascular aneurysm therapy. Klin Neuroradiol 2009;19(1):73–81

Henkes H, Fischer S, Weber W, et al. Endovascular coil occlusion of 1811 intracranial aneurysms: early angiographic and clinical results. Neurosurgery 2004;54(2):268–280, discussion 280–285

Jones RG, Davagnanam I, Colley S, West RJ, Yates DA. Abciximab for treatment of thromboembolic complications during endovascular coiling of intracranial aneurysms. AJNR Am J Neuroradiol 2008;29(10):1925–1929

Park JH, Kim JE, Sheen SH, et al. Intraarterial abciximab for treatment of thromboembolism during coil embolization of intracranial aneurysms: outcome and fatal hemorrhagic complications. J Neurosurg 2008;108(3):450–457

Ries T, Siemonsen S, Grzyska U, Zeumer H, Fiehler J. Abciximab is a safe rescue therapy in thromboembolic events complicating cerebral aneurysm coil embolization: single center experience in 42 cases and review of the literature. Stroke 2009;40(5):1750–1757

van Rooij WJ, Sluzewski M, Beute GN, Nijssen PC. Procedural complications of coiling of ruptured intracranial aneurysms: incidence and risk factors in a consecutive series of 681 patients. AJNR Am J Neuroradiol 2006;27(7):1498–1501

CASE 10

Case Description

Clinical Presentation

A 22-year-old woman presents with a diffuse subarachnoid hemorrhage (SAH) with focal thick clot on initial CT. She is found to have both a right middle cerebral artery (MCA) aneurysm and a right posterior communicating artery aneurysm. These are treated surgically, and the patient has an uneventful postoperative course. On the ninth day after presentation, she experiences left-sided arm and face weakness. CTA shows vasospasm of the supraclinoid internal carotid artery (ICA) and the right middle cerebral and right anterior cerebral arteries. The patient remains symptomatic despite best medical treatment.

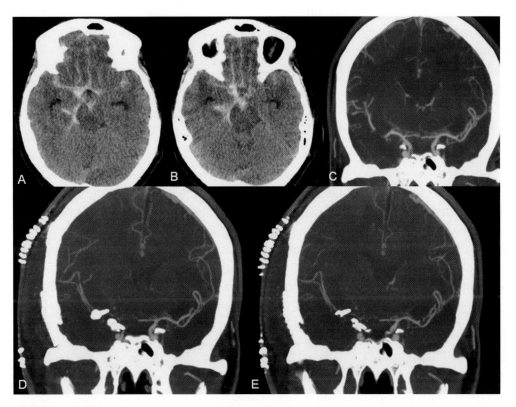

Fig. 10.1 **(A,B)** Initial CT and **(C)** CTA on admission reveal SAH located predominantly in the right basal cisterns. Normal caliber of the intracranial arteries is observed. **(D,E)** Follow-up CTA on day 9 shows markedly reduced calibers of the right ICA and right MCA. Metallic densities are seen, representing surgical aneurysm clips.

Radiologic Studies

CT/CTA

CT on admission demonstrated a thick clot of SAH in her right basal subarachnoid cisterns. CTA on admission demonstrated normal-caliber vessels and a broad-based aneurysm of the right MCA and posterior communicating artery (**Fig. 10.1 A–C**). CTA repeated on day 9 demonstrated significant vasospasm in the right ICA and MCA (**Fig. 10.1 D,E**). The patient proceeded to DSA.

55

DSA

On injection of the right ICA, severe vasospasm of the supraclinoid carotid and the A1 and M1 segments was confirmed. There was a tiny residual aneurysm at the level of the right posterior communicating artery. Injection on the left side showed minimal vasospasm with good filling of the A2 segments bilaterally (**Fig. 10.2**).

Diagnosis

Symptomatic vasospasm following SAH

Treatment

EQUIPMENT

- Standard 6F access (puncture needle, 6F vascular sheath)
- A 6F multipurpose catheter (Envoy; Cordis, Warren, NJ) with continuous flush and a 0.035-in hydrophilic guidewire (Terumo, Somerset, NJ)
- Voyager balloon RX with 2-mm width, 8-mm length (Abbott Vascular, Redwood City, CA) with a 0.014-in guidewire (Synchro 14; Boston Scientific, Natick, MA)
- Microcatheter (Excelsior SL 10; Boston Scientific)
- Contrast material
- Heparin
- Verapamil 5 mg

DESCRIPTION

The 6F multipurpose catheter was placed in the right ICA. A 2-mm Voyager balloon was then advanced over a Synchro 14 guidewire. Sequential gentle angioplasty was performed, starting at the supraclinoid ICA and advancing into the M1 segment in a proximal-to-distal direction. Control angiography after this showed significant resolution of the vasospasm through the supraclinoid carotid and M1 segment of the MCA. There was still distal spasm in the M2 segment and also the A1 segment. We therefore used an Excelsior SL10 microcatheter and dripped a total of 5 mg of verapamil in the supraclinoid carotid and the distal M1 segment (**Fig. 10.3**). This resulted in a reduction in the degree of distal narrowing.

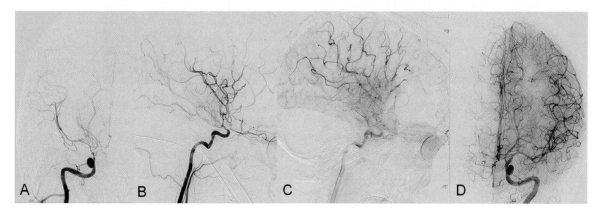

Fig. 10.2 DSA. Right ICA angiogram in **(A)** AP and lateral views in **(B)** early and **(C)** late phases confirms severe vasospasm of the supraclinoid carotid artery and the right A1 and M1 segments. **(D)** The left ICA angiogram in AP view shows minimal vasospasm with good filling of the A2 segments bilaterally through the anterior communicating artery.

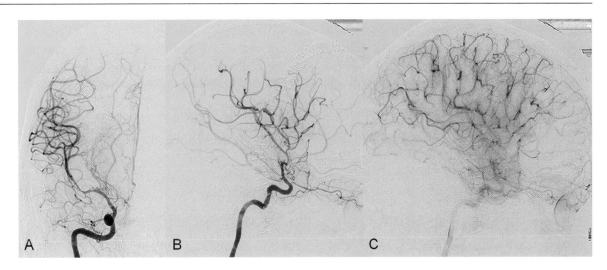

Fig. 10.3 DSA. Right ICA angiogram in **(A)** AP and lateral views in **(B)** early and **(C)** late arterial phases after mechanical and medical treatment for vasospasm demonstrates improvement of the distal perfusion.

Discussion

Background

Symptomatic vasospasm is present in approximately one-third of patients with aneurysmal SAH and results in a combined morbidity and mortality rate of 14%. It classically occurs between days 5 and 14 after the SAH, with a peak around days 7 through 10. Angiographic vasospasm, on the other hand, is present in nearly twice as many patients (60%). The mortality rate of vasospasm is believed to be ~7%, with another 7% of individuals having devastating neurologic deficits. Vasospasm usually does not occur in perimesencephalic, nonaneurysmal, traumatic, or arteriovenous malformation–related SAH. The pathologic mechanism is unknown, but a prolonged contraction of smooth muscle induced by oxyhemoglobin and mediated by nitric oxide, endothelin, or cytokines has been proposed. The following factors make the occurrence of vasospasm more likely: young age, female gender, previous cigarette smoking, and large amount of blood on initial CT (with clots or thick layers of blood more likely to cause vasospasm than diffuse or intraventricular blood). There is no significant difference between the rate of angiographic or symptomatic vasospasm in patients treated with clipping and the rate in patients treated with coiling.

Noninvasive Imaging Workup

PHYSICAL EXAMINATION

- Clinically, confusion, aggressive behavior, and a decreased level of consciousness are the first symptoms of vasospasm, followed by global or focal neurologic deficits.

TRANSCRANIAL DOPPLER ULTRASOUND

- Transcranial Doppler ultrasound is the least invasive "bedside" test to detect vasospasm and can guide further diagnostic imaging, such as CTA, when increases in flow rates of more than 50 cm/s are demonstrated. Peak systolic velocities above 120 cm/s indicate mild-to-moderate vasospasm, and peak systolic velocities above 200 cm/s indicate severe vasospasm.

CT/CTA

- CTA and CT perfusion techniques can be used to detect and quantify vasospasm. Their specificity for large-vessel vasospasm is good; however, the sensitivity for mild-to-moderate or distal vasospasm is low. In addition, they are of limited use in vessels close to metal hardware.

MR/MRA

- Given the usually sick and confused patient, MRI is of limited use in the acute setting of vasospasm.

Invasive Imaging Workup

- Angiography is considered the gold standard; however, it cannot be used as a screening method. Therefore, in most institutions it is used when the clinical findings and noninvasive test results suggest that vasospasm may be amenable to treatment. Angiography is then performed in the same setting as the endovascular treatment. The angiographic workup must include all arteries supplying the brain and indicate the cerebral circulation time and the site (proximal, distal, or both) and severity of vasospasm.

Differential Diagnosis

- The clinical differential diagnosis for neurologic deterioration after SAH includes hydrocephalus and procedure-related complications (e.g., delayed venous infarction or edema due to brain retraction in surgical cases; thromboembolic complications after coiling).
- Narrowing of the vessel can occur as a consequence of the treatment (coils or clips may lead to compromise of the distal circulation) or can be a congenital variation (unilateral hypoplasia of an A1 or P1 segment is commonly seen).

Treatment Options

CONSERVATIVE OR MEDICAL MANAGEMENT

- The first step in the treatment of vasospasm is medical therapy with hypervolemia, hypertension, and hemodilution (triple-H therapy) and additional Ca^{2+} antagonists (nimodipine). Obviously, triple-H therapy is dependent on complete occlusion of the aneurysm from the circulation.
- Hypervolemia and hemodilution are maintained with intravenous fluids (3 L/d) and monitoring of the central venous pressure (8–12 mm Hg, with a pulmonary wedge pressure of 14–18 mm Hg). The goal of hemodilution is to keep the hematocrit at 30 to 32% to reduce the viscosity of the blood while maintaining the oxygen-carrying capacity. Hypertension is achieved with vasopressors (dopamine and dobutamine); an arterial pressure of at least 30 mm Hg above baseline is maintained.
- Ca^{2+} antagonists inhibit the contractile properties of smooth-muscle cells and seem to have neuroprotective effects. When they are administered orally, the dosage is 60 mg every 4 hours.

ENDOVASCULAR TREATMENT

- The intra-arterial injection of vasodilators and balloon angioplasty, or a combination of the two, are the endovascular treatment options currently available.
- In our practice, endovascular options are employed only if the following criteria are fulfilled: new neurologic deficit not explained by other causes, no CT evidence of established cerebral infarction, failure of maximal medical therapy, and angiographic evidence of vasospasm in the same distribution as the neurologic deficit.

- If intra-arterial vasodilators are given, the dosages for the drugs described in the literature are as follows:
  - Papaverine HCl is available in a 3% concentration (30 mg/mL); 300 mg of papaverine is diluted with 100 mL of saline to obtain a 0.3% concentration and is administered at a rate of 3 mL/min.
  - Nimodipine doses are 1 to 3 mg diluted with 15 to 45 mL of saline to obtain a 25% concentration, which is infused over 10 to 30 minutes. A maximum of 5 mg can be given.
  - Nicardipine and verapamil doses should not exceed 5 mg; classically, these drugs are diluted with saline to a concentration 0.1 mg/mL and administered as a slow infusion.
  - Milrinone is diluted with 0.9% saline to a 25% concentration and infused at a rate of 1 mL/min to a total dose of 5 to 15 mg.
  - Fasudil (30 mg) is dissolved in 20 mL of saline, and 15 to 45 mL of this solution is infused at a rate of 1.5 mL/min.
- Balloon angioplasty is performed with either short, undersized coronary balloons 2 mm in diameter and 9 mm in length (Maverick; Boston Scientific) or softer, more compliant balloons used for balloon remodeling (HyperGlide 4 × 10 or HyperForm 4/7 × 7; ev3, Plymouth, MN). Although the HyperGlide balloon is very compliant and soft, the HyperForm balloon shape is better suited to the shape of the vessel. Given the maximum diameter of both balloons, care must be taken not to overinflate them. The balloons are either slowly inflated over a prolonged period or gradually inflated in increments of 25% of the maximum vessel diameter. Balloons should be inflated with a 50:50 mixture of iodinated contrast at a concentration of 300 mg/mL and saline.

Possible Complications

- If not treated properly, vasospasm can result in ischemic deficits.
- Intra-arterially injected vasodilators may cause an increase in intracranial pressure (ICP) and a decrease in heart rate and blood pressure, and their effect usually ceases after 24 hours.
- Overaggressive balloon inflation, on the other hand, may lead to dissection or even rupture of the vessel, with a usually fatal outcome.

Published Literature on Treatment Options

Concerning the oral use of nimodipine, a Cochrane Review revealed a significant effect in reducing the chances of poor outcome, ischemia, or infarction: relative risk (RR) of poor outcome, 0.69 (95% confidence interval [CI], 0.58–0.84); RR of ischemic deficit, 0.67 (95%CI, 0.59–0.76); RR of infarction, 0.80 (95%CI, 0.71–0.89). Therefore, nimodipine is strongly recommended. Triple-H therapy is also recommended, although the level of evidence is not as compelling as that for nimodipine. For patients with symptomatic vasospasm in whom these medical treatments fail, endovascular options have to be discussed, either intra-arterial infusion of drugs, transluminal balloon angioplasty, or a combination of both.

Vasodilators that have been used to treat SAH-induced vasospasm in larger studies are papaverine, nimodipine, nicardipine, verapamil, milrinone, and fasudil. These drugs are administered via slow infusion over a microcatheter or guidewire and in ~40% to 75% of treated patients lead to an initial clinical improvement. No matter which drug used, it is common, though, for clinical vasospasm to recur 12 to 24 hours after the initial response to the agent. Increased ICP, bradycardia, hypotension, and cardiac responses may be present, depending on the injected agent. Repeated treatments may be necessary, although recurrence seems to be less common with the newer drugs (milrinone and fasudil).

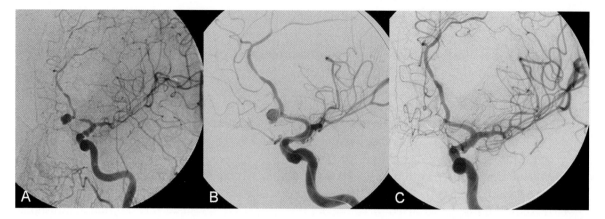

Fig. 10.4 This patient with an anterior communicating artery aneurysm came to our institution on day 6 following an SAH. **(A)** Significant vasospasm was present on the initial left ICA angiogram. In these cases, surgery is not recommended because surgical manipulation of the already spastic vessels may increase the vasospasm. Treatment of the aneurysm is, however, necessary to be able to employ triple-H therapy and oral nimodipine. Following a gentle transluminal angioplasty of **(B)** the spastic A1 segment, **(C)** embolization was performed, resulting in complete obliteration of the aneurysm. The patient had a good clinical outcome.

Angioplasty is a safe and effective treatment for symptomatic vasospasm, and when used early (< 24 hours), it leads to clinical improvement. It can be performed on the proximal vessels, and a slow or staged inflation technique should be employed. The rate of overall clinical improvement is slightly higher than with intra-arterial medical treatment (60–90%), and the results seem to be more durable compared with those of medical treatment. Drawbacks of this technique are the more difficult access and the inability to treat distal vessel segments, which is why in cases of severe proximal and distal vasospasm with no significant improvement of perfusion after proximal balloon angioplasty, combination therapy with the addition of intra-arterial medical treatments is required.

When patients with ruptured aneurysms that have not yet been treated present with vasospasm (e.g., because of belated arrival in the hospital), endovascular therapies are recommended: very gentle (undersized) transluminal balloon angioplasty (**Fig. 10.4**) followed by rapid coiling and subsequent additional angioplasty if spasm persists.

PEARLS AND PITFALLS

- The techniques used for aneurysm repair (clipping and coiling) do not differ with respect to risk for cerebral vasospasm and its consequences.
- Endovascular treatment should be contemplated if the site of angiographic vasospasm corresponds to the neurologic deficit and if all medical therapies fail to ameliorate the neurologic deficit.
- Distal vasospasm may be more amenable to intra-arterial vasodilator injection, whereas proximal vasospasm may be treated by gentle and slow balloon angioplasty.

Further Reading

Bejjani GK, Bank WO, Olan WJ, Sekhar LN. The efficacy and safety of angioplasty for cerebral vasospasm after subarachnoid hemorrhage. Neurosurgery 1998;42(5):979–986, discussion 986–987 de Oliveira JG, Beck J, Ulrich C, Rathert J, Raabe A, Seifert V. Comparison between clipping and coiling on the incidence of cerebral vasospasm after aneurysmal subarachnoid hemorrhage: a systematic review and meta-analysis. Neurosurg Rev 2007;30(1):22–30, discussion 30–31

Eddleman CS, Hurley MC, Naidech AM, Batjer HH, Bendok BR. Endovascular options in the treatment of delayed ischemic neurological deficits due to cerebral vasospasm. Neurosurg Focus 2009;26(3):E6

Harrod CG, Bendok BR, Batjer HH. Prediction of cerebral vasospasm in patients presenting with aneurysmal subarachnoid hemorrhage: a review. Neurosurgery 2005;56(4):633–654, discussion 633–654

Mindea SA, Yang BP, Bendok BR, Miller JW, Batjer HH. Endovascular treatment strategies for cerebral vasospasm. Neurosurg Focus 2006;21(3):E13

Mocco J, Zacharia BE, Komotar RJ, Connolly ES Jr. A review of current and future medical therapies for cerebral vasospasm following aneurysmal subarachnoid hemorrhage. Neurosurg Focus 2006;21(3):E9

Polin RS, Coenen VA, Hansen CA, et al. Efficacy of transluminal angioplasty for the management of symptomatic cerebral vasospasm following aneurysmal subarachnoid hemorrhage. J Neurosurg 2000;92(2):284–290

Sayama CM, Liu JK, Couldwell WT. Update on endovascular therapies for cerebral vasospasm induced by aneurysmal subarachnoid hemorrhage. Neurosurg Focus 2006;21(3):E12

CASE 11

Case Description

Clinical Presentation

A 63-year-old woman has progressive visual loss with no light perception in her right eye and progressive loss in her left eye (20/200). CT and subsequently MRI are performed.

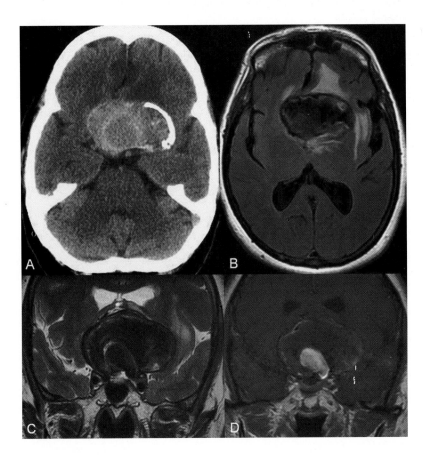

Fig. 11.1 (A) Unenhanced axial CT shows a large hyperdense suprasellar mass lesion with rim calcification. **(B)** Axial FLAIR, **(C)** coronal T2-weighted, and **(D)** T1-weighted contrast-enhanced MR sequences demonstrate a partially thrombosed giant aneurysm. The centrally located enhancing portion represents the nonthrombosed part of the aneurysm.

Radiologic Studies

CT AND MRI

CT and MRI revealed a partially thrombosed giant aneurysm arising from the left suprasellar internal carotid artery (ICA). The aneurysm was partially calcified and had significant mass effect on the chiasm. The adjacent brain exhibited perifocal edema (**Fig. 11.1**). Balloon test occlusion and DSA were performed to evaluate treatment options.

DSA

Injection in the left ICA demonstrated a supra-ophthalmic aneurysm with an opacified lumen that was significantly smaller than the size of entire aneurysm. Elevation of both A1 segments was seen. An anterior communicating artery aneurysm was also visualized. Balloon test occlusion demonstrated a carotid termination aneurysm on the right side and delayed capillary blush while the patient remained neurologically intact (**Fig. 11.2**). For details on how to perform a test occlusion, see Case 45.

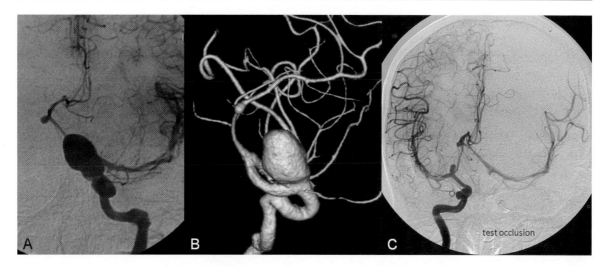

Fig. 11.2 DSA. Left ICA angiograms in **(A)** AP view and **(B)** 3D reconstruction show a large supra-ophthalmic aneurysm and elevation of the left A1 segment by mass effect. A smaller anterior communicating artery aneurysm is also noted. **(C)** Right ICA during balloon test occlusion demonstrates another right carotid termination aneurysm with delayed venous phase of the left cerebral hemisphere (> 4 seconds).

Diagnosis

Giant partially thrombosed supra-ophthalmic ICA aneurysm

Treatment

EQUIPMENT

- Standard 6F access (puncture needle, 6F vascular sheath)
- A 6F multipurpose catheter (Envoy; Cordis, Warren, NJ) with continuous flush and a 0.035-in hydrophilic guidewire (Terumo, Somerset, NJ)
- Marksman microcatheter (Chestnut Medical Technologies, Menlo Park, CA) with a 0.014-in guidewire (Transend 14; Boston Scientific, Natick, MA)
- Two pipeline flow-diverting stents 4.25 mm × 18 mm and 4.25 mm × 12 mm (ev3, Plymouth, MN)
- Contrast material
- Heparin

DESCRIPTION

In view of the delay in circulation time demonstrated at the test occlusion and the presence of both an anterior communicating artery and a carotid termination aneurysm, which would be exposed to a higher flow following sacrifice of the parent vessel, treatment with a flow-diverting stent was chosen. The patient was pre-treated with acetylsalicylic acid and clopidogrel for 3 days and was fully heparinized. After the femoral artery was accessed, a 6F guiding catheter was placed into the left ICA. Under roadmap control, we placed the Marksman microcatheter into the M1 segment of the left middle cerebral artery (MCA) with the aid of a Transend Soft Tip wire. Through the microcatheter, we placed a 4.25 × 18.0-mm pipeline stent into the supraclinoid left ICA. The stent was deployed just proximal to the anterior choroidal artery on the left. The proximal end of this stent was placed in the C4 segment of the left ICA. Control angiogram showed a significant reduction in flow toward the aneurysm. The microcatheter was then advanced again into the M1 segment of the left MCA, and a second stent was deployed within the first stent and placed over the neck of the aneurysm. Control angiogram showed near-absence of persistent flow into the aneurysm and stagnation of contrast material in the patent lumen (**Fig. 11.3**). No narrowing of the parent vessel adjacent to the aneurysm or distal thromboembolic events were noted. No new neurologic deficits developed. Follow-up MRI 4 months after the procedure demonstrated complete occlusion of the aneurysm with unchanged appearance of the mass effect (**Fig. 11.4**).

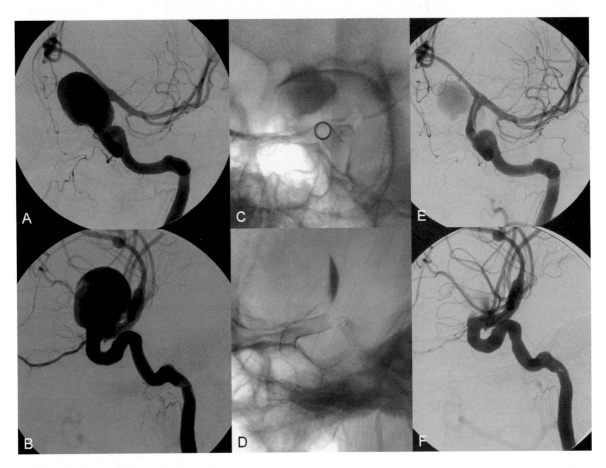

Fig. 11.3 Left ICA angiograms in the working projection **(A,B)** before and **(E,F)** after flow diversion. **(C,D)** Plain radiography demonstrates the position of the stent and stagnation of the contrast within the aneurysm sac.

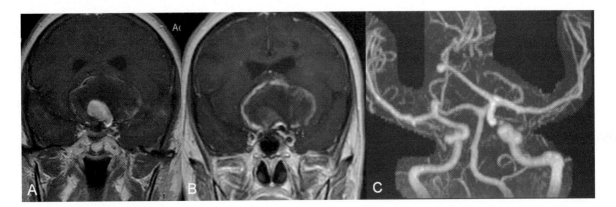

Fig. 11.4 T1-weighted contrast-enhanced MR sequences **(A)** before and **(B)** at 4 months after the procedure and **(C)** MRA show complete occlusion of the aneurysm with enhancement of the central portion no longer seen. The mass effect, however, is essentially unchanged.

Discussion

Background

Partially thrombosed aneurysms are not simply large saccular aneurysms with some clot along the wall. They demonstrate distinct clinical and imaging features and are likely caused by different pathologic mechanisms, so that different treatment approaches are required. Partially thrombosed aneurysms typically present with mass effect, and on imaging, thrombus of different ages in an onion skin pattern surrounds a smaller patent lumen. They usually continue to grow, probably secondary to recurrent subacute intramural dissections and repeated subadventitial bleeding from the vasa vasorum.

Noninvasive Imaging Workup

PHYSICAL EXAMINATION

- Partially thrombosed aneurysms typically present with progressive symptoms due to mass effect. They seldom present with subarachnoid hemorrhage (SAH). If there is SAH with this type of aneurysm, it usually arises at the neck of the aneurysm, presumably because of a transmural dissection at this site.

CT/CTA/MRI/MRA

- Neuroimaging studies of partially thrombosed aneurysms show evidence of intramural hemorrhage of different ages. Typically, CT and MRI show fresh clot at the periphery of the thrombosed portion of the aneurysm, with no apparent connection between the clot and the patent lumen of the aneurysm. The oldest thrombus is close to the patent lumen, indicating that the aneurysm has grown from the periphery.
- Surrounding edema is seen in nearly all cases. Contrast-enhanced studies may show a sickle-shaped zone or a complete ring of contrast enhancement at the periphery of the aneurysm.
- The aneurysm wall is vascularized by a dense network of vasa vasorum that behaves like the membrane of a chronic subdural hematoma. Intramural hemorrhages appear to be the main cause of the continued growth.
- In patients with giant thrombosed aneurysms, serial neuroimaging may demonstrate growth of the thrombosed portion as the consequence of hemorrhage into the thrombus and/or wall. In these cases, new intramural hemorrhage is seen distal to the patent lumen and close to the periphery of the aneurysm, suggestive of dissection between the layers of the aneurysm wall at the periphery of the thrombus.
- Partially thrombosed aneurysms may continue to grow, even when the lumen of the aneurysm is completely occluded or thrombosed. This is likely caused by ongoing hemorrhages within the vessel wall.

Invasive Imaging Workup

- Because angiography visualizes the lumen but not the other parts of an aneurysm, it will underestimate the size of these lesions. Evaluation of mass effect on adjacent structures, including the veins, is of importance.
- Potential collateral pathways for subsequent therapies, including patent anterior and posterior communicating arteries, must be visualized. Compression series, or even balloon test occlusion, may be necessary to estimate whether parent vessel sacrifice is possible.
- An underlying disease of the vessel wall may be present and should be sought.

Differential Diagnosis

- Given the significant mass effect, perifocal contrast enhancement, and edema, the differential diagnosis includes brain tumors (e.g., craniopharyngeomas, high-grade gliomas). The extra-axial location and the presence of pulsation artifacts within the mass should, however, lead to the correct diagnosis.

Treatment Options

CONSERVATIVE OR MEDICAL MANAGEMENT

- If not treated, these aneurysms will continue to grow and lead to mass effect, with compression of the brainstem, cavernous sinus, or supratentorial region of the brain, depending on their location. Although the risk for SAH is not high, the risk for progressive neurologic deficits with significant morbidity and mortality is high.
- Steroids may be indicated to reduce acute mass effect due to edema and to reduce inflammation.

SURGICAL TREATMENT

- Given the pathologic mechanism, complete surgical excision should be the best therapy for these lesions; however, given their size and the predictably considerable difficulties encountered in reconstructing the neck, they are challenging from a surgical perspective.

ENDOVASCULAR TREATMENT

- Flow diversion, flow reversal, parent vessel occlusion, and protective coiling are techniques that can be employed in these challenging lesions.

Possible Complications

- Persistent or increasing mass effect due to rapid thrombus formation and subsequent enlargement of the aneurysm
- Difficulties in navigating distal to the aneurysm, given its broad neck

Published Literature on Treatment Options

The term *partially thrombosed aneurysm* is misleading and may imply that the thrombus is located within the aneurysm lumen. Neuroimaging, surgery, and histology indicate that clot of different ages is located within the vessel wall, not the lumen. These lesions can be regarded as a proliferative disease of the vessel wall, with growth induced by extravascular (presumably partly inflammatory) activity. Mural thrombosis may act as a chronic trigger for perivascular growth factors, which then stimulate the further proliferation of vessels, both within the clot and within the vessel wall. Because their pathologic mechanism is markedly different from that proposed for nonthrombosed or saccular aneurysms, these lesions may be regarded as a separate clinical and pathologic entity.

Because of the specific histologic considerations discussed above, the ideal treatment should be complete surgical excision of the lesion; however, this procedure may be possible only after distal and proximal vessel wall occlusion (trapping) and is associated with a high periprocedural risk, given the significant mass effect, the often calcified aneurysm wall, and the wide neck. Therefore, endovascular options are to be considered. We do not think that endovascular repair of these aneurysms with coils is a durable treatment option. Clinical observations of such aneurysms treated with coils shows aneurysm regrowth over time, possibly due to compaction of the coil mass or to continuation of the pathologic process in the vessel wall. However, amelioration of symptoms with decreased perifocal edema may be seen, presumably as a consequence of a decrease in aneurysm pulsatility. "Protective" coiling may therefore be regarded as a palliative treatment option (**Fig. 11.5**).

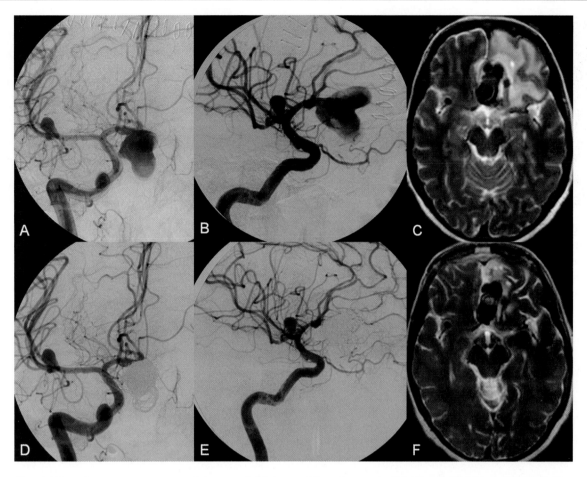

Fig. 11.5 Right ICA angiogram in **(A)** AP and **(B)** lateral views and **(C)** axial T2-weighted MR sequence reveal a giant partially thrombosed aneurysm of the anterior communicating artery complex with significant perifocal edema. A smaller right MCA aneurysm is also noted. Right ICA angiogram in **(D)** AP and **(E)** lateral views following protective or palliative coiling demonstrates occlusion of the aneurysm sac with coils. **(F)** Axial T2-weighted MR sequence at 6 months after embolization demonstrates significant reduction in perifocal edema.

Occlusion of the parent vessel may be a treatment option because (especially in the ICA territory) the vasa vasorum arise from the ICA itself and are thus occluded. However, for these kinds of aneurysms, the results of parent vessel occlusion are not predictable, and it has been shown that aneurysms can continue to grow even after their parent vessels have been sacrificed. Again, we presume that this is because of persistence of the vessel wall disease. Parent vessel occlusion (with or without additional surgical bypass) has been shown to reduce the aneurysm size over time (**Fig. 11.6**).

Flow reversal is a third endovascular treatment alternative, especially in the posterior circulation if sufficiently large posterior communicating arteries are present. Bilateral occlusion of the vertebral arteries below the posterior inferior cerebellar artery will lead to reversal of the flow direction in the basilar artery, which alters the inflow pressure and may lead to aneurysm shrinkage over time (**Fig. 11.7**).

As shown in this case, flow diversion may be a fourth alternative. At present, it seems that this technique yields excellent angiographic results, with preservation of flow in the distal territory and complete occlusion of the aneurysm. Additionally, the complication rate is very low. However, long-term clinical results are still missing (i.e., true size reduction of the aneurysm over time, delayed in-stent stenosis). Nonetheless, based on our initial experience and that of other groups, we are optimistic that this technique will be of help in treating these challenging lesions.

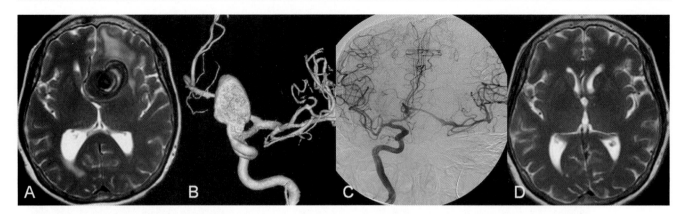

Fig. 11.6 **(A)** Axial T2-weighted MR sequence and **(B)** 3D reconstruction of the left ICA angiogram reveal a giant partially thrombosed aneurysm of the left ICA in a 65-year-old patient presenting with cognitive decline. **(C)** Right ICA angiogram following treatment with parent vessel occlusion after a balloon test occlusion shows good collaterals to the left cerebral hemisphere without a delayed venous phase. **(D)** Axial T2-weighted MR sequence 6 months following the parent vessel occlusion demonstrates significant regression of the perifocal edema and mass effect.

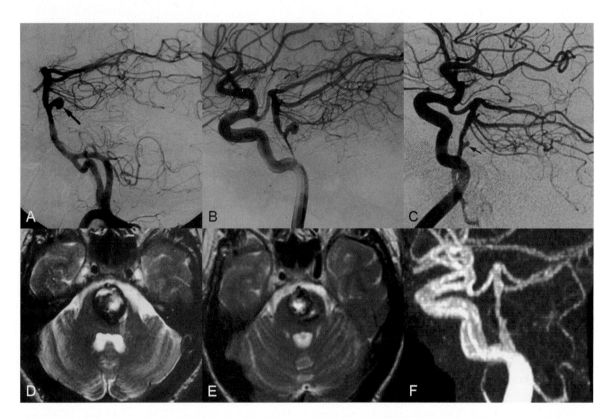

Fig. 11.7 Treatment of a partially thrombosed aneurysm of the basilar artery. **(A)** Left vertebral angiogram before treatment and left ICA angiogram **(B)** directly after and **(C)** 1 year after bilateral vertebral artery occlusion demonstrate reduction in size of the midbasilar aneurysm over time (arrows). **(D)** Axial T2-weighted MR sequences before and **(E)** 4 years after treatment show the size reduction. **(F)** MRA 4 years after treatment reveals occlusion of the aneurysm. The patient is neurologically intact.

PEARLS AND PITFALLS

- The imaging features of "partially thrombosed aneurysms" are peripheral hemorrhage within the "thrombosed" part of the aneurysm far from the patent lumen, a strongly enhancing rim, and an edematous reaction of the adjacent brain parenchyma.
- Treatment strategies include parent vessel occlusion, flow reversal, palliative "protective" coiling, and flow diversion.

Further Reading

Boardman P, Byrne JV. Giant fusiform basilar artery aneurysm: endovascular treatment by flow reversal in the basilar artery. Br J Radiol 1998;71(843):332–335

Krings T, Alvarez H, Reinacher P, et al. Rupture mechanism of partially thrombosed aneurysms. Interventional Neuroradiology 2007;13(2):117–126

Krings T, Piske RL, Lasjaunias PL. Intracranial arterial aneurysm vasculopathies: targeting the outer vessel wall. Neuroradiology 2005;47(12):931–937

Lylyk P, Miranda C, Ceratto R, et al. Curative endovascular reconstruction of cerebral aneurysms with the pipeline embolization device: the Buenos Aires experience. Neurosurgery 2009;64(4):632–642, discussion 642–643, quiz N6

Sorteberg A, Bakke SJ, Boysen M, Sorteberg W. Angiographic balloon test occlusion and therapeutic sacrifice of major arteries to the brain. Neurosurgery 2008;63(4):651–660, 660–661

van Rooij WJ, Sluzewski M. Endovascular treatment of large and giant aneurysms. AJNR Am J Neuroradiol 2009;30(1):12–18

van Rooij WJ, Sluzewski M. Unruptured large and giant carotid artery aneurysms presenting with cranial nerve palsy: comparison of clinical recovery after selective aneurysm coiling and therapeutic carotid artery occlusion. AJNR Am J Neuroradiol 2008;29(5):997–1002

CASE 12

Case Description

Clinical Presentation

A 60-year-old man presents with the sudden onset of headaches that start in his neck and then extend over his entire head. He has nausea and vomiting and is not fully oriented to place and time when seen in the emergency department. CT and CTA are performed.

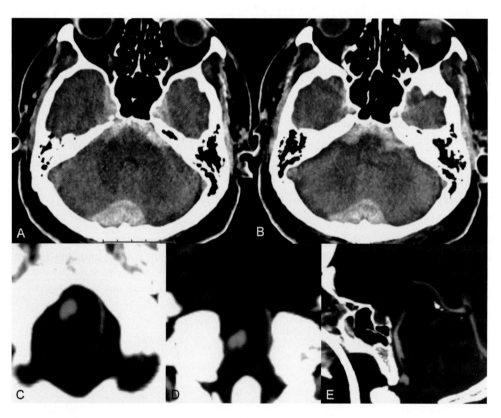

Fig. 12.1 (A,B) Unenhanced axial CT demonstrates SAH, predominantly in the posterior fossa. CTA in **(C)** axial, **(D)** coronal, and **(E)** sagittal views reveals a fusiform dilatation of the right VA, suggesting a dissection.

Radiologic Studies

CT/CTA

CT demonstrated a subarachnoid hemorrhage (SAH) that was dominant at the level of the posterior fossa, with blood in the inferior vermian cistern and surrounding the entire brainstem. CTA performed during the same session demonstrated a fusiform dilatation of the right vertebral artery (VA) suggestive of an acute hemorrhagic VA dissection (**Fig. 12.1**).

DSA

On injection in the left VA, the right V4 dissecting aneurysm was visualized via V4-to-V4 cross-filling. A small bleb was present in the fusiform aneurysm. An extradural origin of the right posterior inferior cerebellar artery (PICA) and the anterior spinal artery arising from the right distal VA were also noted (**Fig. 12.2**).

Diagnosis

Acute hemorrhagic dissecting aneurysm of the right VA

Treatment

EQUIPMENT

- Standard 6F access (puncture needle, 6F vascular sheath)
- A 6F multipurpose catheter (Guider Soft Tip; Boston Scientific, Natick, MA) with continuous flush and a 0.035-in hydrophilic guidewire (Terumo, Somerset, NJ)
- Straight and 90-degree angled microcatheters with a 1.7F tip and a 0.065-in inner lumen (Excelsior SL 10; Boston Scientific) with a 0.014-in guidewire (Synchro 14; Boston Scientific)
- Coil selection: two GDC 360-degree coils 3 mm × 6 cm; for subsequent filling, three GDC HyperSoft 2 mm × 4 cm for both the proximal and distal coil mesh (Boston Scientific)
- Contrast material
- Heparin

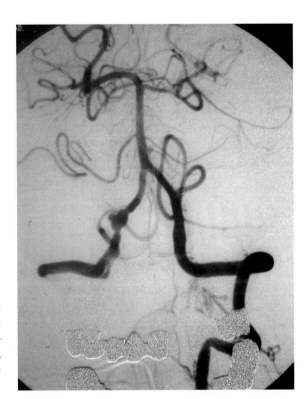

Fig. 12.2 DSA. Left vertebral angiogram in AP view shows irregularity and fusiform dilatation of the V4 right VA with a small bleb, in keeping with a hemorrhagic vertebral dissecting aneurysm. An extradural origin of the right PICA was observed. The anterior spinal artery arises from the distal right VA.

DESCRIPTION

The 6F multipurpose catheter was placed in the distal right VA. Under roadmap conditions, the straight microcatheter was advanced distal to the PICA just proximal to the stenotic portion of the dissection, and a dense coil mesh was deployed. A control from the right side demonstrated complete occlusion of the proximal portion with preservation of the PICA. Subsequently, the left VA was selected again. Injection demonstrated persistent filling of the dissected segment and mild widening at the level of the dissection. Because proximal occlusion of the dissection did not completely exclude the dissection from the arterial circulation, the potential for rebleeding was still present. In addition, the dissected segment did not include the PICA or the anterior spinal artery. Therefore, it was decided to occlude the distal entry zone into the dissection following catheterization of the right V4 segment from the left VA with the aid of a 90-degree angled microcatheter. Rebleeding from a proximally occluded "dissection aneurysm" can be anticipated when the dissection aneurysm does not collapse but increases in size after proximal occlusion, which is what happened in this case. A dense coiling mesh was deployed, and a subsequent control series demonstrated complete occlusion of the dissected portion from the flow with persistent flow in the anterior spinal artery and the right PICA (**Fig. 12.3**).

Discussion

Background

Of all intracranial nontraumatic cases of SAH, 1 to 10% are caused by a ruptured intracranial dissection. In children, the rate may be even higher. The majority of hemorrhagic intracranial dissections are located in the posterior circulation, possibly because on histology, the intradural VA has a thin media and adventitia with relatively few elastic fibers. Apart from the VA, the posterior cerebral artery (PCA) at the P2-P3 transition may be affected (presumably by repetitive microtrauma of the PCA at the free margin of the tentorium). The basilar artery, the distal cerebellar arteries, and the middle cerebral artery are less commonly affected. Although syphilis, fibromuscular dysplasia, col-

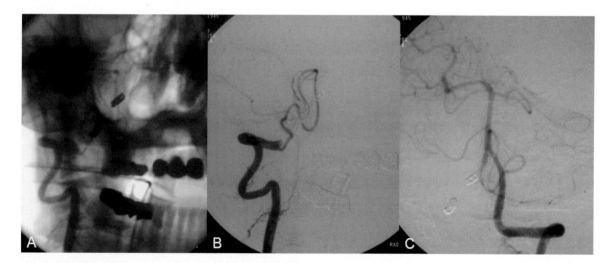

Fig. 12.3 **(A)** Unsubtracted right vertebral angiogram in AP view shows the two coil meshes in the right VA, proximal and distal to the dissection. DSA. **(B)** Right vertebral and **(C)** left vertebral angiograms in AP view demonstrate complete occlusion of the dissecting aneurysm with preservation of the right PICA and the anterior spinal artery originating from the right V4 segment.

lagen disease, and trauma are associated with dissection, the pathogenesis for most dissections is still unclear. On histopathology, sudden disruption of the internal elastic lamina with subsequent penetration of circulating blood into the media, transmural rupture, and SAH is the primary mechanism underlying cerebral dissecting aneurysms.

Noninvasive Imaging Workup

CT/CTA

- The predominant blood distribution in the posterior fossa in VA dissections should raise suspicion of a dissection because up to 30% of posterior fossa SAHs are caused by a dissection.
- The CTA should be scrutinized for focal stenotic portions of the vasculature because a fusiform aspect may not be present in all patients with a hemorrhagic VA dissection.

MR/MRA

- In the acute setting, MRI usually does not play a role unless the dissection is associated with ischemia rather than hemorrhage. In chronic dissections with associated mural hematoma, MRI can better visualize the pathology within the vessel wall, whereas DSA or CTA merely demonstrates the "luminal" aspect of the vessel.

Invasive Imaging Workup

- The most frequent angiographic demonstration in this series was regular or irregular eccentric fusiform dilatation associated with slight luminal narrowing proximal and distal to the dilatation. However, ruptured dissections may not have an obvious "aneurysmal" dilatation, and narrow vessel segments may also lead to hemorrhagic events.
- Angiography will demonstrate the origin of the dissection, which in most instances is a focal stenosis in relation to the PICA, anterior spinal artery, and potential brainstem perforators. Although in most instances brainstem perforators to the dorsolateral medulla oblongata arise from the PICA, the more distal the PICA origin on the VA, the more likely it is that these perforators will arise from the VA.
- Dissections can be bilateral, and as in all cases of SAH, the angiographic evaluation needs to include an evaluation of all four arteries supplying the brain.

Treatment Options

CONSERVATIVE OR MEDICAL MANAGEMENT

- Given the very high rebleeding rate, conservative management is not favored in most centers for acutely symptomatic patients. In the subacute stage (1 month following the dissection), however, conservative treatment may be contemplated.
- In the chronic stage (an asymptomatic patient with an incidentally found fusiform dolicho segment), conservative management with follow-up to rule out growth is recommended.

SURGICAL TREATMENT

- Surgical treatment options described in the literature are trapping, hunterian ligation, bleb clipping, and wrapping of the aneurysm.
- Rates of treatment-related morbidity and mortality are high, given the frequent posterior fossa location. Lower cranial nerve and respiratory complications predominate in most series.

ENDOVASCULAR TREATMENT

- Parent vessel occlusion, endovascular trapping, and stent-assisted treatments have to be discussed, depending on the size of the VA involved, the location of the dissection, and its relationship to the anterior spinal artery, PICA, and brainstem perforators.

Possible Complications

- Local brainstem perforator ischemia due to parent vessel occlusion
- Thromboembolic complications during parent vessel occlusion
- Extensive thrombosis into the distal VA following parent vessel occlusion
- High risk for repeated rupture of the dissected segment
- It is difficult to manage basilar artery vasospasm if the treated (sacrificed) VA was the dominant supply (and access) to the posterior fossa circulation.

Published Literature on Treatment Options

Acutely ruptured dissections are unstable and have a tendency to rebleed. The rebleeding rate has been reported to be as high as 70%, with a 50% mortality rate. The shorter the time elapsed after initial hemorrhage, the higher the risk for rebleeding in the acute phase, with up to 70% of repeated ruptures occurring within the first 24 hours. However, the rebleeding rate decreases considerably after the first week following initial hemorrhage, and unlike saccular aneurysms, ruptured dissections may completely heal via vessel wall repair mechanisms. Conservative management may therefore be adopted when patients are referred in the subacute stage (> 1 month after the initial event).

Surgical options for acute hemorrhagic intracranial dissection include trapping, hunterian ligation, bleb clipping, and wrapping, the latter method being rather historical given the extremely high risk for repeated hemorrhage. Based on the described pathologic mechanism, bleb clipping may also be regarded as insufficient; the dissection may still grow or rupture because in most instances the endoluminal entry point of blood into the vessel wall is not treated. Ligation and trapping are therefore considered the surgical therapies of choice. Depending on the location of the dissection, a surgical approach may be difficult, and because the VA is the most common site of dissection, rates of lower cranial nerve palsy are reported to be as high as 75% and those of respiratory complications as high as 20%, which is why endovascular treatment modalities are favored in most centers.

When contemplating endovascular treatments, one has to remember that because of their inherent capability to heal, dissections can resolve spontaneously; therefore, the aim of treatment is to prevent more blood from entering the dissected vessel segment. Endosaccular coiling (with or without stent assistance) may not necessarily achieve this goal, given the more proximal entry point of the dissection, and rebleeding rates with this treatment strategy are known to be high. Therefore, treatment options to be favored are the following: (1) parent vessel occlusion of the dissected segment by trapping, (2) flow reversal over the dissected segment with proximal vessel occlusion (**Fig. 12.4**), and (3) apposition of the dissected intimal flap to the vessel wall with a stent. The obvious advantage of the latter treatment strategy is the reconstitution of flow through the dissected vessel; however, this treatment strategy can work only if a stent with a dense mesh and a sufficiently high radial force is employed. The new generation of flow diversion stents, discussed in Case 11, are in the author's opinion well suited for this purpose; however, problems with acute in-stent thrombosis, the need for aggressive antiplatelet management in the acute phase of an SAH, and the risk for rebleeding if the dissection is not sufficiently apposed have to be weighed against the risks and benefits of the

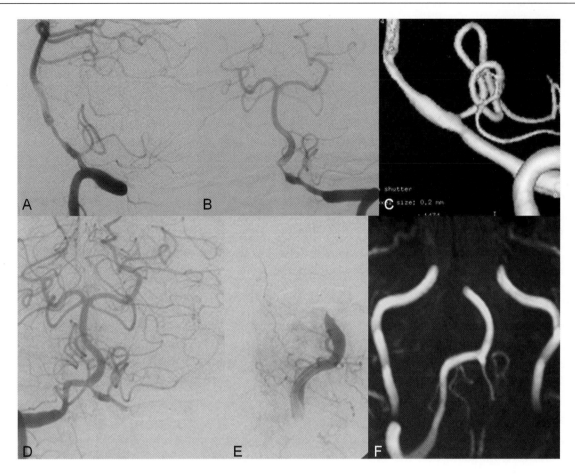

Fig. 12.4 Left vertebral angiogram in **(A)** AP and **(B)** lateral views and **(C)** 3D reconstruction demonstrates irregularity of the distal left VA, corresponding to dissection that also involves the origin of the PICA. Therefore, only a proximal occlusion was performed, with flow reversal from the contralateral VA into the PICA. **(D)** Right and **(E)** left vertebral angiograms in AP view show obliteration of the proximal part of the dissection. Although flow was still visible through the distal dissected lumen after proximal occlusion, **(F)** follow-up MRA reveals remodeling of the dissection to a normal luminal structure, and no perforator ischemia is noted.

established treatment options (i.e., parent vessel occlusion or flow reversal). Because the choice of treatment will depend on the individual vascular anatomy and the site of the dissection, only general guidelines about the management of these challenging cases can be given.

PEARLS AND PITFALLS _____

- Dissections cause up to 10% of all nontraumatic cases of SAH.
- The posterior circulation is more often involved than the anterior circulation because of thinner vessel walls with less elastic fibers.
- On histopathology, the elastic lamina is destroyed.
- The rebleeding rate is as high as 70% in the first 24 hours and 80% in the first week. Rebleeding is associated with a mortality rate of up to 50%.
- At angiography, a focal stenosis is often seen proximal to a fusiform dilatation.

- Treatment choices are dependent on the individual anatomy and include parent vessel occlusion, flow reversal, and trapping. Coiling of the fusiform dilatation (with or without stent assistance) is associated with high periprocedural repeated rupture rates.
- The role of stents for the treatment of acute dissections is a matter of debate. If the stent is able to reposition the flap against the vessel wall without further penetration of blood into the dissected segment, treatment is complete; however, only stents with a very dense mesh and high radial forces will be able to accomplish this. Problems with acute in-stent thrombosis may occur.

Further Reading

Anxionnat R, de Melo Neto JF, Bracard S, et al. Treatment of hemorrhagic intracranial dissections. Neurosurgery 2003;53(2):289–300, discussion 300–301

Hamada J, Kai Y, Morioka M, Yano S, Todaka T, Ushio Y. Multimodal treatment of ruptured dissecting aneurysms of the vertebral artery during the acute stage. J Neurosurg 2003;99(6):960–966

Jin SC, Kwon DH, Choi CG, Ahn JS, Kwun BD. Endovascular strategies for vertebrobasilar dissecting aneurysms. AJNR Am J Neuroradiol 2009;30(8):1518–1523

Mizutani T, Aruga T, Kirino T, Miki Y, Saito I, Tsuchida T. Recurrent subarachnoid hemorrhage from untreated ruptured vertebrobasilar dissecting aneurysms. Neurosurgery 1995;36(5):905–911, discussion 912–913

Mizutani T, Kojima H, Asamoto S, Miki Y. Pathological mechanism and three-dimensional structure of cerebral dissecting aneurysms. J Neurosurg 2001;94(5):712–717

Peluso JP, van Rooij WJ, Sluzewski M, Beute GN, Majoie CB. Endovascular treatment of symptomatic intradural vertebral dissecting aneurysms. AJNR Am J Neuroradiol 2008;29(1):102–106

Schievink WI, Wijdicks EF, Piepgras DG, Chu CP, O'Fallon WM, Whisnant JP. The poor prognosis of ruptured intracranial aneurysms of the posterior circulation. J Neurosurg 1995;82(5):791–795

Zhao WY, Krings T, Alvarez H, Ozanne A, Holmin S, Lasjaunias P. Management of spontaneous haemorrhagic intracranial vertebrobasilar dissection: review of 21 consecutive cases. Acta Neurochir (Wien) 2007;149(6):585–596, discussion 596

CASE 13

Case Description

Clinical Presentation

A 46-year-old woman is admitted for sudden headaches with confusion. No posterior fossa neurologic symptom is noted, considering the interference of confusion with the clinical examination. Outside CT shows a subarachnoid hemorrhage (SAH) without associated intraparenchymal hemorrhage, and the patient is referred to us for further angiographic workup.

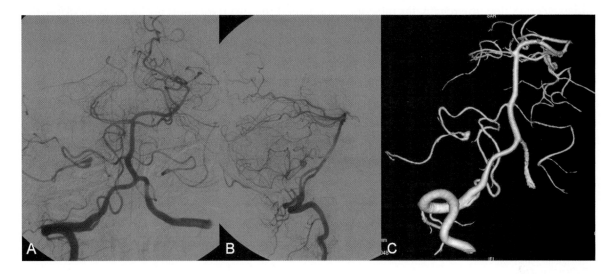

Fig. 13.1 DSA. Right vertebral angiogram in **(A)** AP and **(B)** lateral views and **(C)** 3D reconstruction demonstrates a fusiform aneurysm of the right post-labyrinthine AICA.

Radiologic Studies

DSA

A complete four-vessel angiography was performed. Vertebral artery (VA) injection demonstrated a fusiform aneurysm of the distal right anterior inferior cerebellar artery (AICA). There was no evidence of an associated vascular malformation. Proximal to the fusiform segment, focal narrowing of the vessel lumen was demonstrated (**Fig. 13.1**).

Diagnosis

Acutely ruptured dissecting distal AICA aneurysm

Treatment

EQUIPMENT

- Standard 5F access (puncture needle, 5F vascular sheath)
- A 5F multipurpose catheter (Guider Soft Tip; Boston Scientific, Natick, MA) with continuous flush and a 0.035-in hydrophilic guidewire (Terumo, Somerset, NJ)

- A 0.012-in flow-directed microcatheter (Magic; Balt International, Montmorency, France) with a 0.008-in guidewire (Mirage; ev3, Plymouth, MN)
- A 10% glucose solution
- Histoacryl/Lipiodol (1 mL/1 mL))
- Contrast material
- Steroids
- Heparin

DESCRIPTION

After distal catheterization of the dominant VA with a multipurpose guiding catheter, which was continuously flushed, a flow-directed microcatheter was advanced into the AICA and carefully advanced toward the distal post-labyrinthine portion. A guidewire was introduced into the microcatheter and advanced without exiting the microcatheter to make it easier to push the microcatheter. Superselective slow microcatheter injections confirmed the distal location of the catheter. After the microcatheter had been flushed with the glucose solution, a mixture of 1 mL of glue with 1 mL of Lipiodol was injected that allowed complete occlusion of the diseased segment without significant penetration of the liquid embolic agent into the distal circulation (**Fig. 13.2**). The microcatheter was removed, and control runs demonstrated complete occlusion of the diseased segment, with distal revascularization by leptomeningeal collaterals. The patient was given heparin and steroids for 24 hours. MRI following the procedure showed focal and scattered areas of distal AICA territory ischemia without involvement of the deep cerebellar nuclei, and postural instability was noted clinically. One-year follow-up imaging did not demonstrate any remnant or recurrence of the aneurysm. The clinical course was favorable; the patient's postural instability remained but did not interfere with her daily activities.

Discussion

Background

Intracranial posterior circulation aneurysms account for ~10% of all intracranial aneurysms. Within this group, fewer than 5% are in a peripheral location. In most instances, these aneurysms are caused by distal dissections (i.e., transmural damage secondary to microtrauma, underlying vessel wall disease associated with Ehlers-Danlos syndrome or Marfan syndrome, immune or inflammatory changes). The morbidity and mortality rates of these lesions, which may be associated with subarachnoid and intraparenchymal hemorrhage, are high. Assuming that the outpouching seen on angiography is related to a transmurally dissected vessel, the aneurysmal pouch should be regarded as a false sac or extravascular space.

Noninvasive Imaging Workup

PHYSICAL EXAMINATION

- Because distal dissecting aneurysms can be present in patients with underlying vessel wall diseases such as fibromuscular dysplasia, Marfan syndrome, and Ehlers-Danlos syndrome, a physical examination conducted before an invasive diagnostic workup should include the family history, a history of hypertension or kidney disease (for fibromuscular dysplasia), a history of hypermobile joints, heart valve problems, and retinal detachment (for Marfan syndrome), and a history of loose joints, easy bruising, abnormal wound healing, and "stretchy" soft skin (for Ehlers-Danlos syndrome).

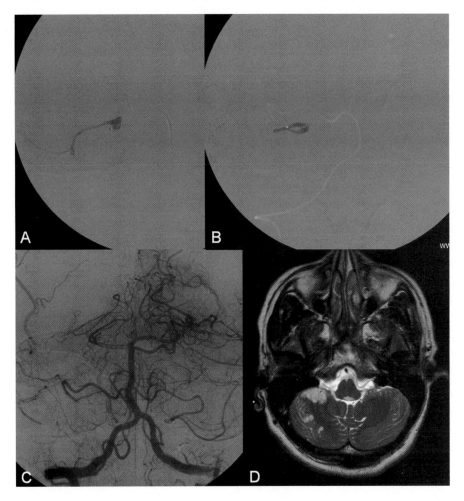

Fig. 13.2 DSA. **(A)** Superselective AICA injection, **(B)** glue cast, and **(C)** right vertebral angiogram in AP view immediately after embolization show complete occlusion of the dissected segment of the right AICA with revascularization of the distal segment by leptomeningeal collaterals. **(D)** Axial T2-weighted MR sequence reveals a small focal area of ischemia without involvement of the deep cerebellar nuclei.

CT/CTA

- CT and CTA in the presence of distal SAH should include the area of bleeding and not be confined to the proximal circle of Willis. Especially in cases in which the dissection is fusiform without a clear aneurysmal outpouching, the diagnosis can be challenging, and an invasive diagnostic workup will be required.

MRI/MRA

- Although MRI and MRA usually do not play a role in the acute setting, they may be helpful to detect and/or exclude entities in the differential diagnosis (see below) for distal SAH.
- In addition, contrast-enhanced MRI with vessel wall imaging can help to identify the cause of distal aneurysms of inflammatory origin.

Invasive Imaging Workup

- Angiography is the method of choice to detect the distal aneurysm and to assess the various treatment options, which depend on the collateral circulation distal to the diseased segment.

- In patients with suspected underlying vasculopathy, extreme caution must be exercised during catheterization of the vessels.
- The disease process classically starts with a focal stenosis proximal to the outpouching; this focal stenosis is believed to represent the origin of the dissection (i.e., the point where blood from the true lumen enters the subendothelial space).

Differential Diagnosis

- Recent trauma (as far back as 4 weeks, especially in children) is suggestive of a traumatic origin of the aneurysm. Endocarditis with septicemia favors an inflammatory origin.
- Distal aneurysms may be present in patients with arteriovenous shunting lesions.
- Apart from distal aneurysms, the following entities must be included in the differential diagnosis for distal SAH: traumatic SAH, vasculitis, Call-Fleming syndrome (reversible cerebral vasoconstriction syndrome), sinus thrombosis, and amyloid angiopathy.
- Incidentally discovered fusiform vessels may represent "healed" remote dissections and in our opinion do not require treatment.

Treatment Options

CONSERVATIVE OR MEDICAL MANAGEMENT

- Given the high rebleeding rate of acute dissections, in our opinion, early treatment is indicated. On the other hand, if a fusiform arterial segment is seen in a patient without symptoms of a recent hemorrhage, no treatment is performed.

SURGICAL TREATMENT

- Surgical treatment is indicated if a space-occupying intraparenchymal hemorrhage is associated with the distal dissection.
- Bypass surgery may be necessary in patients who are not likely to have sufficient collateral circulation and are therefore likely to have neurologic deficits following parent vessel occlusion.
- Treatment of the dissection by surgery is, depending on its location, challenging, and the rate of repeated rupture during decompressive craniotomy and surgical exploration can be high. Therefore, endovascular therapies are the first line of treatment in most centers.

ENDOVASCULAR TREATMENT

- Given the distal location of these types of dissections, stents do not play a role in their treatment.
- Parent vessel occlusion, either with coils or with liquid embolic material, is the therapy of choice.
- Protective coiling to prevent recurrence of hemorrhage is an alternative treatment strategy, as outlined below.

Possible Complications

- The major risks are due to the dissecting process in a distal vessel and therefore related to vessel fragility; hemorrhage may recur because of wire penetration or the forceful injection of contrast or other liquids.
- Distal thromboembolic or ischemic complications may occur during parent vessel occlusion.

- In patients with underlying vessel wall disease, vigorous catheterization may lead to dissections of the proximal vessels.

Published Literature on Treatment Options

Because the majority of distal fusiform aneurysms that present acutely with an SAH are due to a dissecting process, treatment strategies have to be adapted to the presumed pathologic mechanism. The aneurysmal dilatation seen on angiography is the visible part of the dissecting disease, which actually involves the entire segment of the parent artery. The therapeutic approach for these distal dissections may vary. Surgical options that have been proposed are aneurysmal resection, trapping, wrapping, neck clipping, and proximal occlusion; however, high rates of rebleeding have been reported in aneurysms treated by neck clipping or wrapping alone, which may be explained by an incomplete exclusion of the dissecting process. The deep location of the aneurysms, their proximity to the brainstem and cranial nerves, and their fragile vessel walls make surgery challenging, and surgical morbidity and mortality rates of up to 66% have been reported, mainly due to cranial nerve impairment.

Traditional endovascular techniques for the treatment of aneurysms—coiling with or without parent artery occlusion—can be an alternative treatment option. However, the artery that has to be catheterized may be too small to accommodate the microcatheters used for coiling. Moreover, even if coils can be repositioned and retrieved, the fragility of the walls of the vessels precludes repeated mechanical maneuvers, and periprocedural ruptures may occur. Coiling with parent artery preservation, despite successful occlusion of the pouch, may lead to early rebleeding. However, in certain dissecting aneurysms, such as those in the proximal middle cerebral artery, this may be the only possible treatment options (**Fig. 13.3**). In these cases, preventive coiling is used for protection from early rebleeding, allowing the dissecting process to heal.

In the present case, though, parent vessel occlusion with liquid embolic material was considered the therapy of choice because of the predictably good collateral circulation within the cerebellum, the distal location of the dissection, and the fusiform aspect of the dissection without an identifiable circumscribed outpouching. When liquid embolic agents are used for parent vessel occlusion, distal penetration of the embolic material must be avoided. Additional bypass surgery has to be considered in proximal aneurysms when no significant collaterals are present.

PEARLS AND PITFALLS _____

- Distal aneurysms are not caused by the same diseases that cause "classic saccular" aneurysms. Therefore, a different therapeutic strategy is required.
- Because the common pathologic mechanism in most of these aneurysms is a dissecting process (due to transmural traumatic disruption, inflammatory changes, microtrauma, or congenital vasculopathy), parent vessel occlusion with coils or with liquid embolic material without distal penetration is the method of choice.
- There is risk for aneurysm rupture with the injection of liquid embolic material because of its potential to increase the intravascular pressure. This can be prevented by avoiding intra-aneurysmal injection, a wedged position of the catheter tip, or forceful glue injections. Wire penetration in the dome of the aneurysm may also cause procedural rupture.

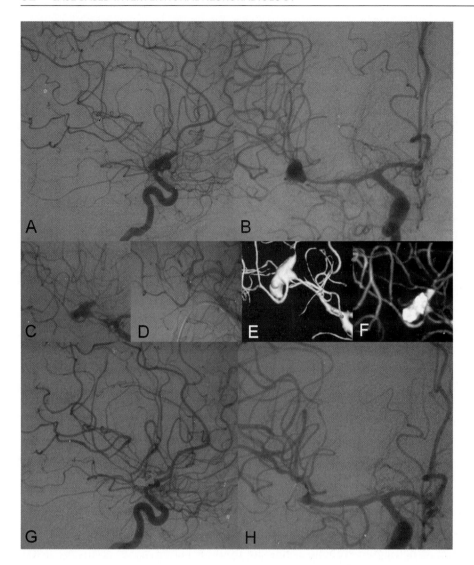

Fig. 13.3 Right ICA angiogram in **(A)** lateral and **(B)** AP views in a patient with SAH demonstrates an acutely ruptured dissecting MCA aneurysm that started at the distal M1 segment and involved three major M2 branches. Parent vessel occlusion was deemed impossible because of the predictably high rate of associated morbidity, and surgery was considered to be associated with a high risk for repeated rupture. **(C,D)** Right ICA angiograms in working projection and **(E,F)** 3D reconstruction **(C,E)** before and **(D,F)** after careful endosaccular coiling with remodeling of the bifurcation without device assistance. Right ICA angiogram in **(G)** lateral and **(H)** AP views at 3 months after the procedure demonstrates healing of the dissecting process and remodeling of the vessel. The patient remained neurologically intact.

Further Reading

Andreou A, Ioannidis I, Mitsos A. Endovascular treatment of peripheral intracranial aneurysms. AJNR Am J Neuroradiol 2007;28(2):355–361

Cognard C, Weill A, Tovi M, Castaings L, Rey A, Moret J. Treatment of distal aneurysms of the cerebellar arteries by intraaneurysmal injection of glue. AJNR Am J Neuroradiol 1999;20(5):780–784

Lubicz B, Leclerc X, Gauvrit JY, Lejeune JP, Pruvo JP. Endovascular treatment of peripheral cerebellar artery aneurysms. AJNR Am J Neuroradiol 2003;24(6):1208–1213

Zager EL, Shaver EG, Hurst RW, Flamm ES. Distal anterior inferior cerebellar artery aneurysms. Report of four cases. J Neurosurg 2002;97(3):692–696

CASE 14

Case Description

Clinical Presentation

An 11-year-old girl has been hospitalized for 1 week for the treatment of bacterial endocarditis and septicemia. She now presents with the sudden onset of headache and mild aphasia. CT is performed.

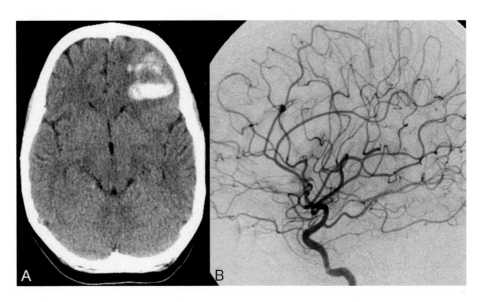

Fig. 14.1 (A) Unenhanced axial CT demonstrates a left frontal hyperdense lesion representing intraparenchymal hemorrhage. **(B)** Left ICA angiogram in lateral view shows a small outpouching at a distal fronto-opercular branch of the left MCA.

Radiologic Studies

CT

CT demonstrated a slightly space-occupying left frontal intraparenchymal hemorrhage abutting the triangular and orbitofrontal portion of the inferior frontal gyrus. There was no evidence of subarachnoid or intraventricular bleeding. No significant midline shift was noted. DSA was performed to elucidate the nature of the hemorrhage.

DSA

After injection in the left internal carotid artery (ICA), a focal outpouching in the distal fronto-opercular branch of the middle cerebral artery (MCA) was detected (**Fig. 14.1**).

Diagnosis

Distal ruptured infectious aneurysm of a distal M3 fronto-opercular branch of the MCA

Treatment

EQUIPMENT

- Standard 5F access (puncture needle, 5F vascular sheath)
- A standard 5F multipurpose catheter (Guider Soft Tip; Boston Scientific, Natick, MA) with continuous flush and a 0.035-in hydrophilic guidewire (Terumo, Somerset, NJ)
- A 0.012-in flow-directed microcatheter (Magic; Balt International, Montmorency, France) with a 0.008-in guidewire (Mirage; ev3, Plymouth, MN)
- A 10% glucose solution
- Histoacryl/Lipiodol (1 mL/1.2 mL)
- Contrast material
- Steroids
- Heparin

DESCRIPTION

Because the aneurysm had ruptured despite sufficient antibiotic therapy, treatment was performed. The 5F multipurpose catheter was placed in the distal ICA, and a flow-directed microcatheter was advanced with the aid of a micro-guidewire into the distal fronto-opercular branch. A careful microcatheter injection demonstrated the fusiform aspect of the aneurysm, with a lateral cortical branch originating from the dome. There was a sufficiently safe distance with respect to the proximal fronto-opercular artery. After the microcatheter had been flushed with the glucose solution, a mixture of 1 mL of glue with 1.2 mL of Lipiodol was injected that allowed occlusion of the aneurysm without reflux into the parent fronto-opercular artery. The patient was given heparin and steroids for 24 hours. Control angiography revealed complete occlusion of the aneurysm and preservation of the proximal fronto-opercular artery (**Fig. 14.2**).

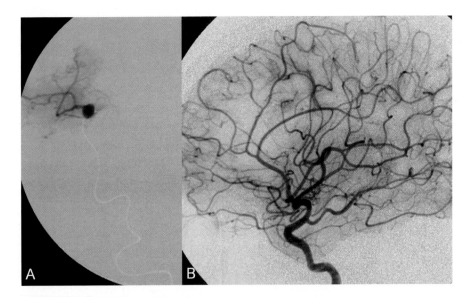

Fig. 14.2 (A) Superselective hand injection and **(B)** left ICA angiogram after the embolization reveal complete occlusion of the aneurysm with preservation of the proximal fronto-opercular artery.

Discussion

Background

Aneurysms associated with an infectious state have historically been termed *mycotic aneurysms.* However, the term *infectious arterial aneurysm* seems more appropriate; although these aneurysms can be caused by fungal infections, they are most often of bacterial origin and account for 1.5 to 9% of all intracranial aneurysms (pediatric and adult) and up to 15% of all pediatric aneurysms. The most common organism is *Staphylococcus aureus*, followed by *Streptococcus viridans* and other gram-negative organisms. Infectious aneurysms can affect distal (small) arteries, or they can have a proximal location close to the skull base and the cavernous sinus region. Consequently, two different pathologic mechanisms have been proposed for aneurysms at the two sites. In distal small arteries, an infectious process is suspected to progress from the lumen to the extravascular space as the infectious agent (i.e., septic emboli) circulates during septicemia and adheres to the endothelium of small arteries. A different mechanism is at work in larger arteries. Here, the infection typically extends from the outside toward the vessel wall and may be caused either by continuous progression of the infection from adjacent structures to the vessel wall (i.e., sphenoid sinus infection with osteomyelitis and cavernous sinus thrombophlebitis extending to the carotid artery) or by involvement with infectious emboli originating in the vasa vasorum. The primary effect of proximal aneurysms is therefore on the adventitia, with infection of the media and intima occurring secondarily. Proximal aneurysms are often bilateral and may increase in size on follow-up. In 20% of cases, infectious aneurysms are multiple, especially in immune-deficient patients and in patients treated with inappropriate antibiotics. Infectious arterial aneurysms typically present with stroke; however, they can also present with intraparenchymal or distal subarachnoid hemorrhage. After involvement with septic emboli, hemorrhage may occur, often within 48 hours.

Noninvasive Imaging Workup

PHYSICAL EXAMINATION

- Endocarditis, septicemia, and sphenoparietal sinus infection with osteomyelitis are the underlying diseases in infectious aneurysms.
- Blood and cerebrospinal fluid cultures will show the suspected causative agent in two-thirds of patients, but no infectious agent can be identified in the other third.

CT/CTA

- CT and CTA can demonstrate the sequelae of intraparenchymal or subarachnoidal blood, associated cortical areas of ischemia, potential involvement of the sinuses, osteomyelitis, and either distal or proximal aneurysms, which are often fusiform in appearance.

MRI/MRA

- MRI is more sensitive for small areas of cortical ischemia; contrast enhancement may speak in favor of cortical septic emboli. Blooming artifacts on susceptibility or T2*-weighted sequences may surround the aneurysms, and vessel wall imaging may demonstrate intense enhancement. In rare cases, edema may be seen surrounding the aneurysms.

Invasive Imaging Workup

- A full angiographic evaluation is necessary to evaluate the extent of involvement in the affected vasculature.
- From an angiographic point of view, infectious arterial aneurysms are often small aneurysms that extend into the hematoma; they may have a fusiform appearance with no neck because they involve the full thickness of the vessel wall, or they may present as false aneurysms, with the "neck" in fact the remnant of the ruptured vessel and the "aneurysm" the hematoma cavity.
- Serial angiography may be necessary to rule out aneurysm growth.

Treatment Options

CONSERVATIVE OR MEDICAL MANAGEMENT

- Appropriate and aggressive antibiotic treatment is the first treatment of choice following identification of the causative agent by blood culture.

SURGICAL TREATMENT

- Surgery is indicated in patients with life-threatening intraparenchymal hemorrhages.
- The surgical exclusion of aneurysms when antibiotic treatment fails may be contemplated if the aneurysms are in very distal and superficial locations that would be difficult to reach via endovascular approaches.

ENDOVASCULAR TREATMENT

- Endovascular options are the least invasive way to exclude infectious aneurysms.
- Because antibiotic treatment is the first choice, patients must be carefully selected, as explained below.

Possible Complications

- Recurrent bleeding from other (untreated) aneurysms
- Ischemic complications due to parent vessel occlusion
- Appearance of "de novo" aneurysms following insufficient antibiotic treatment

Published Literature on Treatment Options

The first line of treatment is appropriate antibiotic treatment following identification of the causative infectious agent. However, endovascular treatment has to be considered for patients (1) responding poorly or not at all to medical treatment, (2) presenting with hemorrhage and aneurysms despite a systemic response to their antibiotic treatment, (3) with aneurysms demonstrating repeated rupture, and (4) with growth of an aneurysm on follow-up despite treatment. Surgery should be reserved for the decompression of associated space-occupying intracranial hemorrhage and for the treatment of aneurysms when parent artery occlusion with a liquid embolic material will predictably lead to infarctions and significant neurologic deficits. Concerning endovascular treatment, the pathologic mechanism described above dictates the treatment of choice (i.e., parent vessel occlusion). Given the distal location of the aneurysms and the small size of the (fragile) vessels, we do not advocate occlusion with coils but rather occlusion with a liquid embolic agent. Migration of the glue should be avoided so that leptomeningeal collaterals can take over the distal vasculature.

PEARLS AND PITFALLS

- Stroke due to septicemia is encountered more often than hemorrhage and hemorrhagic transformation of the ischemic infarct because septic emboli are the most frequent mechanism leading to intracerebral hemorrhage. Mycotic aneurysms are less commonly the source of hemorrhage in septicemia.
- Infectious aneurysms in general are rare; however, they comprise up to 15% of all aneurysms encountered in pediatrics.
- Endovascular therapies are indicated for aneurysms that are symptomatic or growing despite sufficient medical treatment and for aneurysms presenting with repeated rupture.

Further Reading

Barrow DL, Prats AR. Infectious intracranial aneurysms: comparison of groups with and without endocarditis. Neurosurgery 1990;27(4):562–572, discussion 572–573

Chun JY, Smith W, Halbach VV, Higashida RT, Wilson CB, Lawton MT. Current multimodality management of infectious intracranial aneurysms. Neurosurgery 2001;48(6):1203–1213, discussion 1213–1214

Clare CE, Barrow DL. Infectious intracranial aneurysms. Neurosurg Clin N Am 1992;3(3):551–566

Krings T, Lasjaunias PL, Geibprasert S, Pereira V, Hans FJ. The aneurysmal wall the key to a subclassification of intracranial arterial aneurysm vasculopathies. Interv Neuroradiol 2008;14(Suppl 1):315–329

Masuda J, Yutani C, Waki R, Ogata J, Kuriyama Y, Yamaguchi T. Histopathological analysis of the mechanisms of intracranial hemorrhage complicating infective endocarditis. Stroke 1992;23(6):843–850

Peters PJ, Harrison T, Lennox JL. A dangerous dilemma: management of infectious intracranial aneurysms complicating endocarditis. Lancet Infect Dis 2006;6(11):742–748

CASE 15

Case Description

Clinical Presentation

A 42-year-old woman presents with multiple episodes of generalized tonic-clonic seizures that started recently. Despite medication, she experiences up to two seizures per week. Given the adult onset of her seizures, enhanced CT is performed, followed by MRI and angiography.

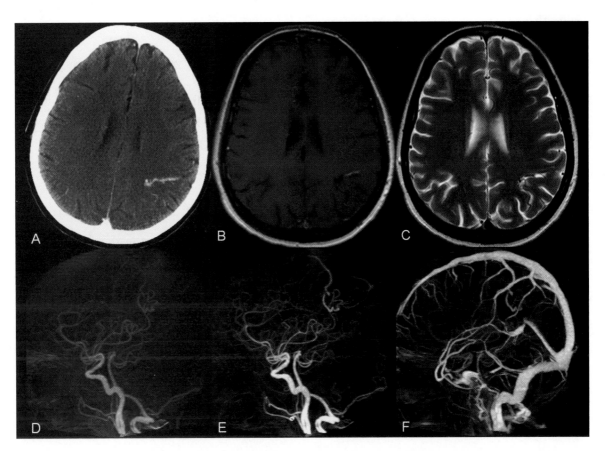

Fig. 15.1 (A) Contrast-enhanced axial CT demonstrates a dilated vessel in the left parietal region. **(B)** Axial T1-weighted contrast-enhanced and **(C)** T2-weighted MR images confirm the presence of an abnormal vascular struc-ture at the left parietal region, seen as flow voids without evidence of a classic caput medusae. Dynamic CTA in **(D)** early arterial, **(E)** late arterial, and **(F)** venous phases show early filling of a cortical vein, indicating an AV shunt.

Radiologic Studies

CT AND MRI

Outside contrast-enhanced CT of the brain demonstrated a dilated vessel in the left parietal region that was also shown by MRI. Because no classic caput medusae was present to suggest a possible developmental venous anomaly, a micro-arteriovenous malformation (AVM) was suspected. CTA demonstrated filling of a cortical vein during the arterial phase, indicating an AV shunt (**Fig. 15.1**).

DSA

Following a complete six-vessel angiographic evaluation, a single AVM was identified in the left parietal region fed solely by the anterior parietal branch of the middle cerebral artery (MCA) and draining into two superficial cortical veins (central and parietal veins) with a long pial course along the surface of the brain. There was evidence of venous ectasia in the central vein proximal to a focal stenosis as the vein reached the superior sagittal sinus. The nidus of the AVM was small (**Fig. 15.2**).

Diagnosis

Small pial AVM with venous ectasia and stenosis

Treatment

EQUIPMENT

- Standard 5F access (puncture needle, 5F vascular sheath)
- A standard 5F multipurpose catheter (Envoy; Cordis, Warren, NJ) with continuous flush and a 0.035-in hydrophilic guidewire (Terumo, Somerset, NJ)
- A 0.012-in flow-directed microcatheter (Magic; Balt International, Montmorency, France) with a 0.008-in guidewire (Mirage; ev3, Plymouth, MN)
- A 10% glucose solution
- Histoacryl/Lipiodol (1 mL/1 mL)
- Contrast material
- Steroids

DESCRIPTION

Following the diagnostic angiography, a 5F multipurpose catheter was placed in the distal infrapetrous internal carotid artery (ICA) and continuously flushed. A flow-directed microcatheter with a steam-shaped 90-degree curve was introduced into the MCA and advanced into the anterior parietal

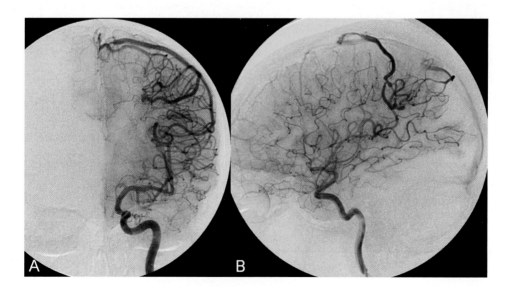

Fig. 15.2 DSA. Left ICA angiogram in **(A)** AP and **(B)** lateral views in arterial phase reveals a small AVM in the left parietal region, supplied by the anterior parietal branch of the left MCA, draining into two superficial cortical veins. A long pial course of the draining veins with a focal stenosis before entry into the superior sagittal sinus is noted.

branch of the MCA. Given the distal tortuosity, a guidewire was introduced into the microcatheter and advanced without exiting the microcatheter to make it easier to push the system and position the microcatheter far distally, just proximal to the nidus as verified by a subsequent microcatheter injection. After the microcatheter had been flushed with the glucose solution, a mixture of 1 mL of glue with 1 mL of Lipiodol was injected that allowed complete occlusion of the nidus without significant venous penetration. The microcatheter was removed, and post-embolization angiogram demonstrated complete occlusion of the AVM without evidence of a missing arterial branch or compromise of the venous flow (**Fig. 15.3**). Immediately after the procedure, 4 mg of dexamethasone was administered.

Discussion

Background

Although there is little discussion about the necessity of treating pial AVMs that have bled because of the significant risk for rebleeding, pial AVMs that have not bled must be further analyzed to select those patients in whom therapy is indicated (i.e., in whom the therapeutic risk is lower than the natural history risk). In our practice, we first classify unruptured AVMs according to their pathologic mechanism and angioarchitecture because hemorrhage is not the only way an AVM may become symptomatic. Second, we try to determine the natural history risk by a careful angioarchitectonic evaluation of the AVM in relation to risk factors for future hemorrhage. Epilepsy is one of the more common presenting symptoms of AVMs, and it may be related to (1) venous congestion (due to a long pial course of a superficial draining vein, as in this case), (2) mass effect of a venous pouch, or (3) perinidal gliosis. Venous outflow obstructions (especially if already associated with venous ectasia, as in this case) are regarded in our practice as a possible risk factor for future hemorrhage related to an increase in intranidal pressure.

Noninvasive Imaging Workup

PHYSICAL EXAMINATION

- AVMs may be clinically silent; however, a thorough neurologic evaluation has to be performed to detect subtle neurologic deficits that may add to the understanding of the pathologic mechanism of the AVM.

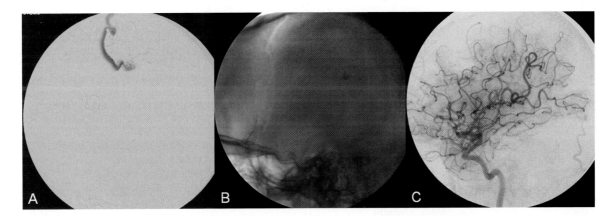

Fig. 15.3 (A) Superselective microcatheter injection and **(B)** plain radiography in lateral view demonstrate deposition of the glue cast within the AVM nidus. **(C)** Left ICA angiogram in lateral view after embolization shows complete occlusion of the AVM.

CT/CTA

- AVMs that do not present with hemorrhage may be detected incidentally during a workup for seizures, headaches, or neurologic deficits. CT and CTA can demonstrate an abnormal tangle of vessels in the parenchyma. Attention should be paid to calcifications, which may suggest long-standing venous congestion.

MRI/MRA

- On MRI, T2-weighted images will show intra-axial and subarachnoidal rounded flow voids within the brain parenchyma. On T1-weighted images, the signal within the AVM is unpredictable because of flow turbulence, blood degradation products, and the flow rate in the veins. Attention should be paid to perifocal edema, gliosis, or hemosiderin staining because these imaging findings may shed light on the individual pathologic mechanism. Although "static" MRA techniques may well detect the lesion, they do not demonstrate the angioarchitecture, and information about flow-related or intranidal aneurysms or the feeding type of the arteries is unlikely to be obtained by MRI because of restrictions in the spatial resolution. Dynamic MRA techniques will be able to demonstrate early venous opacification.
- In some instances, functional imaging techniques may be helpful to determine the eloquence of the perinidal brain tissue and to further evaluate potential pathologic mechanisms, such as arterial steal and venous congestion.

Invasive Imaging Workup

- In patients with suspected brain AVMs, we classically perform six-vessel angiography to determine all potential feeders to the brain AVM and to determine whether multiple brain AVMs are present.
- For incidentally discovered AVMs, the report should include details about the feeding arteries, such as the presence of flow-related aneurysms and the number and type of feeding arteries (en passage versus direct). Details to be reported about the AVM nidus include the number of compartments, the presence of intranidal aneurysms, and plexiform versus fistulous type of nidus. Finally, concerning the veins, the number of draining veins per compartment, any venous ectasia or pouches, and any venous stenoses need to be evaluated. In addition, the normal brain parenchyma must be analyzed for venous congestion or arterial steal.

Differential Diagnosis

- In small unruptured AVMs, the major entities in the differential diagnosis are developmental venous anomalies and capillary telangiectasia. However, these do not classically demonstrate early venous filling (i.e., a shunt).
- In rare cases, dural AV shunts with cortical venous reflux may mimic micro-AVMs.
- If multiple AVMs are present, hereditary hemorrhagic telangiectasia (HHT) should be strongly considered and appropriate investigations be performed. Metameric syndromes (cerebrofacial arteriovenous metameric syndromes, or CAMS) must also be considered.

Treatment Options

CONSERVATIVE OR MEDICAL MANAGEMENT

- Conservative or medical management should be considered if the treatment risks are estimated to be higher than those of the natural history of the lesion, particularly in elderly patients with minimal symptoms.

RADIOSURGERY

- In young patients with asymptomatic lesions and a large lifelong risk for AVM-related symptoms, radiosurgery should be contemplated, especially if no angioarchitectonic risk factors can be identified. Radiosurgery can result in a high cure rate with a rather low complication rate in well-selected cases when it is performed by a treatment team familiar with this modality for the management of AVMs. However, the long time until a cure is achieved (up to 4 years) may make one decide against this treatment if the risk for hemorrhage or neurologic deficits is considered high.

SURGICAL TREATMENT

- In patients who have superficial small lesions with multiple feeders or en passage supply, surgery may be more suitable than endovascular therapies.

ENDOVASCULAR TREATMENT

- In our practice, endovascular therapy is the method of choice for small AVMs when complete endovascular obliteration seems feasible (i.e., no en passage vessels, small number of feeding arteries and AVM compartments) and when a defined pathologic mechanism that is related to the clinical symptoms can be identified.
- We employ only liquid embolic agents to occlude the most distal arterial segment, the nidus, and the most proximal venous segment of the shunt.
- Periprocedural heparin is recommended if the procedure is anticipated to take longer than 30 minutes.
- In our practice, steroids are given following Histoacryl embolization to compensate for the exothermic effect of the glue.

Possible Complications

- Standard angiographic complications may occur (at the puncture site: bleeding, false aneurysms, fistulae; in catheterized vessels: emboli, dissections; systemically: contrast reaction, renal failure).
- Migration of the embolic agent into the draining vein with potential occlusion (especially in stenosed venous segments) of the draining vein may result in hemorrhage or venous ischemia.
- Proximal occlusion of the arterial feeders may result in delayed recanalization of the nidus.
- Arterial ischemia may develop as the consequence of reflux of the embolic agent into arteries supplying the brain.

Published Literature on Treatment Options

The treatment of incidentally discovered pial AVMs of the brain is controversial. Little is yet known about their natural history, their pathologic mechanisms, and the efficacy and risks of some of the proposed treatments (e.g., Onyx). The annual hemorrhagic risk for unruptured brain AVMs varies between 1 and 5%. It is well-known that only complete exclusion of an AVM can eliminate the risk for hemorrhage, and that the rates of curative endovascular embolization of AVMs with an acceptable periprocedural risk are ~20 to 50%. However, these values do not take into account the individual patient for whom the treatment plan has to be tailored. In the present example, a defined pathologic mechanism could be linked to the patient's symptoms and explained by the angioarchitecture, which could be easily treated with a high probability of complete cure, given the type of feeding artery (terminal feeder), the size of the nidus, and its accessibility. Therefore, treatment strategies, including conservative management as well as all three treatment options and combinations thereof, are discussed in our practice within a multidisciplinary team and tailored to the individual patient.

PEARLS AND PITFALLS

- As with dural AV shunts, a proximal vessel occlusion is *not* sufficient to achieve a permanent cure despite initial angiographic occlusion because the AVM may recruit leptomeningeal collaterals.
- A long pial course seems to be associated with a higher risk for and incidence of epilepsy, especially if associated venous stenoses are present and causing venous congestion along the pial surface.
- In AVMs with venous outflow stenoses, venous penetration must be avoided because it may lead to complete occlusion of the already stenosed venous segment; therefore, the authors use a more concentrated glue mixture under these circumstances.
- Surgical therapies are readily available for superficial sulcus AVMs and should be considered if en passage feeding vessels are present, distal catheterization is impossible, or the safety margin (i.e., the distance from the catheter tip to the closest, upstream brain-supplying artery) is too small.

Further Reading

Krings T, Geibprasert S, Terbrugge K. Interventional therapy of brain and spinal arteriovenous malformations. In: Mast et al, eds. Stroke. Philadelphia, PA: Lippincott Williams & Wilkins. In press.

Ledezma CJ, Hoh BL, Carter BS, Pryor JC, Putman CM, Ogilvy CS. Complications of cerebral arteriovenous malformation embolization: multivariate analysis of predictive factors. Neurosurgery 2006;58(4):602–611, discussion 602–611

Willinsky RA, Goyal M, terBrugge K, Montanera W, Wallace MC, Tymiansky M. Embolization of small (< 3cm) brain arteriovenous malformations. Correlation of angiographic results to a proposed angioarchitecture grading system. Interv Neuroradiol 2001;7:19–27

CASE 16

Case Description

Clinical Presentation

A 21-year-old student presents with increasing memory problems, a decreased attention span, and progressive left hemiparesis and clumsiness of his left hand. On physical examination, he has difficulty performing voluntary motor acts with his left arm and leg, and a hemiapraxia is observed, although the muscle tone is maintained. The function of his left side is not affected in serial automatic motor activities (dressing and walking). A supplementary motor syndrome is therefore diagnosed. In addition, his short-term memory is reduced. MRI and CT perfusion are performed.

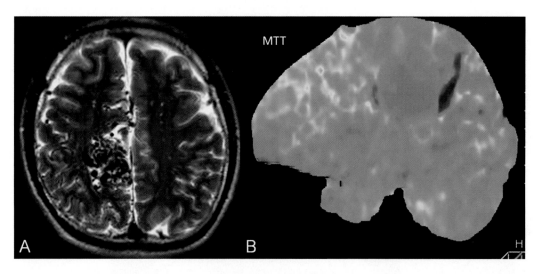

Fig. 16.1 **(A)** T2-weighted MRI demonstrates an abnormal tangle of flow-void structures at the right parasagittal region, corresponding to an AVM. **(B)** Perfusion CTA in a parasagittal view shows a decreased MTT (*blue*) within the AVM caused by rapid shunting and a markedly increased MTT (*yellow* and *orange*) within the SMA and anterior cingulate gyrus region.

Radiologic Studies

MRI AND CT PERFUSION

MRI demonstrated a right parasagittal central arteriovenous malformation (AVM) with leptomeningeal recruitment of middle cerebral artery (MCA) branches. No evidence of recent or remote hemorrhages was found, and no perilesional gliosis was visualized. CT perfusion demonstrated a decreased mean transit time (MTT) within the brain AVM due to a rapid shunt. Most interestingly, a marked increase in the MTT within the supplementary motor area (SMA) and anterior cingulate gyrus region was noted, indicating a prolonged AV transit time due to delayed outflow that resulted in venous congestion remote from the AVM (**Fig. 16.1**).

DSA

Injection in the right internal carotid artery (ICA) demonstrated an AVM that was fed by the pericallosal and callosomarginal arteries. In addition, significant leptomeningeal indirect collaterals were visualized that reconstituted the distal anterior cerebral artery (ACA) territory as well as the AVM, indicating a significant "sump" effect of the AVM (which suggests a high-flow shunt within the AVM nidus). Delayed venous return was visualized in the anterior midline brain parenchyma, indicating venous congestion of the SMA and anterior cingulate gyrus (**Fig. 16.2**).

Diagnosis

Large pial AVM with high-flow shunt and venous congestion associated with progressive neurologic deficits

Treatment

EQUIPMENT

- Standard 5F access (puncture needle, 5F vascular sheath)
- Standard 5F multipurpose catheter (Guider Soft Tip; Boston Scientific, Natick, MA) with continuous flush and a 0.035-in hydrophilic guidewire (Terumo, Somerset, NJ)
- A 0.012-in flow-directed microcatheter (Magic; Balt International, Montmorency, France)
- A 10% glucose solution
- Histoacryl/Lipiodol/tantalum powder (2 mL/0.2 mL/one-half vial)
- Contrast material
- Steroids

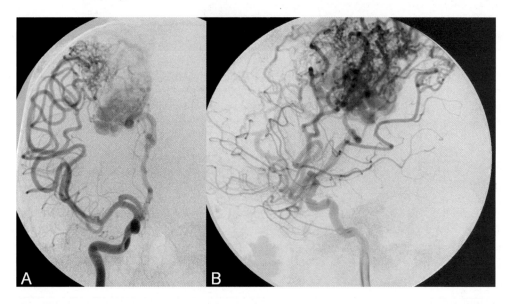

Fig. 16.2 DSA. Left ICA angiogram in **(A)** AP and **(B)** lateral views reveals an AVM supplied mainly by the pericallosal and callosomarginal arteries of the ACA, with significant indirect leptomeningeal collaterals from the MCA branches.

DESCRIPTION

Following diagnostic angiography, a 5F multipurpose catheter was placed in the distal infrapetrous ICA and continuously flushed. A flow-directed microcatheter with a steam-shaped 90-degree curve was introduced into the ACA and advanced into the proximal A2 segment, where microcatheter injections revealed the anticipated fistulous component of the AVM. Because of the high flow in the lesion, no guidewire was required. The microcatheter was placed ~5 mm proximal to the fistula, as verified by a subsequent microcatheter injection with the tip of the catheter pointing against the wall of the artery. After the microcatheter had been flushed with the glucose solution, a mixture of 2 mL of glue with 0.2 mL of Lipiodol and half of a vial of tantalum powder was injected that allowed complete occlusion of the fistulous component of the AVM nidus. Following microcatheter removal, control runs demonstrated significantly altered hemodynamics, with reduced flow through the AVM. Immediately after the procedure, 4 mg of dexamethasone was administered. Follow-up CT perfusion demonstrated improvement in the perfusion of the SMA and anterior cingulate gyrus (**Fig. 16.3**). The patient's neurologic deficits decreased significantly, and he was scheduled for subsequent radiosurgery.

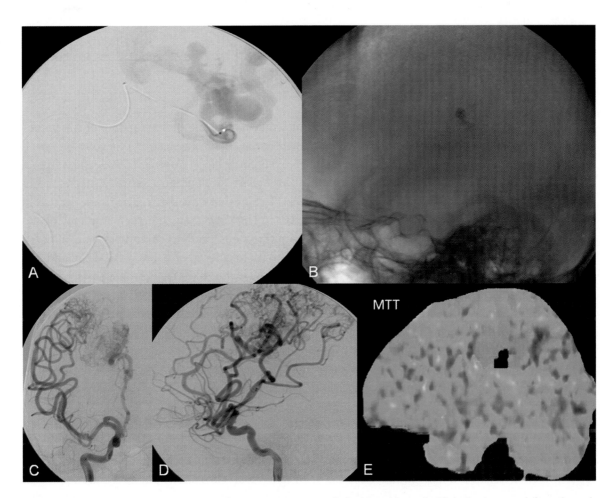

Fig. 16.3 (A) Superselective microcatheter injection reveals a fistula within the AVM nidus. **(B)** Plain radiography demonstrates the location of the glue cast, and left ICA angiogram in **(C)** AP and **(D)** lateral views after embolization shows significantly decreased flow through the AVM. There is better perfusion of the SMA and anterior cingulate gyrus region on the follow-up CT perfusion **(E)**.

Discussion

Background

Venous congestion may be related to decreased outflow (in the case of venous stenoses) or increased inflow (in the case of fistulous AVMs) and can be associated with progressive neurologic symptoms. Even if treatment is not complete following the first embolization session, endovascular treatment may play a role in reducing the shunt to relieve clinical symptoms before definitive treatment of the AVM. The strategy of defining a target (i.e., a pathologic mechanism that is related to a clinical symptom as verified by imaging of the angioarchitecture) before treatment has been termed *partial targeted embolization*. The role of endovascular treatment is therefore to "secure" the AVM, stabilize or ameliorate the symptoms, or reduce the size of the AVM so that additional therapies that may take longer to be effective are made safer. In the present case, the perfusion data, the recruitment of leptomeningeal collaterals from a different vascular territory (MCA) to reconstitute the distal ACA territory, and the progressive neurologic symptoms strongly suggested a fistulous compartment within the AVM, which could then be regarded as the target of embolization.

Noninvasive Imaging Workup

See also Case 15.

PERFUSION IMAGING

- Perfusion imaging can be done with CT or MRI and may add to the understanding of the pathologic mechanisms of brain AVMs. Following the intravenous bolus application of a contrast agent, the time to peak (TTP), mean transit time (MTT), cerebral blood volume (CBV), and cerebral blood flow (CBF) can be determined. TTP indicates the arterial blood flow velocity (decreased in shunts, increased in slow arterial flow), and the MTT represents the AV transit time (decreased in shunts, increased in edema or venous congestion). The CBV is an indirect parameter of the venous outflow (increased CBV indicates venous outflow obstruction). A combination of these parameters may add to our understanding of the remote effects of a brain AVM. In patients with neurologic symptoms, arterial steal and venous congestion have been proposed as potential pathologic mechanisms to explain neurologic deficits. In venous congestion, an increased MTT and a normal or even decreased TTP are seen (as in the present case), whereas in arterial steal, a decreased MTT and TTP will be seen (and therefore, a decreased time during which oxygen can be extracted by tissue and subsequent chronic ischemia). Functional imaging can detect subtle changes before structural imaging, and the results can be correlated with the imaging findings during angiography.

Invasive Imaging Workup

- In patients with suspected fistulous components, neo-angiogenesis surrounding the AVM (due to perinidal arterial steal and chronic ischemia with new vessel formation) but also leptomeningeal collaterals (due to the "sump" effect of the shunting lesion) can be seen. It is important to differentiate these two vessel types from true AVM feeding arteries because they represent a normal vasculature that is (secondarily) abnormally triggered by ischemia or high-flow angiopathy. Following treatment of the proper target (i.e., the fistulous component), these secondarily enlarged or recruited vessels remodel and decrease in size if endovascular treatment has been able to reach the proximal venous site and has not been associated with simply an arterial ligation.
- Long-standing venous congestion leads to a pseudophlebitic aspect of the veins (increased tortuosity) and venous stagnation.

- Neo-angiogenesis can be differentiated from brain AVM feeding vessels only by their nonshunting nature.
- Leptomeningeal collaterals can be identified if the vascular territories are enlarged as a consequence of the sump effect (high-flow angiopathy) and if the distal territories are reconstituted by a network of leptomeningeal superficial vessels.

Treatment Options

See also Case 15.

CONSERVATIVE OR MEDICAL MANAGEMENT

- Although prospective randomized trials are lacking, it is our opinion that conservative management in young patients with neurologic symptoms that can be attributed to a high-flow AVM is not a good option, especially if the risks of treatment are low.

RADIOSURGERY

- Intranidal high-flow or fistulous compartments of AVMs are thought to be less likely to become obliterated following radiosurgery. In addition, because of the longer time needed for obliteration following radiosurgery, a treatment modality with more rapid effects may be necessary.

SURGICAL TREATMENT

- In general, surgical resectability and the clinical outcome depend on the size of an AVM, the drainage pattern, and the eloquence of the brain region that harbors the AVM. Although the flow rate therefore does not seem to play a role in surgical resectability, in everyday practice, most neurosurgeons will appreciate a flow reduction achieved by endovascular means.

ENDOVASCULAR TREATMENT

- In our practice, endovascular therapies are the method of choice for AVMs that harbor fistulous components, in particular when they are perceived to be responsible for the clinical symptoms.
- In most instances, a liquid embolic agent that polymerizes quickly is used (in the present case, 2 mL of N-butyl-cyanoacrylate mixed with 0.2 mL of Lipiodol). To increase the visibility of the embolic agent, tantalum powder is added.
- In our practice, steroids are given following Histoacryl embolization to compensate for the exothermic effect of the glue.

Possible Complications

- Standard angiographic complications may develop at the puncture site (bleeding, false aneurysms, fistulae), in catheterized vessels (emboli, dissections), and systemically (contrast reaction, renal failure).
- Migration of the embolic agent into the draining vein with potential occlusion may result in hemorrhage or venous ischemia, proximal occlusion with delayed reopening, and arterial ischemia due to reflux of the embolic agent into arteries supplying the brain.
- Seizures following successful treatment may result from significant alterations in cerebral hemodynamics.
- Delayed venous thrombosis may develop as a result of significant flow reduction.

Published Literature on Treatment Options

Management strategies will be influenced by local preferences and capabilities; however, results presented in the literature suggest the following therapeutic strategies. Small, superficially located

AVMs (nidus volume < 10 mL) are best operated on; however, a presurgical attempt to cure by embolization may be warranted unless the angioarchitecture is unfavorable. In single feeder–single compartment AVMs or AVMs with large fistulous components, embolization should be the first therapy of choice. Deep-seated, small AVMs should be treated by radiosurgery unless they are suitable for cure by embolization or have angioarchitectonic risk factors (fistulae, intranidal aneurysms, venous stenoses). Large AVMs (nidus volume > 10 mL) may benefit from partial embolization followed by radiosurgery or surgery, depending on the location and angioarchitecture. Finally, very large AVMs (nidus volume > 20 mL) will present a high treatment risk with all modalities and are therefore best managed conservatively. As in the present case, multimodality treatment with endovascular therapy preceding either surgery or radiosurgery is in most centers the therapy of choice. Although the risks of two treatment modalities are combined, there is consensus in the literature that in specific and selected cases, the risks of two treatment modalities are smaller for an individual patient than the risks of a single-modality treatment.

PEARLS AND PITFALLS _____

- The liquid embolic agent must penetrate from the arterial to the venous side to ensure stable obliteration of the fistulous compartment.
- Following an embolization procedure, we generally wait for 6 weeks to 3 months before performing a second embolization procedure to allow the brain vasculature time to remodel.
- If flow changes are significant following embolization, headaches and seizures may develop transiently. If new neurologic symptoms occur, follow-up imaging is necessary to rule out excessive venous thrombosis, which may require anticoagulation and steroid therapies.

Further Reading

Back AG, Vollmer D, Zeck O, Shkedy C, Shedden PM. Retrospective analysis of unstaged and staged gamma knife surgery with and without preceding embolization for the treatment of arteriovenous malformations. J Neurosurg 2008;109(Suppl):57–64

Hartmann A, Mast H, Mohr JP, et al. Determinants of staged endovascular and surgical treatment outcome of brain arteriovenous malformations. Stroke 2005;36(11):2431–2435

Krings T, Hans FJ, Geibprasert S, Terbrugge K. Partial targeted embolization of brain arteriovenous malformations. Eur Radiol June 11, 2010 [Epub ahead of print]

Ledezma CJ, Hoh BL, Carter BS, Pryor JC, Putman CM, Ogilvy CS. Complications of cerebral arteriovenous malformation embolization: multivariate analysis of predictive factors. Neurosurgery 2006;58(4):602–611, discussion 602–611

Natarajan SK, Ghodke B, Britz GW, Born DE, Sekhar LN. Multimodality treatment of brain arteriovenous malformations with microsurgery after embolization with onyx: single-center experience and technical nuances. Neurosurgery 2008;62(6):1213–1225, discussion 1225–1226

Söderman M, Andersson T, Karlsson B, Wallace MC, Edner G. Management of patients with brain arteriovenous malformations. Eur J Radiol 2003;46(3):195–205

Yuki I, Kim RH, Duckwiler G, et al. Treatment of brain arteriovenous malformations with high-flow arteriovenous fistulas: risk and complications associated with endovascular embolization in multimodality treatment. J Neurosurg Oct 16, 2009 [Epub ahead of print]

CASE 17

Case Description

Clinical Presentation

A 28-year-old right-handed woman has had migraine headaches for 3 months, which have progressed in intensity over the last weeks. In addition, she experiences transient ischemic attack (TIA)–like symptoms (motor aphasia) that are not related to the headaches and are not associated with a loss of consciousness. Outside imaging reveals a right parieto-occipital arteriovenous malformation (AVM). Functional MRI and CT perfusion are performed.

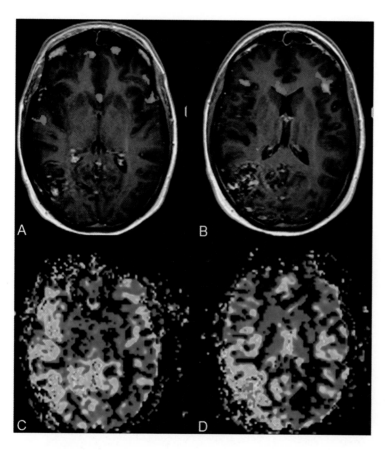

Fig. 17.1 (A,B) Functional MRI during speech production. **(C,D)** Perfusion MRI in axial cuts.

Radiologic Studies

MRI, MR PERFUSION, AND FUNCTIONAL MRI

MRI demonstrated a large right parieto-occipital AVM without evidence of remote hemorrhage or perilesional gliosis. Functional MRI during speech production revealed bilateral representation of the patient's speech areas in the opercular portion of the inferior frontal gyrus (Broca's area). Perfusion MRI revealed a decreased mean transit time not only within the parieto-occipital AVM location, indicating a shunt, but also remote from the AVM in the previously identified speech areas, suggesting arterial steal as the most likely explanation of the patient's recurrent TIA-like symptoms (**Fig. 17.1**).

DSA

Injection in the right ICA demonstrated an AVM that was fed by the angular and the temporo-occipital artery in a terminal fashion. A flow-related aneurysm was present at the bifurcation of the angular artery proximal to the nidus proper. A single massively enlarged posterior parietal vein drained the AVM without signs of distal venous stenosis. A dramatic reduction in flow in the remainder of the middle cerebral artery (MCA) branches on angiography suggested significant arterial steal into the AVM. The AVM nidus measured 19.4 mm^3 (**Fig. 17.2**).

Diagnosis

Large pial AVM with prenidal flow-related aneurysms and arterial steal

Treatment

EQUIPMENT

- Standard 5F access (puncture needle, 5F vascular sheath)
- Standard 5F multipurpose catheter (Guider Soft Tip; Boston Scientific, Natick, MA) with continuous flush and a 0.035-in hydrophilic guidewire (Terumo, Somerset, NJ)
- A 3 × 0.012-in flow-directed microcatheter (Magic; Balt International, Montmorency, France) with a 0.008-in guidewire (Mirage; ev3, Plymouth, MN)
- A 10% glucose solution
- Histoacryl/Lipiodol (1 mL/1.2 mL)
- Contrast material
- Steroids

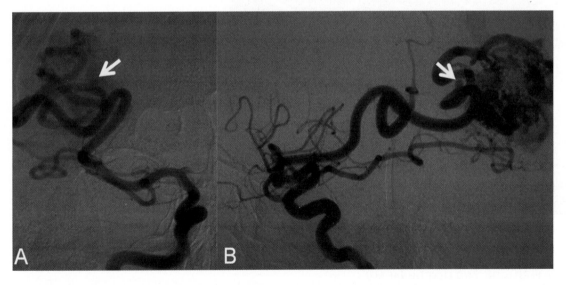

Fig. 17.2 DSA. Right ICA injection in **(A)** AP and **(B)** lateral views, arterial phase. The *arrows* point toward the flow-related prenidal aneurysm.

DESCRIPTION

Following diagnostic angiography, a 5F multipurpose catheter was placed in the distal infrapetrous internal carotid artery (ICA) and continuously flushed. A flow-directed microcatheter with a steam-shaped 45-degree curve was introduced into the MCA and advanced into the proximal angular artery. With the aid of a micro-guidewire that had a short, sharp curve, we passed the arterial segment harboring the prenidal aneurysm. Three pedicles were treated with a mixture of 1 mL of glue and 1.2 mL of Lipiodol, which achieved a significant reduction in size and flow. Immediately after the procedure, 4 mg of dexamethasone was administered. Follow-up angiography after 3 months, before radiotherapy, demonstrated a significant reduction in the size of the AVM and complete regression of the flow-related prenidal aneurysm (**Fig. 17.3**). The patient underwent radiosurgery, resulting in obliteration of the AVM after 2 years. Following embolizaton, the patient no longer experienced headaches and TIA-like symptoms.

Discussion

Background

The purpose of embolization before radiosurgery is either size reduction or targeted embolization of symptomatic or angioarchitectonic weak points. In the present case, the purpose of embolization was (1) size reduction and (2) reduction of the arterial steal; the prenidal flow-related aneurysm was not considered a target. Intranidal aneurysms and pseudoaneurysms in the setting of an acutely ruptured AVM are discussed in Case 18. Proximal flow-related aneurysms in unruptured AVMs by themselves do not seem to alter the natural history of the AVM, and although they may be a marker of generalized increased vessel fragility, they are not a priority target of treatment. Rupture of remote

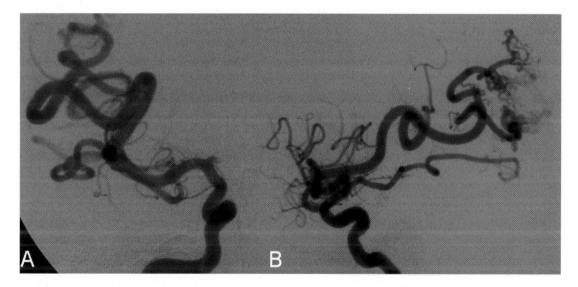

Fig. 17.3 DSA. Right ICA injection in **(A)** AP and **(B)** lateral views, arterial phase, at follow-up after 3 months. The nidus size is markedly reduced, and there is complete regression of the flow-related aneurysm.

flow-related aneurysms following embolization has not been observed in our experience, and flow-related aneurysms typically regress, especially if the aneurysm is close to the nidus and more than 50% of the AVM is obliterated. For embolization before radiosurgery, the following points have to be kept in mind: The size of the AVM determines the dose given and therefore the risk for adverse effects of radiosurgery (i.e., the smaller the AVM, the higher the rate of complete obliteration without side effects). On the other hand, large amounts of radiopaque liquid embolic agent make definition of the residual target difficult and may even reduce the radiation dose delivered because of absorption within the embolic agent. Therefore, a multidisciplinary approach before embolization is of great importance. Irrespective of these considerations, an intranidal deposit of the liquid embolic agent is mandatory to reduce the potential for delayed reopening, which has occurred in embolized and irradiated AVMs.

Noninvasive Imaging Workup

MRI AND CT

- The size of previously untreated AVMs is in our experience best estimated with volumetric contrast-enhanced CT or multiplanar T2-weighted MRI. Still, it may be difficult to differentiate the true nidus from the draining veins and feeding arteries.
- Following embolization, artifacts will be present on both MRI and CT that make it nearly impossible to estimate the residual target volume.
- In most instances, the spatial resolution of high-quality MRA or CTA will allow the detection of prenidal flow-related aneurysms.

FUNCTIONAL IMAGING

- The present case demonstrates that in rare cases, additional information about the "eloquence" of cortical areas may be helpful. The blood oxygenation level–dependent (BOLD) effect can be used to visualize brain regions that are active during the performance of a specified task. However, this visualization is based on hemodynamic changes associated with neuronal activity, so the results have to be regarded with caution in brain regions that are in close contact to the AVM because it is likely that in these regions, the AVM has primarily altered the hemodynamic response. This may lead to false-negative results of the functional MRI results. As indicated in Case 16, a decrease in the mean transit time in a brain region distant from the AVM will decrease the time during which oxygen can be extracted by tissue (i.e., arterial steal with TIA-like symptoms).

Invasive Imaging Workup

- Because flow-related aneurysms may increase slightly the risk associated with an embolization procedure, a working projection that demonstrates the aneurysm and the parent artery is recommended.
- It is helpful to discuss with the radiosurgeon or neurosurgeon the target of embolization (i.e., the volume to be reduced or the compartment to be embolized based on the invasive imaging workup).
- At present, only invasive imaging with DSA can correctly estimate the size of a residual AVM following embolization because artifacts caused by the liquid embolic agent will prevent a correct determination of the size on MRI or CT.
- A waiting period of at least 2 months between embolization and radiosurgery is recommended to ensure stability of the embolization results achieved (i.e., before the next invasive imaging workup is contemplated for planning radiosurgery).

Treatment Options

CONSERVATIVE OR MEDICAL MANAGEMENT

- For very large AVMs, any treatment or combination of treatments is associated with a high risk, and conservative management may very well be the best choice. However, in the present case of a young patient with a large, symptomatic AVM, treatment was deemed feasible, with an acceptable risk and a high likelihood of improving the natural history of the disease.

RADIOSURGERY

- The volume of healthy tissue irradiated around large lesions is rather significant, necessitating a reduction of radiation doses to avoid complications. As a consequence, obliteration rates in large and very large AVMs may be poor. To circumvent dose volume problems with large AVMs, repeated treatments in addition to dose and volume fractionation schemes have been proposed; however, these therapeutic schemes have lower obliteration rates and higher complication rates. Therefore, a combined treatment with prior size reduction by embolization is recommended for large AVMs.

SURGICAL TREATMENT

- In this particular case, surgery would have been a good therapeutic choice in view of the superficial location, the absence of deep venous drainage, and the size. However, the potential bilateral speech representation and the patient's strong wish for a "less invasive" treatment prompted the described approach.

ENDOVASCULAR TREATMENT

- Pre-radiosurgical size reduction is best achieved by means of endovascular embolization with liquid material. A close interdisciplinary discussion with the radiosurgeon is recommended.
- The liquid embolic agent must enter the nidus to ensure stable results. Therefore, to ensure good penetration in the present case, we opted for a mixture of 1 mL of N-butyl-cyanoacrylate and 1.2 mL of Lipiodol.
- In the present case, two factors slightly increased the risk of embolization therapy: the single venous drainage despite at least three different arterial feeders and the flow-related aneurysm.

Possible Complications

- In single-draining veins, extreme caution must be taken that the glue does not migrate or occlude the vein in partial embolization because this may lead to hemorrhage.
- Flow-related aneurysms may rupture during vigorous catheterization.
- In multimodality treatment, the risks of the different methods are combined.
- Reopening may be delayed if the glue does not penetrate the nidus.

Published Literature on Treatment Options

Concerning radiosurgery for very large AVMs, rather low peripheral doses (< 15 Gy) have been proposed that do not obliterate the AVM but may diminish its size after treatment. Higher doses may then be reapplied to any residual nidus after an appropriate follow-up period. In volume fractionation, AVMs are divided into smaller segments, with target volumes of 5 to 15 mL treated on separate occasions, thereby minimizing the amount of radiation delivered to surrounding brain tissue. Fewer adverse radiologic effects have been reported with fractionated radiosurgery than with standard radiosurgery. However, the rate of obliteration is lower, and during the extended latency period between treatment and occlusion, the patient is at risk for hemorrhage. Therefore, pre-radiosurgical embolization for size reduction remains of interest (**Fig. 17.4**).

The goals of endovascular therapies for presurgical embolization are the following: elimination of deep feeding arterial supply, occlusion of intranidal fistulous compartments, and general reduction of flow through the nidus. The latter can be established by "ligation" embolization (i.e., proximal occlusion without the need to penetrate the nidus because the nidus proper will be removed subsequently at surgery). If nidal penetration occurs, mobilization of the AVM at the time of resection may be slightly more difficult, which is why we recommend a highly concentrated glue for ligation embolization, to avoid delayed nidal polymerization. AVMs that are located in the phylogenetic and vascular border zone between the leptomeningeal and lenticulostriate arteries will harbor both types of arterial supply (i.e., superficial and deep). In these instances, embolization of the lenticulostriate arterial supply will be helpful for further surgical therapies (**Fig. 17.5**).

PEARLS AND PITFALLS

- In AVMs with multiple feeders but a single draining vein, caution must be taken not to occlude the draining vein with the liquid embolic agent. If this happens, either complete obliteration in the same setting or surgical intervention with complete excision of the AVM may be necessary.

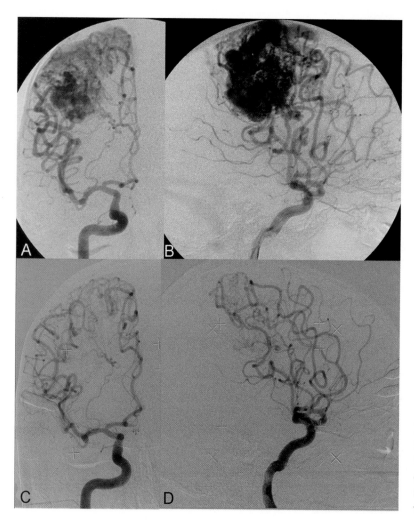

Fig. 17.4 DSA. Right ICA injection in **(A)** AP and **(B)** lateral views **(C)** before embolization and **(D)** after embolization demonstrating dramatic size reduction after embolization and before radiosurgery.

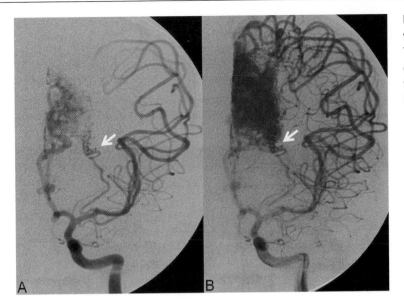

Fig. 17.5 DSA. Left ICA injection in AP view in **(A)** early and **(B)** late phases. There is evidence of superficial and deep supply. For presurgical embolization, the deep supply (*arrows*) should be targeted.

- Although in our experience flow-related aneurysms do not rupture spontaneously, they are slightly more likely to rupture during therapy because flow-directed microcatheters tend to enter the aneurysm. A good roadmap and navigation with a guidewire are employed in our practice to prevent this complication.
- We do not treat flow-related aneurysms first, even if the aneurysm is larger or more proximally located. The treatment of prenidal aneurysms is, however, considered if they do not regress within 6 months following significant flow reduction in the AVM.
- The target of embolization (number and location of AVM compartments to be occluded for sufficient volume reduction or safe surgery) should be discussed before the procedure with the radiosurgeon or neurosurgeon, who will manage the expected remainder of the AVM.
- Surgery must follow "ligation" embolization (i.e., proximal arterial embolization) within 3 weeks, which is not sufficient for pre-radiosurgical embolization (because of delayed reconstitution of the nidus via leptomeningeal collaterals). Pre-radiosurgical embolization is helpful only if the liquid embolic material penetrates the nidus. The authors wait for at least 3 months between embolization and radiosurgery to ensure stable conditions of the AVM and to prevent the reopening of (insufficiently) embolized compartments.

Further Reading

Andrade-Souza YM, Ramani M, Beachey DJ, et al. Liquid embolisation material reduces the delivered radiation dose: a physical experiment. Acta Neurochir (Wien) 2008;150(2):161–164, discussion 164

Andrade-Souza YM, Ramani M, Scora D, Tsao MN, terBrugge K, Schwartz ML. Embolization before radiosurgery reduces the obliteration rate of arteriovenous malformations. Neurosurgery 2007;60(3):443–451, discussion 451–452

Back AG, Vollmer D, Zeck O, Shkedy C, Shedden PM. Retrospective analysis of unstaged and staged Gamma Knife surgery with and without preceding embolization for the treatment of arteriovenous malformations. J Neurosurg 2008;109(Suppl):57–64

Hartmann A, Mast H, Mohr JP, et al. Determinants of staged endovascular and surgical treatment outcome of brain arteriovenous malformations. Stroke 2005;36(11):2431–2435

Jones J, Jang S, Getch CC, Kepka AG, Marymont MH. Advances in the radiosurgical treatment of large inoperable arteriovenous malformations. Neurosurg Focus 2007;23(6):E7

Natarajan SK, Ghodke B, Britz GW, Born DE, Sekhar LN. Multimodality treatment of brain arteriovenous malformations with microsurgery after embolization with onyx: single-center experience and technical nuances. Neurosurgery 2008;62(6):1213–1225, discussion 1225–1226

CASE 18

Case Description

Clinical Presentation

A 78-year-old woman presents to the emergency department with the acute onset of headaches, nausea, and ataxia. She is awake, although slightly confused and not fully oriented to time and place. Emergency CT is performed.

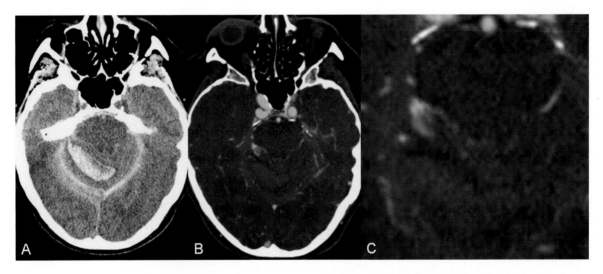

Fig. 18.1 **(A)** Unenhanced axial CT and CTA in **(B)** axial and **(C)** magnified images demonstrate subarachnoid and intraparenchymal hemorrhage and the presumed cause (i.e., a false aneurysm within the AVM).

Radiologic Studies

CT AND CTA

Unenhanced CT demonstrated a subarachnoid and intraparenchymal hemorrhage centered in the posterior fossa. The intraparenchymal component was located in the superior lobule of the right cerebellar hemisphere. CTA performed in the acute setting to evaluate an underlying cause of the hemorrhage demonstrated a tangle of enlarged abnormal vessels in close vicinity to the hemorrhage, indicating an arteriovenous malformation (AVM) in the cerebellum. Evidence was found of a focal aneurysmal dilatation that pointed directly into the hemorrhagic cavity and was in close spatial relation to the subarachnoid space (**Fig. 18.1**).

DSA

Injection in the left dominant vertebral artery demonstrated a small plexiform AVM fed by the lateral hemispheric branch of the right superior cerebellar artery and draining via the lateral perimesencephalic vein cranially and the petrosal vein laterally. Superselective injection confirmed the intranidal aneurysmal outpouching in the dorsal and superior aspects of the AVM (**Fig. 18.2**).

Diagnosis

Ruptured cerebellar AVM with intranidal (pseudo)aneurysm

Treatment

EQUIPMENT

- Standard 5F access (puncture needle, 5F vascular sheath)

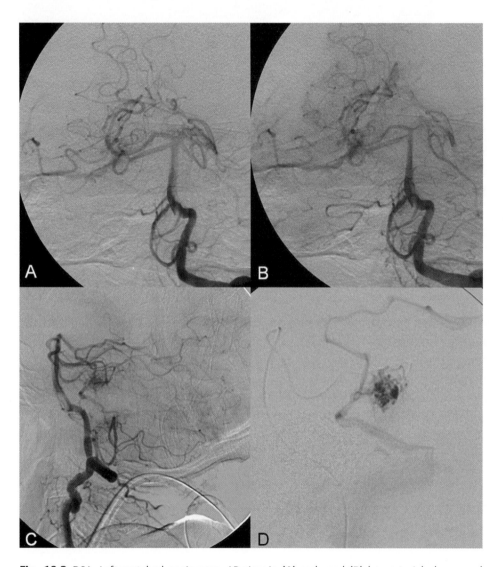

Fig. 18.2 DSA. Left vertebral angiogram, AP view in **(A)** early and **(B)** late arterial phases and **(C)** lateral view, shows a small, diffuse AVM nidus, supplied by the lateral hemispheric branch of the right superior cerebellar artery and draining via the lateral perimesencephalic and petrosal veins. **(D)** Superselective injection into the superior cerebellar artery reveals a small intranidal outpouching in the dorsal superior aspect of the AVM.

- Standard 5F multipurpose catheter (Envoy; Cordis, Warren, NJ) with continuous flush and a 0.035-in hydrophilic guidewire (Terumo, Somerset, NJ)
- A 2 × 0.012-in flow-directed microcatheter (Magic; Balt International, Montmorency, France) with a 0.008-in guidewire (Mirage; ev3, Plymouth, MN)
- A 10% glucose solution
- Histoacryl/Lipiodol (1 mL/1.2 mL)
- Contrast material
- Steroids

DESCRIPTION

Following diagnostic angiography, a 5F multipurpose catheter was placed in the distal vertebral artery and continuously flushed. A flow-directed microcatheter with a steam-shaped 45-degree curve was introduced into the superior cerebellar artery and advanced into the lateral hemispheric branch with the aid of a micro-guidewire. The intranidal aneurysm was identified as the point of rupture and treated with a mixture of 1 mL of glue and 1.2 mL of Lipiodol, which achieved complete occlusion of the aneurysm; however, because glue penetrated the petrosal vein, it was decided to occlude the remainder of the AVM as well. Follow-up angiography demonstrated complete occlusion of the AVM (**Fig. 18.3**), and 4 mg of dexamethasone was administered. Follow-up CTA demonstrated the glue cast within the aneurysmal outpouching (not shown).

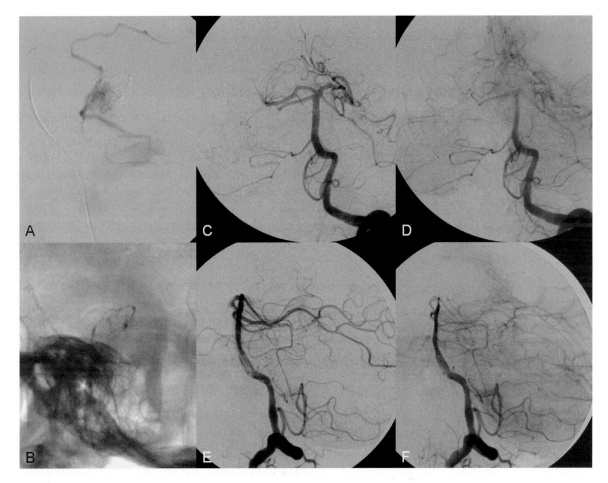

Fig. 18.3 (A) Superselective injection before the second embolization and **(B)** plain radiography demonstrate the final glue cast. A small amount of glue in the petrosal vein prompted further embolization of the entire AVM. Left vertebral angiograms in **(C,D)** AP and **(E,F)** lateral views after embolization reveal complete obliteration of the small AVM.

Discussion

Background

There are few indications for the acute treatment of ruptured brain AVMs. In our opinion, treatment is indicated if angiography demonstrates an intranidal (pseudo)aneurysm or outpouching, an aneurysm that has enlarged since previous examinations, or a venous pseudoaneurysm, especially in the presence of venous outlet stenosis or venous stagnation. Although the natural history of pseudoaneurysms is not known, they represent in our opinion a significant feature of instability and warrant active intervention. The risk for rebleeding is higher in patients with intranidal aneurysms; however, early rebleeding is rare, and therefore an aggressive early endovascular intervention may compromise recovery from the primary hemorrhagic insult. If, on the other hand, emergency surgical evacuation of a blood clot or emergency shunting procedures have to be performed, interdisciplinary discussion with the neurosurgeon is necessary to determine the associated risk for rebleeding in the setting of decompressive interventions. Therefore, no general guidelines can be given with respect to the timing of the intervention after the initial hemorrhagic event, and treatment decisions must take into account the patient's clinical state, extent of the hemorrhage, and individual angioarchitectonic features of the AVM.

Noninvasive Imaging Workup

PHYSICAL EXAMINATION

- A neurologic evaluation is necessary to prompt the emergency evacuation of a space-occupying hematoma or, in the presence of intraventricular blood, emergency extraventricular drainage.

CT/CTA, MR/MRA

- In the acute setting, CT is the method of choice to determine the location and amount of hemorrhage, potential mass effect, perilesional edema, and associated hydrocephalus.
- During the same scanning session, CTA should be performed to evaluate the cause of the hemorrhage. CTA can demonstrate dilated vessels or an intraparenchymal tangle of vessels, and it may also demonstrate the cause of the rupture (i.e., an intranidal aneurysm or venous stenosis). In most instances, this information will be sufficient for emergency management.
- MR and MRA may have to be performed to rule out other causes of "atypical" intraparenchymal hemorrhage (i.e., hemorrhage in a young patient, in a location distant from the basal ganglia or cerebellum, or in a patient with no known risk factors for hypertensive hemorrhage).

Invasive Imaging Workup

- Six-vessel angiography is classically performed to determine all the feeders potentially associated with a vascular malformation and the transdural supply. Careful analysis of the nidus (especially if an intranidal aneurysm is present) and the venous outflow routes (venous stensosis, redirection of venous flow) is required.
- Microcatheterization may be beneficial to evaluate the microanatomy of the vascular lesion and determine whether small intranidal aneurysms are present.
- Although in the acute phase the size of an AVM may be underestimated because of mass effect, an early angiographic evaluation is in our opinion of importance if a sudden deterioration in the patient's clinical status should necessitate emergency surgery.

Differential Diagnosis

- The differential diagnosis for intraparenchymal hemorrhage is vast and beyond the scope of this book. However, because in most instances at least CTA is available, an abnormal tangle of vessels should suggest the diagnosis of a vascular malformation. However, a developmental venous anomaly with an associated cavernoma, a hemorrhagic presentation of moyamoya disease with increased vessels within the basal cisterns, or a dural arteriovenous shunt with cortical venous reflux and a hemorrhagic presentation may mimic a true AVM.

Treatment Options

CONSERVATIVE OR MEDICAL MANAGEMENT

- Previous rupture of an AVM is a major risk factor for subsequent repeated hemorrhage. Therefore, conservative treatment is not recommended in ruptured AVMs. However, the timing of intervention in relation to the first hemorrhagic event is a matter of debate and will depend mainly on the clinical status of the patient and the individual AVM morphology.

RADIOSURGERY

- Because radiosurgery takes longer to be effective in preventing repeated hemorrhage, treatment strategies that produce faster results are recommended over radiosurgery.
- Radiosurgery plays a role, though, in combination with prior embolization, which can secure the AVM in the acute phase and reduce risks for subsequent hemorrhage if angioarchitectonic weak points can be identified and eliminated.

SURGICAL TREATMENT

- Surgery is indicated for acutely ruptured AVMs when significant mass effect warrants early clot removal during the same session.
- For patients with superficial, previously bled lesions, surgery may be a better choice than embolization if multiple small feeders, en passage feeders, or a large nidus is present; these will make complete cure rates with embolization less likely.
- In some instances, presurgical ligation embolization may be helpful.

ENDOVASCULAR TREATMENT

- There are three major indications for embolization of a previously bled AVM: (1) in the acute phase if the cause of the hemorrhage can be identified and is felt to be curable by embolization, in which case a partial targeted embolization is performed; (2) in the subacute setting if it is felt that the AVM can be cured completely by endovascular means alone (i.e., small AVM with few feeders), in which case the aim is curative embolization; and (3) in the subacute setting to secure the AVM before radiosurgery, in which case endovascular microcatheter exploration may be necessary to evaluate whether morphologic weak points are present that should be targeted before radiosurgery.
- If noninvasive imaging techniques demonstrate pseudoaneurysms or intranidal aneurysms, microcatheterization may be indicated in the acute setting to prevent early rebleeding. In these instances, complete cure of the AVM is not the aim of treatment, and embolization should be performed only if the target can be reached.
- We choose a liquid embolic agent depending on the pathologic mechanism. If the patient has an intranidal aneurysm, a mixture that does not polymerize immediately is chosen to penetrate

the compartment harboring the false aneurysm (N-butyl-cyanoacrylate/Lipiodol 1 mL/1.5 mL), whereas if the patient has a venous stenosis with outflow restriction, a mixture that polymerizes faster is chosen (N-butyl-cyanoacrylate/Lipiodol 1 mL/1 mL).

- If no cause of the hemorrhage is found, the embolization of one compartment may change the hemodynamics and increase flow into another (potentially ruptured) compartment and is therefore not recommended.

Possible Complications

- In the acute setting, early aggressive embolization may compromise recovery from the initial hemorrhage. In addition, embolization may not be complete because compartments of the AVM can be compressed by mass effect and reopening delayed.
- If no cause of the hemorrhage is found, simple embolization of part of the AVM may increase the risk for repeated hemorrhage from the untreated part of the AVM that contained the source of bleeding.
- Forceful microcatheter injections close to pseudoaneurysms may increase the risk for repeated hemorrhage.

Published Literature on Treatment Options

The risk for future bleeding from a brain AVM has been the subject of many studies. In 1983, Graf et al published their results concerning risks for future hemorrhage, which were calculated to be 37% in 20 years for unruptured AVMs and 47% for ruptured AVMs. Crawford et al found similar 20-year cumulative risks for hemorrhage (33% for unruptured and 51% for ruptured AVMs); however, they added that older age was a major risk factor, with patients older than 60 years having a risk for rupture of 90% in 9 years. In a prospective series published by Mast et al in 1997, the risk for hemorrhage of previously ruptured brain AVMs was calculated to be 17% per year; in unruptured AVMs, the risk for hemorrhage was 2% per year. Finally, in a recent study by our group, DaCosta et al described an annual risk for repeated hemorrhage of 7.5% in AVMs that presented with hemorrhage, which was approximately twofold the risk for nonruptured AVMs to hemorrhage.

Specific angioarchitectonic features of AVMs can be regarded as "weak points" and may predispose to hemorrhage. These angioarchitectonic weak points are (1) intranidal aneurysms and venous ectases, and (2) venous stenosis. The first authors to state that specific angioarchitectonic features in brain AVMs make them more prone to future hemorrhage were Brown et al in 1988, who found that the annual risk for future hemorrhage was 3% in brain AVMs without aneurysms and 7%/year in brain AVMs with associated aneurysms. Meisel et al found that among 662 patients with brain AVMs, 305 patients had associated aneurysms, and there was a significant increase in episodes of rebleeding in brain AVMs that harbored intranidal aneurysms ($p < 0.002$). In the Toronto series of 759 brain AVMs published by Stefani et al, the presence of aneurysms was statistically significantly ($p = 0.015$) associated with future bleeding. It may be difficult to discern intranidal arterial aneurysms from intranidal venous ectases, which is why these two angioarchitectonic features are grouped as one entity in most series. Venous stenoses, on the other hand, are a separate angiographic weak point and lead to an imbalance of pressure in various compartments of the AVM, which may induce subsequent rupture of the AVM.

Given the high risk for repeated hemorrhage and the defined angioarchitectonic risk factors, we classically opt for either surgery to completely exclude the AVM (if this is unlikely to be achieved by embolization) or embolization to eliminate the described risk factors and thereby secure the AVM for subsequent radiosurgery.

PEARLS AND PITFALLS

- The size of an acutely ruptured AVM may be underestimated because of associated mass effect with compression of the AVM compartments.
- In rare cases of small AVMs, the associated mass effect may "cure" the AVM through venous stenosis and subsequent occlusion of the nidus.
- Choroidal AVMs with vessel outpouchings into the ventricles are in our experience more prone to early rebleeding, especially if extraventricular drainage is performed.
- If no weak point is identified at global angiography in an acutely ruptured AVM, it may be necessary to perform microcatheterization, in particular if CT demonstrates a potential pseudoaneurysm. If no weak point is identified, even at microcatheterization, then it is safer not to embolize at all to prevent hemodynamic redirection into a potentially more harmful AVM compartment.

Further Reading

Brown RD Jr, Wiebers DO, Forbes G, et al. The natural history of unruptured intracranial arteriovenous malformations. J Neurosurg 1988;68(3):352–357

Crawford PM, West CR, Chadwick DW, Shaw MD. Arteriovenous malformations of the brain: natural history in unoperated patients. J Neurol Neurosurg Psychiatry 1986;49(1):1–10

da Costa L, Wallace MC, Ter Brugge KG, O'Kelly C, Willinsky RA, Tymianski M. The natural history and predictive features of hemorrhage from brain arteriovenous malformations. Stroke 2009;40(1):100–105

Graf CJ, Perret GE, Torner JC. Bleeding from cerebral arteriovenous malformations as part of their natural history. J Neurosurg 1983;58(3):331–337

Mast H, Young WL, Koennecke HC, et al. Risk of spontaneous haemorrhage after diagnosis of cerebral arteriovenous malformation. Lancet 1997;350(9084):1065–1068

Meisel HJ, Mansmann U, Alvarez H, Rodesch G, Brock M, Lasjaunias P. Cerebral arteriovenous malformations and associated aneurysms: analysis of 305 cases from a series of 662 patients. Neurosurgery 2000;46(4):793–800, discussion 800–802

Stefani MA, Porter PJ, terBrugge KG, Montanera W, Willinsky RA, Wallace MC. Angioarchitectural factors present in brain arteriovenous malformations associated with hemorrhagic presentation. Stroke 2002;33(4):920–924

CASE 19

Case Description

Clinical Presentation

A 39-year-old woman presents with gradually progressive headaches that began 4 months earlier and the new onset of seizures 3 months earlier. CT was performed after her first seizure, followed by MRI.

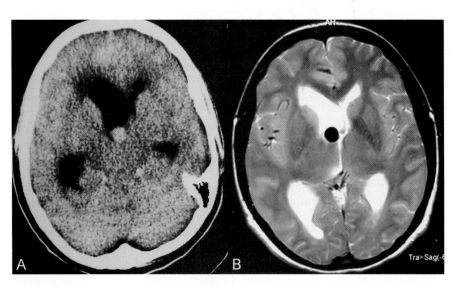

Fig. 19.1 (A) Unenhanced axial CT and **(B)** T2-weighted MRI show a dilated vessel within the right frontal horn at the level of the foramen of Monro with unilateral right lateral ventricular dilatation. Periventricular hypodensity suggestive of transependymal edema was also observed.

Radiologic Studies

CT AND MRI

Outside nonenhanced CT of the brain demonstrated a dilated vessel in the right frontal horn close to the foramen of Monro and right-sided ventricular dilatation with associated increased transependymal resorption of cerebrospinal fluid (CSF). A pathologic tangle of vessels was demonstrated in the right parasagittal region. MRI verified the diagnosis of right-sided parasagittal arteriovenous malformation (AVM) with drainage predominantly into the right thalamostriate vein. Massive enlargement of the vein was causing unilateral blockage of the right foramen of Monro (**Fig. 19.1**).

DSA

Following injections into the right and left internal carotid arteries (ICAs), a frontocallosal and cingulate diffuse nidus type of AVM was revealed, with superficial drainage toward the superior sagittal sinus via midline veins and deep drainage into the right thalamostriate vein, which drained into the internal cerebral veins (**Fig. 19.2**).

116

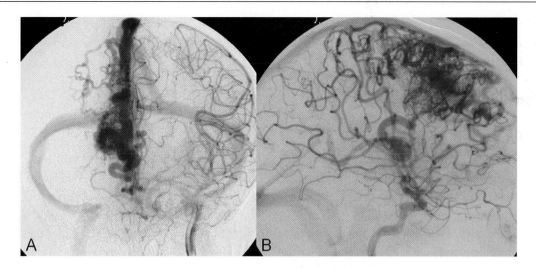

Fig. 19.2 DSA. Left ICA angiogram in **(A)** AP and **(B)** lateral views reveals a diffuse nidus type of AVM at the right frontocallosal and cingulate regions. Multiple arterial feeders from both the anterior cerebral artery and middle cerebral artery are observed, with superficial drainage toward the superior sagittal sinus and deep venous drainage into the right thalamostriate vein and further drainage into the internal cerebral veins.

Diagnosis

Frontocallosal and cingulate AVM with venous ectasia causing hydrocephalus

Treatment

EQUIPMENT

- Standard 5F Access (puncture needle, 5F vascular sheath)
- Standard 5F multipurpose catheter (Guider Soft Tip; Boston Scientific, Natick, MA) with continuous flush and a 0.035-in hydrophilic guidewire (Terumo, Somerset, NJ)
- Three 0.012-in flow-directed microcatheters (Magic; Balt International, Montmorency, France) with a 0.008-in guidewire (Mirage; ev3, Plymouth, MN)
- A 10% glucose solution
- Histoacryl/Lipiodol (1 mL/1 mL)
- Contrast material
- Steroids

DESCRIPTION

The 5F multipurpose catheter was placed in the distal infrapetrous ICA and continuously flushed. A flow-directed microcatheter with a steam-shaped 45-degree curve was introduced into the pericallosal artery and advanced to the portion of the AVM draining solely into the thalamostriate vein. The microcatheter was positioned proximal to the nidus, as verified by microcatheter injections. After the microcatheter had been flushed with the glucose solution, a mixture of 1 mL of glue with 1 mL of Lipiodol was injected. This procedure was repeated three times in different deep compartments of the AVM, which finally resulted in partial embolization of the inferior aspects of the AVM and reduced deep venous drainage. Following the procedure, the patient was free of headaches. A follow-up CT after 4 weeks demonstrated the glue case in the inferior aspect of the AVM and a reduced size of the draining vein as well as reduced ventricular volume (**Fig. 19.3**). Given its diffuse nature, the remainder of the AVM was treated with radiosurgery.

Discussion

Background

The most common cause of hydrocephalus in a patient with a pial brain AVM is rupture with intraventricular or subarachnoid hemorrhage and subsequent blockage of the arachnoid villi or cisterns surrounding the brainstem. A less common cause in unruptured AVMs is overproduction of CSF, which has been reported in choroidal AVMs. Distant venous outflow obstruction can lead to venous congestion and hydrocephalus, especially in young children. Obstruction of the ventricles is an extremely rare cause of hydrocephalus and may be caused by the AVM nidus itself or, more commonly, by its draining veins. In the latter case, the obstruction can occur at the level of the foramen of Monro or at the aqueduct. Therefore, only AVMs draining into the deep venous system cause ventricular obstruction as a consequence of their close proximity to the CSF pathways. The veins responsible for this obstruction may be the enlarged thalamostriate–internal cerebral vein complex or the vein of Galen; therefore, supratentorial AVMs causing this symptom will demonstrate a dominant venous outlet into the deep venous system, whereas infratentorial AVMs will be associated with a dilated vein of Galen.

Noninvasive Imaging Workup

PHYSICAL EXAMINATION

- Headaches in patients with AVMs may be the presenting symptoms for a variety of reasons, including, as in this case, hydrocephalus. However, a more common cause of headaches is mass effect due to the AVM nidus or an associated dilated venous pouch. In addition, transdural supply can lead to headaches. Finally, occipital AVMs are more likely to present with headaches, and posterior cerebral artery supply is supposed to be responsible for these symptoms.

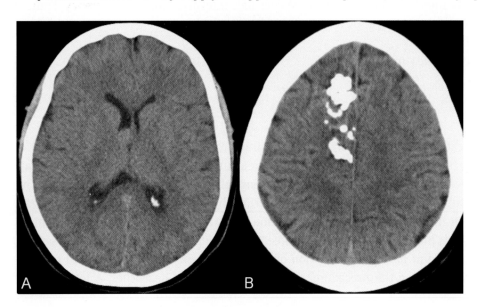

Fig. 19.3 Unenhanced axial CT following embolization demonstrates **(A)** reduced ventricular size and **(B)** the hyperdense glue cast within the AVM nidus.

CT/MRI

- The classic findings for hydrocephalus are a discrepancy between the width of the ventricles and the width of the sulci, dilatation of the ventricles, and increased transependymal CSF resorption with edema surrounding first the frontal and later also the temporal and occipital horns. Cross-sectional imaging can identify the cause and location of obstructive hydrocephalus in most instances.

Invasive Imaging Workup

- If hydrocephalus is due to venous dilatation, an invasive imaging workup must be performed to identify the compartment that drains into the vein. Subsequent embolization must target this structure to reduce the venous size and pressure on the brain structures.

Differential Diagnosis

- A dilated vein as the cause of obstructive hydrocephalus has been observed in rare cases of complex and large developmental venous anomalies with a collecting vein located in a critical area, as described above.
- The more common causes of hydrocephalus in brain AVMs must be considered first: previous rupture, choroidal AVMs with CSF overproduction, and venous congestion.

Treatment Options

RADIOSURGERY

- Radiosurgery may be a treatment option because it will also reduce the shunting volume and therefore the size of the draining veins; however, this may take longer than either surgery or embolization and should therefore be used judiciously, depending on the severity of the symptoms and the severity of the imaging findings of hydrocephalus. Radiosurgery, however, may play a role following embolization and flow reduction for treatment of the AVM rather than the hydrocephalus.

SURGICAL TREATMENT

- Because most AVMs presenting with hydrocephalus are due to deep venous drainage, risks associated with surgery are generally considered relatively high. Surgical options for the treatment of hydrocephalus have to be considered and are discussed below.

ENDOVASCULAR TREATMENT

- Endovascular therapies are an elegant way to reduce flow through the AVM and secondarily the size of the draining vein. The effects of embolization are fast, and patients may be saved from additional craniotomy for CSF drainage.
- Caution must be taken to embolize preferably the compartment that drains into the deep vein rather than a compartment with superficial drainage so as not to increase flow through the wrong compartment.

Possible Complications

- Migration of the embolic agent into the draining vein or "ballooning" of the draining vein with large amounts of liquid glue must be avoided.

Published Literature on Treatment Options

If patients with hydrocephalus related to a brain AVM are treated with ventriculoperitoneal or ventriculoatrial shunts, potentially harmful overdrainage may occur, increasing the transmural pressure gradient of the AVM vessels and potentially causing slit ventricles or subdural effusions. Overdrainage reduces ventricular size until slit ventricles provoke chronic subdural hematomas. On the other hand, contact between the ventricular walls and the shunt may lead to shunt occlusion, which may explain the high rate of complications associated with shunts reported in the literature in these patients. Therefore, besides endovascular reduction of the AVM flow and therefore the size of the vein, the surgical therapy of choice for dealing with obstructive hydrocephalus is endoscopic third ventriculostomy for aqueductal compression, as long as no AVM vessels are located near the shunt trajectory. For unilateral blockage of the foramen of Monro, endoscopic septum pellucidostomy can be proposed. In the emergency setting of a patient with symptoms of acute hydrocephalus, the surgical options are the fastest treatment and may therefore be required. However, in patients with mild-to-moderate hydrocephalus and no neurologic deficits, the aim of treatment (irrespective of the modality chosen) should be reduction of the arteriovenous flow and subsequent reduction of the size of the vein causing the obstruction rather than elimination of the "secondary" effect (i.e., the hydrocephalus).

PEARLS AND PITFALLS

- Hydrocephalus due to an unruptured AVM is rare and may be related to different pathologic mechanisms, including increased CSF production, compression of the foramen of Monro or the aqueduct, or venous congestion.
- Treatment by embolization can reduce the flow and therefore the size of the draining vein, which can reduce the compressive effect of the draining vein.

Further Reading

Chimowitz MI, Little JR, Awad IA, Sila CA, Kosmorsky G, Furlan AJ. Intracranial hypertension associated with unruptured cerebral arteriovenous malformations. Ann Neurol 1990;27(5):474–479

Geibprasert S, Pereira V, Krings T, Jiarakongmun P, Lasjaunias P, Pongpech S. Hydrocephalus in unruptured brain AVMs: pathomechanical considerations, therapeutic implications, and clinical course. J Neurosurg 2009;110(3):500–507

Willinsky R, Terbrugge K, Montanera W, Mikulis D, Wallace MC. Venous congestion: an MR finding in dural arteriovenous malformations with cortical venous drainage. AJNR Am J Neuroradiol 1994;15(8):1501–1507

CASE 20

Case Description

Clinical Presentation

A 36-year-old man presented 2 months earlier at an outside institution with an acute onset of headaches followed by loss of consciousness. CT demonstrated an intraventricular hemorrhage and, following contrast enhancement, pathologically dilated vessels in the quadrigeminal cistern. He is referred to our institution for further workup and potential endovascular treatment.

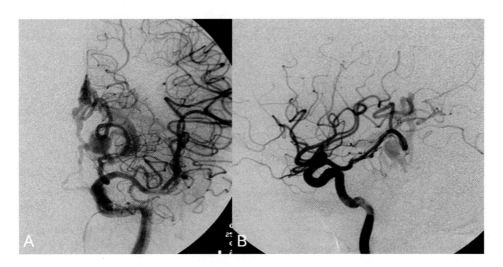

Fig. 20.1 DSA. Left ICA angiogram in **(A)** AP and **(B)** lateral views demonstrates a fistulous AVM supplied by the left posterolateral choroidal artery, seen through a dominant left posterior communicating artery, draining directly into ectatic lateral choroidal veins.

Radiologic Studies

DSA

Injection in the left internal carotid artery (ICA) demonstrated a dominant posterior communicating artery feeding the posterior cerebral artery. A fistulous arteriovenous malformation (AVM) was shown to be fed by the posterolateral choroidal artery on the left side, draining without an intervening nidus directly into ectatic lateral choroidal veins, the basal vein of Rosenthal, and the internal cerebral vein system (**Fig. 20.1**).

DIAGNOSIS

Small fistulous pial AVM with venous ectasia

Treatment

EQUIPMENT

- Standard 5F access (puncture needle, 5F vascular sheath)
- Standard 5F multipurpose catheter (Envoy; Cordis, Warren, NJ) with continuous flush and a 0.035-in hydrophilic guidewire (Terumo, Somerset, NJ)

121

- A 0.012-in flow-directed microcatheter (Magic; Balt International, Montmorency, France)
- A 10% glucose solution
- Histoacryl/Lipiodol/tantalum powder (1 mL/0.5 mL/one-fourth vial)
- Contrast material
- Steroids

DESCRIPTION

Following diagnostic angiography, a 5F multipurpose catheter was placed in the distal infrapetrous ICA and continuously flushed. A flow-directed microcatheter with a small steam-shaped hook (120-degree curve) was introduced via the posterior communicating artery into the lateral posterior choroidal artery and advanced proximal to the fistula. A microcatheter injection revealed the anticipated fistulous nature of the shunt. The microcatheter tip was placed facing against the wall of the artery ~5 mm proximal to the fistula. After the microcatheter had been flushed with glucose solution, a mixture of 1 mL of glue with 0.5 mL of Lipiodol and one-fourth of a vial of tantalum powder was injected, achieving complete occlusion of the fistulous AVM nidus. Following microcatheter removal, control runs (from both the ICA and the vertebral artery) demonstrated complete occlusion of the arteriovenous shunt (**Fig. 20.2**).

Discussion

Background

Depending on the angioarchitecture of the AVM, fistulous and "plexiform" (or glomus-type) nidi can be distinguished. In the latter, a network of pathologic vessels is present between the feeding artery and draining vein, whereas in the former, there is a direct transition of the shunts from artery to vein. Depending on the shunt flow, micro- and macrofistulae can be further differentiated. In general, flow in these shunts is faster than in the plexiform nidus type of AVMs, and therefore venous ectases are more often present. Fistulous compartments can coexist with plexiform compartments in the same AVM. It is not known whether fistulous or plexiform AVMs more often cause hemorrhage; however, the fistulous type frequently presents in younger persons, especially in that apart from the hemorrhagic presentation, the high-flow nature of the AVM and associated venous pouches may lead to symptoms related to mass effect or venous congestion.

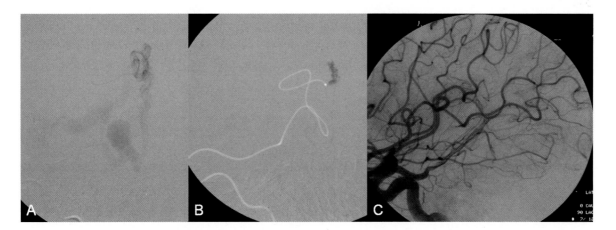

Fig. 20.2 (A) Superselective microcatheter injection and **(B)** glue cast show the fistulous communication. **(C)** Left ICA angiogram in lateral view after embolization shows complete occlusion of the fistulous AVM.

Noninvasive Imaging Workup

See also Case 21.

CT/MRI

- Purely fistulous AVMs can sometimes be identified based on noninvasive imaging alone; pathologic vessels are present in the subarachnoid space, but no tangle of vessels is seen in the brain parenchyma. At the same time, there is dilatation of both feeding pial arteries (which differentiates these shunts from dural arteriovenous fistulae with cortical venous reflux) and draining veins. Often, venous pouches can be detected.

INVASIVE IMAGING WORKUP

- All arteries supplying the brain must be investigated in patients with fistulous arteriovenous shunts because they are one potential phenotype of hereditary hemorrhagic telangiectasia (see Case 57), a disease that can be associated with a multiplicity of arteriovenous shunting lesions in the brain.
- The sequelae of high-flow shunting lesions in adjacent brain and vessels, including neo-angiogenesis surrounding the AVM and leptomeningeal collaterals, have to be differentiated from the fistula proper.
- Of the utmost importance in treatment planning is identification of the transition of the artery into the vein because during endovascular therapy, the goal will be to occlude the most distal part of the artery together with the most proximal part of the vein. Typically, the transition is marked by a sudden change in caliber or an atypical change in the direction of flow (from centrifugal flow to centripetal flow). In some cases, the transition is marked by a venous pouch; however, these can also be present downstream from the true fistulous transition.

Treatment Options

See also Case 21.

CONSERVATIVE OR MEDICAL MANAGEMENT AND RADIOSURGERY

- As discussed in previous cases, patients harboring an AVM and presenting with hemorrhage are at high risk for repeated hemorrhage, which is why we do not recommend conservative treatment. Likewise, the longer time needed for obliteration following radiosurgery may not favor this treatment modality, especially because there is doubt concerning the obliteration rate of fistulous AVMs compared with "plexiform" nidi following radiosurgery. If, as in the present case, angioarchitectonic weak points, such as venous ectases, are also present and the fistula is easily accessible, other treatment options should be preferred.

SURGICAL TREATMENT

- Surgical occlusion of the fistulous point is a safe and definitive treatment option; however, depending on the location of the fistula, it is more invasive than endovascular techniques.

ENDOVASCULAR TREATMENT

- The goal of treatment with the endovascular approach is occlusion of the most distal part of the artery and the most proximal part of the vein with a liquid embolic agent that optimally should not fragment but rather deploy in a "mushroom-shaped" pattern in the venous site.
- Given the higher flow rate in fistulous lesions, a glue with a higher concentration is used in our practice.

- If the glue does not penetrate the vein, the fistula may still be cured as a consequence of subsequent venous thrombosis, and we recommend follow-up imaging with DSA in 3 months.

Possible Complications

- Possible complications include migration of the embolic agent into the draining vein with potential occlusion and hemorrhage or venous ischemia, proximal occlusion with delayed reopening, and arterial ischemia due to reflux of the embolic agent into arteries supplying normal brain.
- Seizures following successful treatment are due to significant alterations in cerebral hemodynamics.
- Delayed venous thrombosis and mass effect of the venous pouches are due to significant flow reduction.

Published Literature on Treatment Options

In the present literature, there is no differentiation between AVM subtypes with respect to their natural history, treatment-related complications, and the superiority of one treatment modality over another. However, it is the experience of most neurointerventionalists that endovascular treatment options are an excellent choice for fistulous AVMs, given their configuration of a single feeding artery and draining vein, easy accessibility, and frequently symptomatic presentation.

PEARLS AND PITFALLS _____

- The liquid embolic agent must penetrate from the arterial to the venous side; however, because only a single feeder and a single vein are present in these purely fistulous lesions, even arterial ligation may lead to durable results because subsequent venous thrombosis may result in stable occlusion of the fistula.
- Patients with fistulous AVMs may have an underlying disease, such as hereditary hemorrhagic telangiectasia.
- Following embolization, headaches and seizures may develop transiently. If new neurologic symptoms occur, follow-up imaging is necessary to rule out excessive venous thrombosis, which may require anticoagulation and steroid therapy.

Further Reading

Krings T, Chng SM, Ozanne A, Alvarez H, Rodesch G, Lasjaunias PL. Hereditary hemorrhagic telangiectasia in children: endovascular treatment of neurovascular malformations: results in 31 patients. Neuroradiology 2005;47(12):946–95416163493

Krings T, Ozanne A, Chng SM, Alvarez H, Rodesch G, Lasjaunias PL. Neurovascular phenotypes in hereditary haemorrhagic telangiectasia patients according to age. Review of 50 consecutive patients aged 1 day–60 years. Neuroradiology 2005;47(10):711–72016136265

Yuki I, Kim RH, Duckwiler G, et al. Treatment of brain arteriovenous malformations with high flow arteriovenous fistulas: risk and complications associated with endovascular embolization in multimodality treatment. J Neurosurg Oct 16, 2009 [Epub ahead of print]

CASE 21

Case Description

Clinical Presentation

A 41-year-old woman presents with progressive weakness of her left lower and upper extremities and a recent generalized seizure. MRI and subsequently angiography are performed.

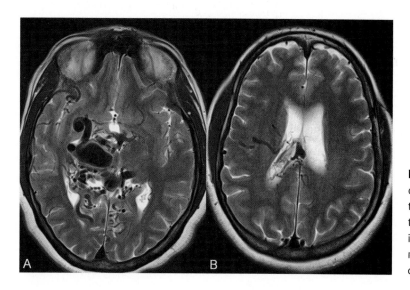

Fig. 21.1 **(A)** T2-weighted MRI demonstrates a large venous pouch within the right ambient cistern compressing the right cerebral peduncle. **(B)** There is dilatation of the right-sided transmedullary veins, suggestive of venous congestion.

Radiologic Studies

MRI

On MRI, T2-weighted sequences demonstrate a large venous pouch within the right ambient cistern compressing the right cerebral peduncle. Multiple dilated vessels are seen along the tentorium and also supratentorially, with right-sided dilated transmedullary veins (**Fig. 21.1**). The presence of dilated veins distant from the nidus is suggestive of venous congestion, due either to a high-flow shunt or to venous outlet obstruction.

DSA

There is evidence of a high-flow arteriovenous malformation (AVM) that is fed predominantly by both posterior cerebral arteries via the lateral posterior choroidal arteries, which are massively enlarged. In addition, multiple small transependymal feeders from the tip of the basilar artery and from the P1 segments also contribute to the feeding of this choroidal type of high-flow AVM, presumably as a secondary "sump" effect. On the arterial side, there is significant arterial remodeling, with widening of both posterior cerebral arteries and evidence of flow-related aneurysms at the left superior cerebellar artery and at the right P1 segment just anterior to the right posterior communicating artery. The nidus has both fistulous and plexiform compartments. Multiple venous pouches are present, both within the nidus and distal to the AVM. There is significant venous rerouting because despite the location of the AVM in the midline, there is no visible drainage via the straight sinus or the vein of Galen. The drainage occurs predominantly via the basal vein of Rosenthal, which demonstrates a venous pouch ~4 cm in size directly adjacent to the cerebral peduncle; drainage from there is via transtemporal veins but also via the superficial middle cerebral vein and the sphenoparietal sinus toward the superficial venous drainage system. In addition, drainage occurs via median parietal and median frontal veins toward the superior sagittal sinus bilaterally. There is a significant amount of venous congestion with a pseudophlebitic aspect of the draining veins. It is only in the late phases of angiography that filling of cerebellar veins is demonstrated, suggesting a significant amount of venous congestion also at the level of the posterior fossa. Injection in the internal carotid arteries demonstrates a pseudophlebitic aspect of the draining veins in the late venous phase and significant cross-filling of the AVM via the right posterior communicating artery (**Fig. 21.2**).

Diagnosis

High-flow fistulous choroidal AVM with venous remodeling

Treatment

EQUIPMENT

- Standard 5F access (puncture needle, 5F vascular sheath)

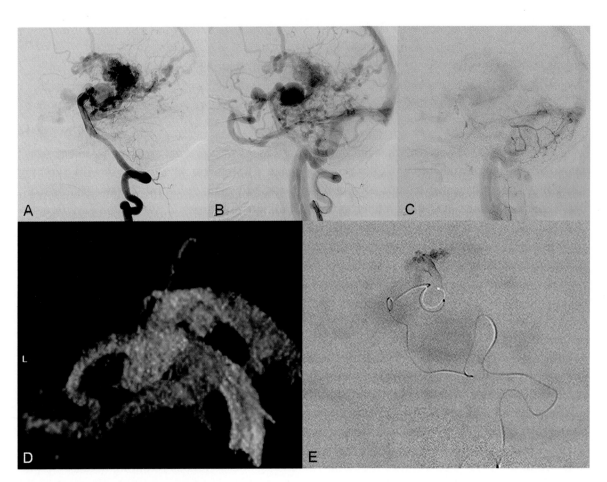

Fig. 21.2 DSA. Left vertebral angiogram in lateral view. **(A)** Early, **(B)** late arterial, and **(C)** venous phases demonstrate a high-flow AVM supplied predominantly by the lateral posterior choroidal arteries from the posterior communicating arteries. **(D)** 3D reconstruction of the basilar tip shows flow-related aneurysms at the origin of the left superior cerebellar artery and at the right P1 segment just anterior to the right posterior communicating artery. **(E)** Superselective microcatheter injection before embolization reveals a fistula within the AVM nidus.

- Standard 5F multipurpose catheter (Envoy; Cordis, Warren, NJ) with continuous flush and a 0.035-in hydrophilic guidewire (Terumo, Somerset, NJ)
- A 2 × 0.012-in flow-directed microcatheter (Magic; Balt International, Montmorency, France)
- A 10% glucose solution
- Histoacryl/Lipiodol/tantalum powder (2 mL/0.2 mL/one-half vial)
- Contrast material
- Steroids

DESCRIPTION

We intended to approach the AVM through the posterior communicating artery in an effort to avoid prenidal aneurysms at the superior cerebellar origin and the posterior basilar apex. A flow-directed microcatheter with a small, steam-shaped, 90-degree curve was introduced via the posterior communicating artery into the lateral posterior choroidal artery and advanced to the fistulous portion of the AVM, as verified by microcatheter injections. A mixture of 2 mL of glue, 0.2 mL of Lipiodol, and half of a vial of tantalum powder was injected, achieving occlusion of the fistulous compartment and significant flow reduction in the basal vein of Rosenthal and its venous pouch (**Fig. 21.3**). Partial embolization slowed the flow through the AVM, providing a measure of symptomatic relief and secondarily reducing the size of the nidus in an effort to make the lesion amenable to gamma knife radiosurgery, which was planned for the patient.

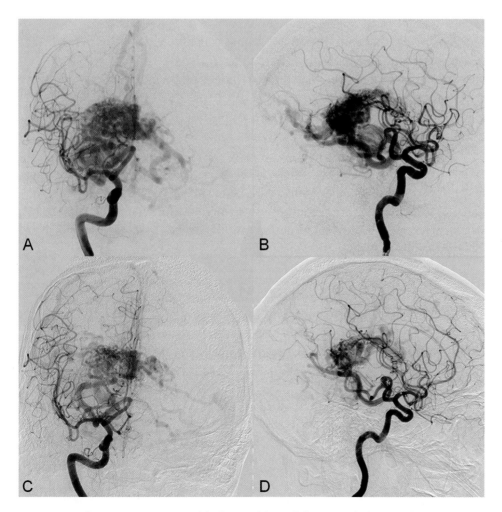

Fig. 21.3 Right ICA angiogram **(A,B)** before and **(C,D)** following embolization shows reduction in flow and size of the AVM.

Discussion

Background

The patient in the present case had an AVM with mixed fistulous and plexiform compartments. Given the high-flow nature, it is in most instances the fistulous component that is responsible for symptoms, which may include epileptic seizures, neurologic deficits, headaches, and hemorrhage. The presumed pathologic mechanisms of these symptoms include mass effect of the venous pouches and venous congestion, which may be due either to the high flow rate or secondary venous outflow obstruction. The combination of cross-sectional imaging clues, angioarchitectonic features, and clinical symptoms is of importance to understand the primary pathologic mechanism and define a treatment strategy. In our experience, a discrepancy between the predicted venous drainage pattern and the actually observed venous drainage pattern points toward an unstable situation in which the normal venous outflow routes are no longer used—for example, as a result of high-flow venous angiopathy. The onset of seizures in a previously healthy individual harboring an AVM suggests changes in hemodynamics (i.e., rerouting of drainage from the AV shunt toward veins that normally drain normal brain).

Noninvasive Imaging Workup

See also Case 20.

CT/MR

- Cross-sectional imaging findings that are suggestive of venous congestion are dilated veins distant from the predicted anatomic outflow route of the AVM nidus.
- Dilated venous pouches and associated flow-related arterial aneurysms are indicative of high-flow shunts.

Invasive Imaging Workup

- In fistulous AV shunts, the venous phase can reveal (1) whether rerouting of the outflow tracts has occurred and (2) how the normal brain drains and whether this drainage is compromised.
- Compartments harboring the fistulous connections must be targeted during embolization before other AVM compartments to avoid additional rerouting toward the fistulous compartments.

Treatment Options

See also Case 20.

RADIOSURGERY

- Radiosurgery is commonly used following embolization of a high-flow compartment to eliminate the plexiform compartments of an AVM with multiple compartments. It is not recommended as the primary treatment modality under such circumstances.

SURGICAL TREATMENT

- Because of the high-flow nature of the fistula and the large size of the concomitant nidus, surgery may be associated with a higher risk for complications than a combination therapy of embolization and radiosurgery.

ENDOVASCULAR TREATMENT

- In fistulous AVMs, the catheter should point against the wall before embolization, especially when a catheter with a small inner diameter is used, to avoid venous penetration. If possible, catheters with a larger inner diameter (which are therefore also stiffer and more difficult to navigate through tortuous anatomy) may be used.
- Treatment has to be carried out in our experience in multiple sessions to avoid too abrupt a change in hemodynamics, which may provoke seizures, headaches, or excessive venous thrombosis with mass effect of the thrombosed pouch.
- In selected cases, coils may be delivered into the venous pouch before glue embolization to reduce the flow; however, overly dense packing of these coils may cause a mass effect and should be avoided.
- To date, there is ongoing debate about what kind of liquid embolic agent to use. The personal experience of the authors and published data indicate a higher rate of complete obliteration with Onyx (40–60%), but with a significantly increased treatment-associated risk for permanent morbidity and mortality (8–12%).

Possible Complications

- Embolization may increase the mass effect as the consequence of acute thrombosis within the venous pouches and secondary worsening of neurologic symptoms. If the flow is reduced extensively, treatment with heparin over a period of 1 week may be required.

Published Literature on Treatment Options

Venous outflow obstruction in brain AVMs may lead to the rerouting of arterialized blood into veins that normally drain the brain or even the spinal cord and will therefore interfere with function of the brain remote from the shunt proper. This can result in progressive neurologic symptoms. It has been argued that venous outflow obstruction may be caused by the high-flow situation in the veins and is therefore more likely to occur in fistulae; however, longitudinal studies to prove this hypothesis are missing. In addition to venous outflow obstruction, venous pouches can lead to mass effect, with concomitant neurologic deficits or seizures. In both instances, the target of treatment must be reduction of flow, which is best accomplished with embolization.

PEARLS AND PITFALLS _____

- Both plexiform and fistulous compartments may be present within one AVM.
- In most instances, the fistulous compartments are related to the patient's symptoms, can be targeted with embolization, and should be embolized before other treatment modalities are used.
- Patients are symptomatic because of a disequilibrium between the AVM and its host (i.e., changes in the cerebral hemodynamics).

Further Reading

Gault J, Sarin H, Awadallah NA, Shenkar R, Awad IA. Pathobiology of human cerebrovascular malformations: basic mechanisms and clinical relevance. Neurosurgery 2004;55(1):1–16, discussion 16–17

Nishizawa S, Ryu H, Yokoyama T, Kitamura S, Uemura K. Intentionally staged operation for large and high-flow cerebral arteriovenous malformation. J Clin Neurosci 1998;5(Suppl):78–83

Valavanis A, Yaşargil MG. The endovascular treatment of brain arteriovenous malformations. Adv Tech Stand Neurosurg 1998;24:131–214

Yuki I, Kim RH, Duckwiler G, et al. Treatment of brain arteriovenous malformations with high flow arteriovenous fistulas: risk and complications associated with endovascular embolization in multi-modality treatment. J Neurosurg Oct 16, 2009 [Epub ahead of print]

CASE 22

Case Description

Clinical Presentation

A previously healthy 11-year-old boy presents with the acute onset of headaches, nausea, and ataxia and is brought to the emergency department. CT and then MRI and angiography are performed.

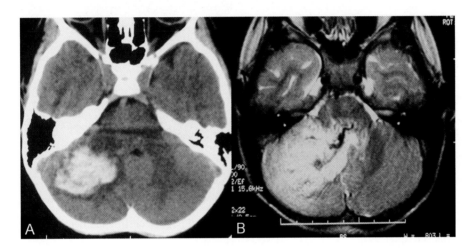

Fig. 22.1 **(A)** Unenhanced axial CT and **(B)** T2-weighted MRI demonstrate an intraparenchymal cerebellar hemorrhage and a dilated vascular with a classic caput medusae appearance draining toward the fourth ventricle.

Radiologic Studies

CT AND MR

Unenhanced CT demonstrated an intraparenchymal hemorrhage in the right cerebellum with no significant mass effect and no subarachnoid component. MRI demonstrated a vascular structure traversing the hemorrhage with a classic caput medusae appearance of dilated venous channels. Although it was felt that the most likely diagnosis was an acutely ruptured cavernoma with an associated developmental venous anomaly (DVA), angiography was performed to rule out an arteriovenous (AV) shunt (**Fig. 22.1**).

DSA

Injection in the left dominant vertebral artery demonstrated early venous filling of a large cerebellar DVA, the classic shape of which could be better appreciated on the late venous phases and 3D rotational angiography of the venous phase. The shunt was fed by the superior cerebellar artery, and drainage was via one of the collector veins of the caput medusae and subsequently via the DVA draining vein (**Fig. 22.2**).

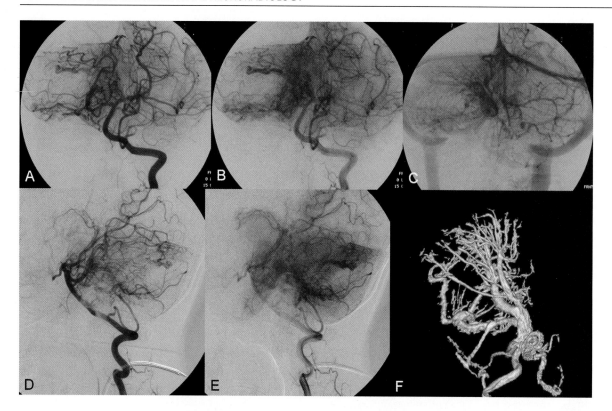

Fig. 22.2 DSA. Left vertebral angiogram in **(A–C)** AP and **(D,E)** lateral views and **(F)** 3D reconstruction demonstrates an AV shunt draining into a large cerebellar DVA.

Diagnosis

Ruptured microshunt draining into a cerebellar DVA

Treatment

EQUIPMENT

- Standard 5F access (puncture needle, 5F vascular sheath)
- Standard 5F multipurpose catheter (Guider Soft Tip; Boston Scientific, Natick, MA) with continuous flush and a 0.035-in hydrophilic guidewire (Terumo, Somerset, NJ)
- A 2 × 0.012-in flow-directed microcatheter (Magic; Balt International, Montmorency, France) with a 0.008-in guidewire (Mirage; ev3, Plymouth, MN)
- A 10% glucose solution
- Histoacryl/Lipiodol (1 mL/1 mL)
- Contrast material
- Steroids

DESCRIPTION

A 5F multipurpose catheter was placed in the distal vertebral artery and continuously flushed. A flow-directed microcatheter with a steam-shaped 45-degree curve was introduced into the superior cerebellar artery with the aid of a micro-guidewire and advanced distally. Microcatheter injections revealed two distinct shunting zones; these were subsequently treated with a mixture of 1 mL of glue and 1 mL of Lipiodol, which achieved complete occlusion of the shunts without penetration of the DVA (**Fig. 22.3**). Follow-up angiography demonstrated complete occlusion of the shunt and preservation of the DVA.

Discussion

Background

DVAs, which were previously called venous angiomas, are extreme variations of normal transmedullary veins, which are necessary for the drainage of white and gray matter. They consist of converging dilated medullary veins that drain centripetally and radially into a transcerebral collector, which opens into either the superficial subcortical or deep pial veins. DVAs have no proliferative potential and normally harbor no direct AV shunts. Normal brain parenchyma is found between the dilated veins. DVAs serve as normal drainage routes of the brain tissue because the usual venous drainage of their territory is absent. Their etiology and mechanism of development are unknown, but it is currently accepted that they act as a compensatory system of cerebral parenchyma venous drainage after early failure, abnormal development, or intrauterine occlusion of normal capillaries or small transcerebral veins. DVAs are benign anatomic variations and are therefore usually incidentally discovered. Most hemorrhages that are encountered when a DVA is present are related to associated cavernomas rather than to the DVA. Epilepsy is due to associated cortical dysplasia, and pseudotumoral effects can be secondary to associated lymphatic malformations. Because a DVA represents a venous system that is not fully developed, it may be prone to hemorrhage when it serves as the outflow route of a shunt. This was the pathologic mechanism in the present case.

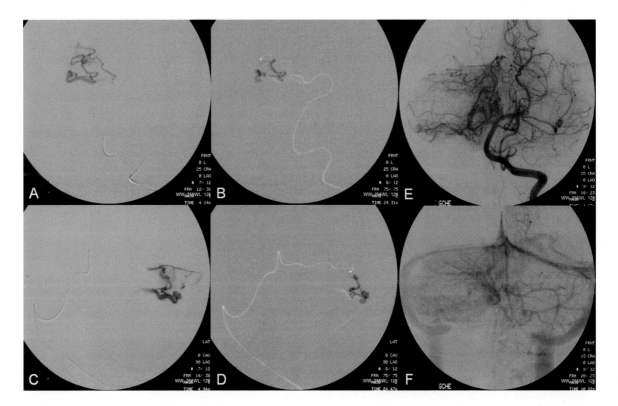

Fig. 22.3 Superselective hand injections and glue cast during **(A,B)** first and **(C,D)** second embolization procedures. **(B)** Minimal penetration of the glue into the petrosal vein prompted embolization of the entire AV shunt. Left vertebral angiogram in AP view in **(E)** arterial and **(F)** venous phases reveals complete obliteration of the shunt with preservation of the DVA.

Noninvasive Imaging Workup

PHYSICAL EXAMINATION

- Radiologic and autopsy series have demonstrated DVAs in 2.5 to 3% of the population. DVAs are the most common vascular "malformation" of the central nervous system, constituting ~60% of all vascular malformations; capillary telangiectases account for 20%, cavernomas 10%, arteriovenous malformations (AVMs) 9%, and dural AV shunts 1% in larger autopsy series. They have been seen or diagnosed in patients presenting with symptoms such as seizures, vertigo, syncope, tinnitus, and headaches; however, because these symptoms are among the ones that most often lead to MRI investigation, a direct relationship cannot be established, and it is currently accepted that DVAs are an incidental finding in the vast majority of cases.

CT/CTA, MRI/MRA

- On contrast-enhanced CT, the venous collector of the DVA is readily detectable as a linear or cur-vilinear focus of enhancement, typically coursing from the deep white matter to a cortical vein or a deep vein or to a dural sinus.
- On MRI, DVAs typically exhibit a trans-hemispheric flow void on both T1- and T2-weighted images. After the administration of gadolinium, because of the slow flow, significant enhancement of the caput medusae of the medullary veins and venous collector is observed.
- Associated cavernomas and/or cortical dysplasias must be ruled out by MRI once a DVA is identified.
- Further invasive diagnostic workup is necessary only when a DVA presents with hemorrhage without an associated cavernoma or when the differential diagnosis of a complex DVA and a true AVM is unclear.

Invasive Imaging Workup

- DSA is rarely necessary to diagnose a DVA. The classic angiographic appearance is that of a caput medusae of transmedullary veins, visualized during the early to middle venous phase, draining into a large venous collector, which can extend to either the superficial or deep venous system, depending on the type of DVA.
- DVAs are classified as deep (i.e., draining into deep subependymal veins and the galenic system) or superficial (i.e., draining into cortical veins). Complex DVAs can have multiple collectors, drain a large area, and be associated with both a deep and a superficial drainage.
- Early opacification of a DVA may be seen with an associated capillary blush. In most cases, this represents a rapid capillary transit time rather than true AV shunting; however, the shunt of an AVM into a DVA or microshunts must be ruled out if the patient has presented with hemorrhage.
- AVMs associated with DVAs are more likely to cause symptoms because of the reduced flexibility and capacity to adjust to changes in venous pressure within DVAs.

Differential Diagnosis

- In most instances, when a DVA is diagnosed in the acute setting of a hemorrhage, an underlying cavernoma is likely to be the cause of the bleeding.
- Complex DVAs with an extensive capillary blush must be differentiated from DVAs that harbor true AV shunts; this sometimes requires microcatheter exploration, which we deem necessary only in patients who present with hemorrhage without an associated cavernoma.
- Telangiectases may mimic DVAs on cross-sectional imaging; however, they do not demonstrate shunting compartments or early venous drainage on DSA.

Treatment Options

CONSERVATIVE OR MEDICAL MANAGEMENT

- In acutely ruptured AVMs, the necessity of treatment has been pointed out previously. However, we also favor the treatment of incidental AVMs whose outflow route is a DVA because the DVA as an anatomic variation of the venous drainage may be less flexible to changes of the venous pressure. Therefore, a superimposed AV shunt may be associated with a higher rate of complications.

RADIOSURGERY

- As described previously, radiosurgery takes longer to effectively prevent repeated hemorrhage and is in our opinion less suited for the developing brain, which is why we tend to use alternate treatment strategies in children, especially when they present with an acute hemorrhage.
- Identification of the target may be more difficult in patients with an AVM that drains into a DVA because this may lead to dilatation of the caput medusae veins and an overestimation of the true nidus.

SURGICAL TREATMENT

- Surgery is indicated for acutely ruptured AVMs when significant mass effect warrants early clot removal during the same session.
- The differentiation of dilated transmedullary veins from a true AVM may be difficult on surgical inspection. However, because preservation of the DVA proper is of the utmost importance to avoid delayed venous ischemic problems in adjacent brain, this is necessary and may be better achieved by endovascular means.

ENDOVASCULAR TREATMENT

- In complex DVAs and DVAs that have presented with hemorrhage without evidence of an associated cavernoma, microcatheter exploration may prove helpful to identify potential microshunts.
- Endovascular treatment must preserve the draining vein and the collector vein; therefore, a liquid embolic agent that polymerizes fast is chosen in our practice.
- Treatment is recommended even for a nonruptured AVM that is associated with a DVA, as described above.

Possible Complications

- In the hyperacute setting, mass effect of the hematoma may compress parts of the AVM; follow-up is therefore necessary.
- Penetration into the venous collector must be avoided to preserve the integrity of the DVA.

Published Literature on Treatment Options

DVAs are in most cases incidental and nonsymptomatic. They may become symptomatic through a variety of pathologic mechanisms; it has been reported that the collecting vein can cause mechanical compression of intracranial structures. Hydrocephalus due to venous vascular compression of the aqueduct or cranial nerves may ensue and is best treated by ventriculocisternostomy and microvascular decompression. Second, the venous drainage of a DVA may become restricted (because of stenosis or thrombosis of the DVA or its drainage vein or because of a "functional" obstacle such as an increase in the venous pressure secondary to a distant AV shunt). If the outflow of a DVA is restricted, venous congestion may occur in the territory normally drained by the DVA. The treatment of choice for this condition is to reconstitute the normal flow through the DVA (in cases of thrombosis, this is best accomplished with anticoagulation). The third pathologic mechanism of a DVA (the one in the present case) is increased inflow into the DVA.

When the DVA is the outflow route of an AV shunt, the venous collector may be overloaded and likely to become symptomatic because the chronically increased pressure within the DVA may increase the risk for venous rupture in an already fragile venous outlet. The association of an AVM with a DVA is presumably coincidental; however, we believe that the risk for hemorrhage and complications is increased. Therefore, in our practice, we may perform preventive treatment even in an asymptomatic patient with a shunt draining into a DVA. Treatment options include radiosurgery, surgery, or endovascular means, as in all other AVMs; however, it is of the utmost importance to preserve the DVA proper and treat only the shunt because the DVA will be needed to drain normal adjacent brain. It may sometimes be difficult to differentiate a true shunt from a DVA (with its associated dilated medullary veins), so that definition of the target for radiosurgery may be challenging, and we prefer endovascular means to try to obliterate the shunt, given the better visualization of a shunt during microcatheter injections.

PEARLS AND PITFALLS

- DVAs are considered to be stable and benign; however, as an anatomic variation, they occur in atypical locations and may be less able to respond to changes of the intracranial venous equilibrium. Because the flexibility and capacity to adjust to changes in the venous pressure is reduced in DVAs, superimposed AV shunts may increase the risk for venous infarction or hemorrhage.
- Treatment is indicated and should be aimed at occluding the shunt with preservation of the draining vein.

Further Reading

Komiyama M, Yamanaka K, Iwai Y, Yasui T. Venous angiomas with arteriovenous shunts: report of three cases and review of the literature. Neurosurgery 1999;44(6):1328–1334, discussion 1334–1335

Lasjaunias P, Burrows P, Planet C. Developmental venous anomalies (DVA): the so-called venous angioma. Neurosurg Rev 1986;9(3):233–242

Pereira VM, Geibprasert S, Krings T, et al. Pathomechanisms of symptomatic developmental venous anomalies. Stroke 2008;39(12):3201–3215

Valavanis A, Wellauer J, Yaşargil MG. The radiological diagnosis of cerebral venous angioma: cerebral angiography and computed tomography. Neuroradiology 1983;24(4):193–199

Wilms G, Bleus E, Demaerel P, et al. Simultaneous occurrence of developmental venous anomalies and cavernous angiomas. AJNR Am J Neuroradiol 1994;15(7):1247–1254, discussion 1255–1257

CASE 23

Case Description

Clinical Presentation

A 44-year-old man presents to the emergency department with the acute onset of severe headaches and dysphasia. His wife reports that the patient has had unusual headaches for the last 3 weeks. Emergency CT is performed, followed by dynamic CTA and angiography.

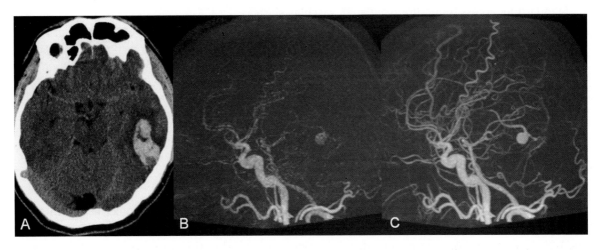

Fig. 23.1 (A) Unenhanced axial CT demonstrates a hyperdense lesion at the left temporal lobe, representing intraparenchymal hemorrhage, with surrounding hypodense brain edema and mild mass effect. Dynamic CTA in **(B)** early and **(C)** late arterial phases in lateral view shows early arterial filling of a venous pouch and cortical vein.

Radiologic Studies

CT

Plain CT of the brain demonstrated an intraparenchymal hemorrhage in the left temporal lobe measuring 4.5 × 1.8 cm and surrounded by edema. It caused a mild mass effect on the atrium of the left lateral ventricle with no significant midline shift. There was also a small subdural component at the left temporofrontal region. On CTA, an enlarged venous pouch measuring 8 mm in diameter was noted at the posterior aspect of the parenchymal hemorrhage. Dynamic CTA demonstrated early arterial filling of the venous pouch, corresponding to a shunting lesion (**Fig. 23.1**).

DSA

Injection of the left external carotid artery (ECA) showed an arteriovenous fistula fed by the petrosquamous branch of the middle meningeal artery and the auricular branch of the occipital artery in the absence of a posterior auricular artery. The two feeding arteries formed a small arterial network just above the level of the sigmoid sinus and then shunted into a pial vein, from which blood refluxed in retrograde fashion into two veins. One of these ran toward the anterior temporal pole and the other ran toward the anterior sylvian fissure, then drained into a frontal cortical vein toward the superior sagittal sinus. This latter vein also filled a branch that ran back to drain into the sigmoid sinus **(Fig. 23.2)**. More importantly, this vein had a venous pouch, which was felt to be responsible for the hemorrhage. The left internal carotid artery (ICA) appeared normal without evidence of venous stagnation or congestion. The remaining territories of both vertebral arteries, the right ICA, and the right ECA were normal.

Diagnosis

Dural arteriovenous fistula (DAVF) with direct communication into a pial vein having an associated venous pouch (Borden type 3)

Treatment

EQUIPMENT

- Standard 5F access (puncture needle, 5F vascular sheath)
- Standard 5F multipurpose catheter (Guider Soft Tip; Boston Scientific, Natick MA) with continuous flush and a 0.035-in hydrophilic guidewire (Terumo, Somerset, NJ)
- A 0.012-in flow-directed microcatheter (Magic; Balt International, Montmorency, France) with a 0.008-in guidewire (Mirage; ev3, Plymouth, MN)
- A 10% glucose solution
- Histoacryl/Lipiodol (1 mL/1.5 mL)
- Contrast material
- Steroids

DESCRIPTION

Following diagnostic angiography, a 5F multipurpose catheter was advanced into the left internal maxillary artery. A flow-directed microcatheter was introduced over a guidewire into the middle meningeal artery and advanced immediately proximal to the shunting zone, as verified by control runs done via the microcatheter. After the microcatheter had been flushed with the glucose solution,

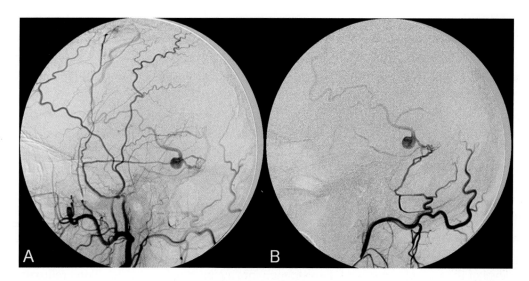

Fig. 23.2 DSA. **(A)** Left internal maxillary and **(B)** left occipital angiograms in lateral view show an AVF supplied by branches of the left middle meningeal artery and left stylomastoid branch originating from the left occipital artery. The AVF drains into an ectatic venous pouch and further drains into two cortical veins.

a mixture of 1 mL of glue with 1.5 mL of Lipiodol was injected and filled the two veins and venous pouch in antegrade fashion, as well as the arterial network and two feeding arteries in retrograde fashion (**Fig. 23.3**). The microcatheter was removed, and control runs were performed of both the internal maxillary artery and the occipital artery. These showed no more filling of the fistula. A control run of the left ICA showed unchanged drainage through the left sigmoid artery without evidence of a compromise of the venous flow. Immediately after the procedure, 4 mg of dexamethasone was administered.

Discussion

Background

DAVFs are abnormal connections between arteries (that would normally feed the meninges, bone, or muscles but *not* the brain) and small venules within the dura mater. They account for 10 to 15% of all intracranial AV shunts. The simplest way to classify these lesions is according to whether they do or do not exhibit corticovenous reflux. Although those without corticovenous reflux are benign fistulae (Borden type 1) that almost never lead to neurologic deficits, those with corticovenous reflux may be regarded as malignant fistulae. They are classified as Borden type 2 (if the shunt is directed into the dural sinuses and subsequently into cortical veins) and Borden type 3 (if the shunt is directed immediately into cortical veins). Malignant DAVFs often have an aggressive clinical presentation, with intracranial hemorrhage (e.g., from rupture of venous pouches), seizures, dementia, alteration of consciousness, and focal nonhemorrhagic neurologic symptoms due to venous congestion. Given the high risk for hemorrhage, complete treatment of *all* malignant DAVFs must be carried out. In most centers, endovascular management is the therapy of choice.

Noninvasive Imaging Workup

PHYSICAL EXAMINATION

- Depending on the location of the DAVF, a bruit may be present.

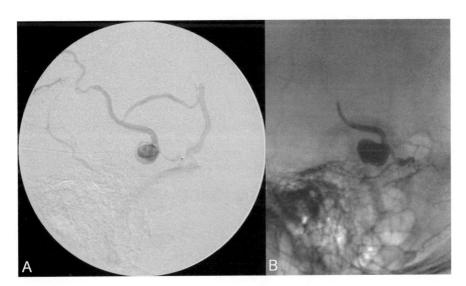

Fig. 23.3 (A) Superselective microcatheter injection within the left middle meningeal artery branch and **(B)** plain radiography demonstrate the glue cast filling the venous pouch and proximal vein after embolization.

CT/CTA

- In patients with otherwise unexplained intraparenchymal hemorrhage, a DAVF must be included in the differential diagnosis, especially if CT demonstrates an associated subdural hematoma, intraparenchymal calcifications, or too many vessels in the subpial space.
- Although static CTA may be negative (or just demonstrate too many dilated subpial vessels), dynamic CTA can demonstrate the early draining vein and therefore confirm the diagnosis.

MRI/MRA

- Like CT, MRI in patients who have a DAVF with cortical venous reflux will show abnormal vessels on the surface of the brain parenchyma. Findings include dilated cortical veins (pseudophlebitic pattern) and abnormally enhancing tubular structures or flow voids within the cortical sulci without a true nidus within the brain parenchyma.
- Hyperintensity on T2-weighted images indicates venous congestion or infarction, which may eventually lead to venous hemorrhage. Focal enhancement of these areas may also be observed as a sign of chronic venous ischemia.
- Static MRA may not be sufficient to diagnose a shunting lesion; a dynamic MRA sequence helps to identify a shunting lesion.

Invasive Imaging Workup

- In a patient with a DAVF, all potential feeders must be evaluated and the venous drainage of the normal brain must be studied; therefore, a six-vessel workup is typically necessary (including both vertebral arteries, both external carotid arteries, and both internal carotid arteries).
- Depending on the location of the fistula, injections of the ascending and deep cervical arteries and selective injections of the ascending pharyngeal arteries may also be required.

Differential Diagnosis

- Moyamoya disease may be associated with intraparenchymal hemorrhage and dilated perforating vessels. However, no early draining vein is present, and dilated perforating vessels compensate for the (classically bilateral) stenoses of the M1 segment and distal ICA.
- Pial AVFs (Cases 21–22) are fistulous lesions fed by arteries that normally feed the brain and can thereby be differentiated from dural AVFs.

Treatment Options

SURGICAL TREATMENT

- If endovascular treatment fails to occlude the fistulous site (including the distal arterial segment[s] and the proximal venous segment [s]), surgery must be performed to obliterate the fistula.
- Surgery may be the method of choice if a space-occupying hemorrhage is present to evacuate the hematoma and occlude the fistula in the same session.
- In our institution, catheter angiography is performed to confirm complete occlusion of the fistula after surgery.

ENDOVASCULAR TREATMENT

- In our practice, endovascular treatment is the method of choice for all patients with "malignant" DAVFs.
- Proximal occlusions and particle embolization procedures are obsolete because they lead to recanalization with a high risk for repeated hemorrhage (up to 16% annually).

- Liquid embolic agents (e.g., Histoacryl, Onyx) should be employed to occlude the distal arterial segment and the proximal venous segment of the shunt.
- Periprocedural heparin is recommended if the procedure is anticipated to take longer than 30 minutes.
- In our practice, steroids are given following Histoacryl embolization to compensate for the exothermic effect of the glue.

Possible Complications

- Standard angiographic complications may develop (at the puncture site: bleeding, false aneurysms, fistulae; in catheterized vessels: emboli, dissections; systemically: contrast reaction, renal failure).
- The embolic agent may migrate into veins that are still functional (i.e., that are used to drain normal brain).
- Proximal occlusion with delayed reopening of the shunt may occur.
- Stroke or cranial nerve palsies are due to extracranial or intracranial anastomoses and embolization and occlusion of arteries that supply the cranial nerves.

Published Literature on Treatment Options

Given that DAVFs with cortical venous reflux carried an annual risk of more than 8% for hemorrhage and 6% for nonhemorrhagic deficits and an annual mortality rate of 10% in the series reported by van Dijk et al from our group, curative treatment is deemed a necessity and should be obtained in a timely fashion. If endovascular treatment is unsuccessful, then surgical treatment should be performed during the same hospital admission. Both surgical and endovascular treatment options follow the same principle (i.e., to occlude the distal arterial site and the proximal venous outflow), and high success rates with low rates of procedure-related morbidity and mortality have been reported.

PEARLS AND PITFALLS

- A proximal arterial occlusion is *not* sufficient, despite angiographic nonopacification of the fistula, because the fistulous site will still be active. With excellent dural collaterals, it will in time recruit other dural supply and reopen.
- Migration of the embolic agent into distal (still functioning) cerebral veins can lead to catastrophic venous infarction.
- If multiple arterial feeders are present, the (1) safest artery with (2) the straightest course should be used.
- Technical failure does not preclude subsequent surgery, which should be considered if arterial access proves to be too difficult.

Further Reading

Borden JA, Wu JK, Shucart WA. A proposed classification for spinal and cranial dural arteriovenous fistulous malformations and implications for treatment. J Neurosurg 1995;82(2):166–179

Cognard C, Gobin YP, Pierot L, et al. Cerebral dural arteriovenous fistulas: clinical and angiographic correlation with a revised classification of venous drainage. Radiology 1995;194(3):671–680

Davies MA, TerBrugge K, Willinsky R, Coyne T, Saleh J, Wallace MC. The validity of classification for the clinical presentation of intracranial dural arteriovenous fistulas. J Neurosurg 1996;85(5):830–837

Geibprasert S, Pereira V, Krings T, et al. Dural arteriovenous shunts: a new classification of craniospinal epidural venous anatomical bases and clinical correlations. Stroke 2008;39(10):2783–2794

van Dijk JM, terBrugge KG, Willinsky RA, Wallace MC. Clinical course of cranial dural arteriovenous fistulas with long-term persistent cortical venous reflux. Stroke 2002;33(5):1233–1236

CASE 24

Case Description

Clinical Presentation

A 63-year-old man presents to the emergency department with the acute onset of seizures. Emergency CT and MRI are performed, followed by angiography.

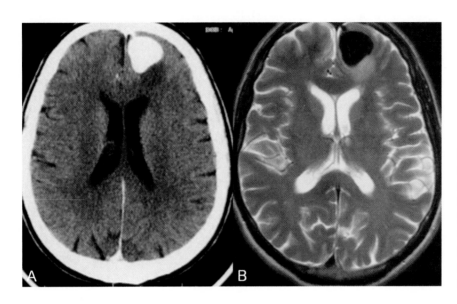

Fig. 24.1 (A) Contrast-enhanced CT and (B) T2-weighted MRI demonstrate a venous pouch with surrounding brain edema. A small flow void adjacent to the venous pouch, corresponding to a dilated cortical vein, is noted on the T2-weighted image.

Radiologic Studies

CT AND MRI

Contrast-enhanced CT of the brain demonstrated a well-defined, intensely enhancing vascular structure at the left frontal lobe, consistent with a venous pouch (**Fig. 24.1**). Surrounding hypodensity indicated brain edema. A T2-weighted image demonstrated similar findings. The tubular flow-void structure adjacent to the venous pouch, corresponding to a dilated cortical vein, and the brain edema were better seen than on the CT scan.

DSA

Injection of the left internal carotid artery (ICA) showed an arteriovenous fistula (AVF) at the level of the anterior cranial fossa floor, supplied mainly by the ethmoidal branches of the left ophthalmic artery (**Fig. 24.2**). There was also minimal supply from branches of the right ophthalmic artery. No significant arterial supply from the external carotid artery (ECA) branches was seen, although the venous pouch was faintly opacified through indirect supply from the nasoethmoidal branches of the left facial artery (not shown). There was direct drainage into the left frontal cortical vein, with a large venous pouch, and further drainage into the superior sagittal sinus.

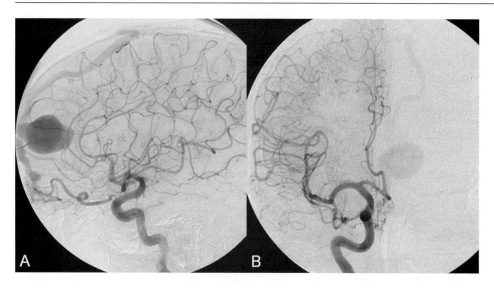

Fig. 24.2 DSA. **(A)** Left ICA injection in lateral view and **(B)** right ICA injection in AP view show an AVF at the anterior cranial fossa, supplied mainly by the ethmoidal branches of **(A)** the left ophthalmic artery with minimal supply from **(B)** the right ophthalmic artery. There is direct drainage into a left frontal cortical vein, which harbors a large venous pouch, before drainage into the superior sagittal sinus.

Diagnosis

Ethmoidal dural arteriovenous fistula (DAVF) with a direct communication into a cortical vein and an associated venous pouch (Borden type 3)

Treatment

EQUIPMENT

- Standard 5F access (puncture needle, 5F vascular sheath)
- Standard 5F multipurpose catheter (Envoy; Cordis, Warren, NJ) with continuous flush and a 0.035-in hydrophilic guidewire
- A 0.012-in flow-directed microcatheter (Magic; Balt International, Montmorency, France) with a 0.008-in guidewire (Mirage; ev3, Plymouth, MN)
- A 10% glucose solution
- Histoacryl/Lipiodol (1 mL/1.5 mL)
- Contrast material

DESCRIPTION

Following diagnostic angiography, a 5F multipurpose catheter was advanced into the left ICA. A flow-directed microcatheter was introduced over a micro-guidewire into the left ophthalmic artery and advanced to a point immediately proximal to the shunting zone. Control runs were done by hand injections via the microcatheter to confirm the position (**Fig. 24.3**). After the microcatheter had been flushed with the glucose solution, a mixture of 1 mL of glue and 2 mL of Lipiodol was injected, penetrating the shunt zone and filling the proximal draining vein without any reflux of the glue. The microcatheter was removed, and control runs were performed of both ICAs and both ECAs, confirming complete closure of the fistula.

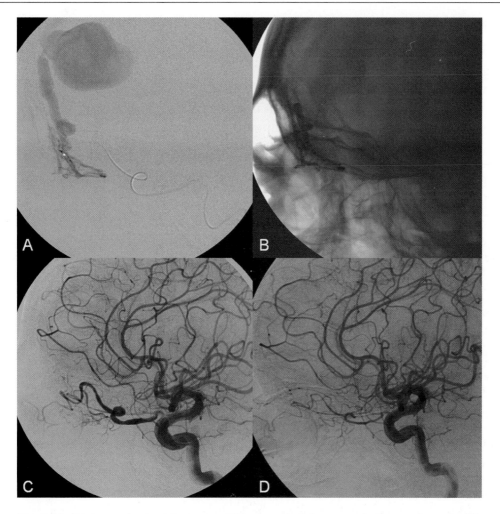

Fig. 24.3 **(A)** Superselective injection and **(B)** glue cast following embolization show glue filling the proximal venous segment. Control left ICA angiograms **(C)** immediately after and **(D)** 3 months after the procedure confirm complete obliteration of the fistula. Note the remodeling of the ophthalmic artery after embolization.

Discussion

Background

DAVFs at the anterior cranial fossa are also known as "ethmoidal" DAVFs. Such DAVFs are rare and can be classified among the DAVFs of the lateral epidural type. Other places where lateral epidural DAVFs are found include the spine (the classic location), foramen magnum, falx (vein of Galen), tentorium (basal vein of Rosenthal and superior petrosal sinus), and cortical veins. Arterial supply to ethmoidal DAVFs is characteristically from the ethmoidal branches of the ophthalmic artery, and venous drainage is through the frontal cortical veins before a sinus (therefore, ethmoidal DAVFs are always Borden type 3 lesions). They are often associated with venous pouches, which frequently rupture and result in intracranial hemorrhage. Transarterial embolization is the treatment of choice in our institution, followed by open surgery when embolization fails to cure the lesion.

Noninvasive Imaging Workup

CT/MRI

- CT and MRI findings may be subtle. Only tubular enhancing structures or flow voids may be seen at the frontal cortical sulci on contrast-enhanced CT and T2-weighted images.
- Occasionally, a venous pouch may be seen, often associated with either subdural or parenchymal hemorrhage or surrounding brain edema, as in the present case.

CTA/MRA

- Both CTA and MRA can be used to confirm the presence of an AV shunt at the level of the anterior cranial fossa as well as the venous pouches.

Invasive Imaging Workup

- The arterial supply arises mainly from the ethmoidal branches of the ophthalmic artery and is usually bilateral. Additional indirect supply from branches of the ECA via small anastomoses may also be seen.

Differential Diagnosis

- Pial AVFs (see Cases 20 and 21) at the frontal lobe are fistulous lesions fed by arteries that would feed the brain. In the present case, the normal frontal branches of the anterior cerebral artery can easily be differentiated from the ethmoidal branches supplying the DAVF.

Treatment Options

SURGICAL TREATMENT

- If endovascular options fail to occlude the fistulous site (including the distal arterial segment[s] and the proximal venous segment[s]), open surgical disconnection is necessary to occlude the fistula.
- Surgery may be the treatment method of choice if a space-occupying hemorrhage is present, to evacuate the hematoma and occlude the fistula in the same session.
- Preoperative embolization with particles in the external carotid feeders is generally not useful because the supply is mainly through the ophthalmic artery.
- In our experience, angiographic confirmation of complete occlusion of the fistula is necessary following surgery.

ENDOVASCULAR TREATMENT

- In our current practice, endovascular therapies are the method of first choice in all patients with "malignant" DAVFs.
- Proximal occlusion and particle embolization procedures are inadequate because they lead to recanalization.
- Permanent liquid embolic agents should be employed to occlude the distal arterial segment and the proximal venous segment of the shunt.
- Periprocedural heparin is recommended.
- The position of the microcatheter *must* be beyond the origin of the central retinal artery (identified through the choroidal blush of the adjacent posterior ciliary arteries in lateral view), and reflux of the embolic material into the ophthalmic artery *must* be avoided.

Possible Complications

- Standard angiographic complications may occur (at the puncture site: bleeding, false aneurysms, fistulae; in catheterized vessels: emboli, dissections; systemically: contrast reaction, renal failure).
- Stroke and blindness may be caused by reflux of the embolic material into the ICA or central retinal artery.
- The embolic agent may migrate too far into frontal cortical veins that are still functional.
- Proximal arterial occlusion with delayed reopening of the fistula may occur.

Published Literature on Treatment Options

Surgery is the most common type of treatment in previous case series, usually with a 95 to 100% cure rate. Operations are typically performed via a frontal or bifrontal craniotomy to identify the dura-based feeding arteries and enlarged draining cortical veins. Subsequent disconnection of the fistula on the venous side is then performed, with a low risk for stroke and blindness. In the past years, an increasing number of case series have reported the successful use of endovascular treatment. In the report by Agid et al, the success rate for transarterial embolization through the ophthalmic artery was ~60%. Embolization through indirect branches of the ECA is usually not successful. Although transvenous approaches have been reported, they are technically more challenging, requiring navigation of the microcatheter to the anterior superior sagittal sinus and then selectively into the draining cortical vein. Coiling of this vein must be done as close as possible to the fistulous site and proximal to the venous pouch to avoid a catastrophic hemorrhage.

PEARLS AND PITFALLS

- The major arterial supply to an ethmoidal DAVF is from the ophthalmic artery, and the drainage is directly into a frontal cortical vein; therefore, these DAVFs are *always* Borden type 3, and treatment is indicated.
- Proximal occlusion of the arterial feeder is insufficient, and occlusion of the proximal vein is necessary.
- If transarterial embolization through the ophthalmic artery is attempted, the microcatheter must be beyond the origin of the central retinal artery, and *no* reflux is permitted.
- Surgical disconnection has a high cure rate and can be done even after failed embolization.

Further Reading

Abrahams JM, Bagley LJ, Flamm ES, Hurst RW, Sinson GP. Alternative management considerations for ethmoidal dural arteriovenous fistulas. Surg Neurol 2002;58(6):410–416, discussion 416

Agid R, Terbrugge K, Rodesch G, Andersson T, Söderman M. Management strategies for anterior cranial fossa (ethmoidal) dural arteriovenous fistulas with an emphasis on endovascular treatment. J Neurosurg 2009;110(1):79–84

Lawton MT, Chun J, Wilson CB, Halbach VV. Ethmoidal dural arteriovenous fistulae: an assessment of surgical and endovascular management. Neurosurgery 1999;45(4):805–810, discussion 810–811

Lv X, Li Y, Wu Z. Endovascular treatment of anterior cranial fossa dural arteriovenous fistula. Neuroradiology 2008;50(5):433–437

CASE 25

Case Description

Clinical Presentation

A 49-year-old man presented 2 years previously with complex partial seizures, which were controlled with medication. Now his seizures are worsening despite increases in his seizure medication. There are no neurologic deficits on clinical examination. A CT scan is performed at an outside hospital, and the patient is referred to our institution for angiography and treatment.

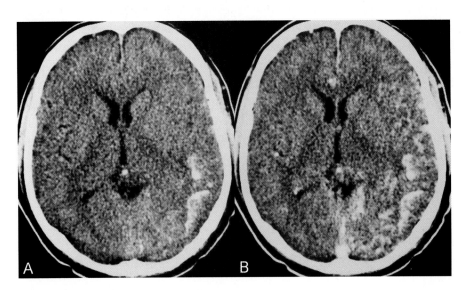

Fig. 25.1 **(A)** Unenhanced and **(B)** post-contrast CT scans demonstrating subcortical calcification at the level of the left temporo-occipital lobe, with enhancing vessels along the cortical surface of the left cerebral hemisphere.

Radiologic Studies

CT

Unenhanced CT scan showed subcortical calcification involving the left temporo-occipital lobe. After the administration of contrast, prominent enhancing vessels along the cortical surface of the left cerebral hemisphere were noted, suggestive of a dural arteriovenous fistula (DAVF) with cortical venous reflux (**Fig. 25.1**).

DSA

Injection of the left external carotid artery (ECA) showed early filling of an irregular left transverse sinus segment, supplied by branches of the left occipital artery and additional supply from the left middle meningeal artery and left posterior meningeal artery. Thrombosis of the proximal left transverse sinus and distal left sigmoid sinus created an isolated sinus segment, resulting in reflux of the venous drainage into the left occipital cortical veins. A pseudophlebitic appearance of the cortical veins in the venous phase of the left internal carotid artery (ICA) injection was noted, suggesting venous congestion (**Fig. 25.2**).

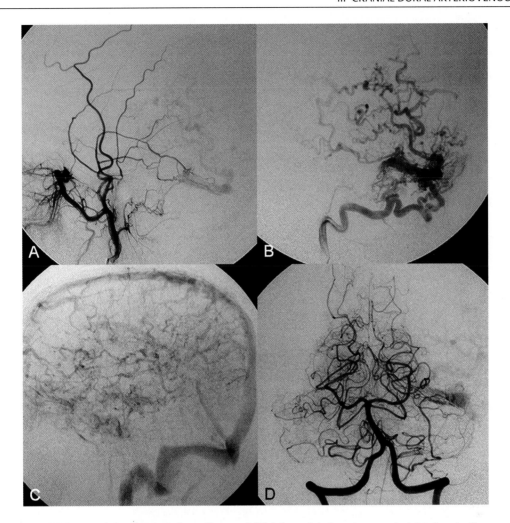

Fig. 25.2 DSA. **(A)** Left internal maxillary and **(B)** left occipital angiograms in lateral projection demonstrate an AV shunt supplied by branches of the left middle meningeal artery and left occipital artery and draining into an irregular venous segment of the left transverse sinus. Occlusion of the left proximal transverse sinus and distal sigmoid sinus segments is noted, causing cortical venous reflux into the left occipital veins. **(C)** Left ICA angiogram in late venous phase shows a pseudophlebitic pattern of the cortical veins with stagnation of the contrast, corresponding to venous congestion. Additional supply to the DAVF from the left posterior meningeal artery of **(D)** the left VA is also noted.

Diagnosis

Aggressive DAVF of the left transverse sinus associated with an isolated sinus (Borden type 2)

Treatment

EQUIPMENT

- Standard 6F access (puncture needle, 6F vascular sheath)
- Standard 6F multipurpose catheter (Envoy; Cordis, Warren, NJ) with continuous flush and a 0.035-in hydrophilic guidewire (Terumo, Somerset, NJ)
- Two 0.015-in over-the-wire microcatheters (Prowler 10; Cordis) with a 0.010-in hydrophilic guidewire (Agility 10; Cordis)
- A 10% glucose solution
- Histoacryl/Lipiodol (1 mL/2 mL)
- Contrast material

DESCRIPTION

Following diagnostic angiography, a 5F multipurpose catheter was advanced into the left occipital artery (**Fig. 25.3**). An over-the-wire microcatheter was introduced over a micro-guidewire into the dural branches originating from the occipital artery in a wedged position as close to the shunt zone as possible. Control runs were done via hand injection through the microcatheter to verify the position. The microcatheter was then flushed with the glucose solution, followed by the injection of glue at 50% concentration in an attempt to fill the venous pouch. The procedure was repeated twice, both times through branches of the occipital artery. Following the second glue embolization, filling of the isolated sinus segment was no longer seen on control angiograms. Follow-up angiogram at 3 months confirmed the complete closure of the DAVF.

Discussion

Background

DAVFs are abnormal AV shunts located within the dura mater comprising the walls of the dural sinuses. The transverse and sigmoid sinuses are the most common location, accounting for ~30 to

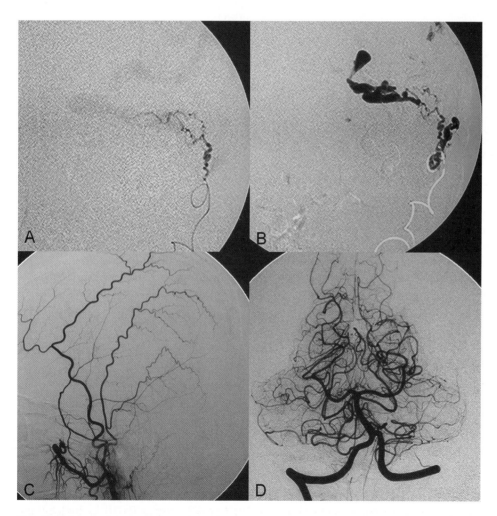

Fig. 25.3 **(A)** Hand injection through a microcatheter wedged within a branch of the left occipital artery in AP view shows filling of the isolated sinus segment, followed by **(B)** the glue injection. **(C)** Follow-up ECA and **(D)** right VA angiograms at 3 months show complete closure of the fistula.

50% of all DAVFs. Lesions in this location are typically benign (Borden type 1, without cortical venous reflux). Exceptions are cases with extensive thrombosis of the venous outflow and those with high-flow shunts, which may result in malignant dural AV shunts *with* cortical venous reflux (Borden type 2). In patients in whom the involved dural sinus is still patent, cure by endovascular means is difficult because in most instances the patent dural sinus is still a normal pathway for brain drainage, and its closure may result in venous infarction.

Ideally, transarterial embolization with permanent liquid material that closes only the AV shunts within the wall of the sinus is desirable, although this can be technically challenging, and a role for Onyx in these special circumstances should be considered. Diluted embolic material is not recommended in these instances because the embolic material will penetrate the sinus, possibly resulting in either closure of the sinus or the formation of pulmonary emboli. A highly concentrated embolic material, on the other hand, may result in proximal occlusion and delayed reopening, as will be the case if a particulate embolic material is used. Although the patient's symptoms may temporarily abate, the shunt will recruit collaterals that are even more difficult to treat. In cases with an isolated sinus segment, the involved sinus segment is not functioning to drain the normal brain; therefore, it can be sacrificed during treatment.

Noninvasive Imaging Workup

CT/MRI

- In benign DAVFs located at the sigmoid and transverse sinuses, CT and MR may yield false-negative results because no dilated cortical vessels are present.
- Malignant DAVFs with cortical venous reflux may show intraparenchymal hemorrhage and subcortical calcification on unenhanced CT scans. Venous congestion may be seen as hypodensity on CT; however, it is better demonstrated by FLAIR sequences on MRI. Contrast-enhanced CT, T2-weighted images, and/or post-gadolinium T1-weighted images best demonstrate the dilated vessels within the cortical sulci.

CTA/MRA

- Early filling of the involved sinus and the cortical venous reflux can both be seen with CTA and MRA; however, angiography is required for a detailed evaluation of the arterial feeders and possible endovascular access.

Invasive Imaging Workup

- Angiography is required in the pre-treatment evaluation of DAVFs and may be performed before or at the same time as the endovascular treatment.
- All potential feeders must be evaluated, including the external carotid arteries ECAs (and occipital arteries), the ICAs, and the vertebral arteries (VAs). A delayed venous phase of both the ICAs and VAs is necessary to evaluate the brain drainage, which may be very prolonged as a consequence of the venous congestion.

Treatment Options

RADIOSURGERY

- The major limitation of radiosurgery is that it takes at least several months before the DAVF closes, and therefore it is usually recommended only for DAVFs without evidence of cortical venous reflux and in locations that are difficult to reach (e.g., vein of Galen, tentorial incisura).

SURGICAL TREATMENT

- Surgical options that have been reported range from simple disconnection of the cortical venous reflux to sinus packing and resection of the diseased sinus segment.
- Preoperative proximal embolization with particles may have a role to decrease surgical blood loss.

ENDOVASCULAR TREATMENT

- Embolization is the preferred treatment of DAVFs.
- Proximal occlusion and particle embolization procedures will lead to recanalization and may be used only as a palliative measure in benign fistulae without cortical reflux.
- If the sinus is still patent, transarterial embolization with a permanent liquid material, aiming to close *only* the AV shunts within the wall of the dural sinus, is the preferred method of treatment. This can be achieved with the use of a slightly diluted concentration of glue in experienced hands, newer embolic materials having a prolonged polymerization time (e.g., Onyx), or temporary venous balloon protection within the dural sinus. Compartmentalized transvenous embolization (with coils) may be used in those patients in whom the DAVF involves only a compartment of the sinus; however, in most instances, preservation of the dural sinus when a transvenous route is used for treatment is not possible.
- In cases with an isolated venous pouch, either transarterial embolization with liquid embolic agents or transvenous embolization with coils and/or liquid embolic agents (employing a blind approach, as discussed in Case 27) may be used to occlude the diseased sinus segment. The choice depends on the angioarchitecture. If a large arterial feeder is present, a transarterial route is preferred; otherwise, a transvenous route can be attempted.
- Although venous penetration of the liquid embolic material is necessary, there is no need to completely fill the isolated sinus segment if glue is used because of its thrombogenic effect. If Onyx is employed, complete filling of the isolated sinus is recommended without reflux into cortical veins.
- Periprocedural heparin is recommended if the procedure is anticipated to take longer than 30 minutes.
- Steroids are not routinely given unless excessive occlusion of the cortical veins with the embolic material occurs.

Possible Complications

- Pulmonary emboli may form, and/or the embolic agent may migrate too far into cortical veins that may still be functional.
- Stroke may occur if embolic material refluxes toward the brain vessels because of failure to recognize the extracranial-to-intracranial anastomoses, which become functional following overzealous injection into the ECA branches.
- Cranial nerve palsies can occur following the inadvertent embolization of arteries that supply the cranial nerves.

Published Literature on Treatment Options

In a large series of DAVFs of the transverse and sigmoid sinuses in 150 patients recently published by Kirsch et al, the occlusion rate of transarterial embolization alone was 30%, and multiple procedures were often required. This is similar to our experience, in which complete occlusion of the DAVF is difficult to obtain, especially if the dural sinus is still patent. Some authors have proposed the use of newer embolic materials with prolonged polymerization times, such as Onyx, and/or the use of transvenous balloon protection within the dural sinus to facilitate closure of the DAVF with preservation of the sinus. Some have proposed the use of transvenous angioplasty and stenting together with transarterial embolization; however, we do not recommend this because of the high rate of in-stent thrombosis within the venous system, which may worsen the situation. Radiosurgery may be a good option for DAVFs without any cortical venous reflux, and a high rate of total or nearly total obliteration has been reported.

PEARLS AND PITFALLS

- In DAVFs of the transverse and sigmoid sinuses in which the involved sinus is still patent, the aim of treatment is to close the AV shunt within the wall and preserve the dural sinus. A transarterial route is preferred to achieve this goal.
- Venous drainage of the normal brain must be evaluated with late venous phases on angiography, and if the involved sinus is a route of drainage for the brain, then the sinus cannot be sacrificed because venous infarction will necessarily occur.
- Most DAVFs at the level of the transverse sinus are benign, and their natural history does not warrant aggressive therapy unless the patient cannot tolerate the clinical symptoms (e.g., bruit). Even so, transarterial therapy is likely to be safer than transvenous deconstructive approaches.

Further Reading

Friedman JA, Pollock BE, Nichols DA, Gorman DA, Foote RL, Stafford SL. Results of combined stereotactic radiosurgery and transarterial embolization for dural arteriovenous fistulas of the transverse and sigmoid sinuses. J Neurosurg 2001;94(6):886–891

Kirsch M, Liebig T, Kühne D, Henkes H. Endovascular management of dural arteriovenous fistulas of the transverse and sigmoid sinus in 150 patients. Neuroradiology 2009;51(7):477–483

Piske RL, Campos CM, Chaves JB, et al. Dural sinus compartment in dural arteriovenous shunts: a new angioarchitectural feature allowing superselective transvenous dural sinus occlusion treatment. AJNR Am J Neuroradiol 2005;26(7):1715–1722

Shi ZS, Loh Y, Duckwiler GR, Jahan R, Viñuela F. Balloon-assisted transarterial embolization of intracranial dural arteriovenous fistulas. J Neurosurg 2009;110(5):921–928

CASE 26

Case Description

Clinical Presentation

A 51-year-old woman presents with chemosis of the right eye, proptosis, and persistent pulsatile tinnitus that has gradually become worse over the last 3 years. The patient undergoes CTA at an outside hospital before being referred to our institution for angiography and treatment.

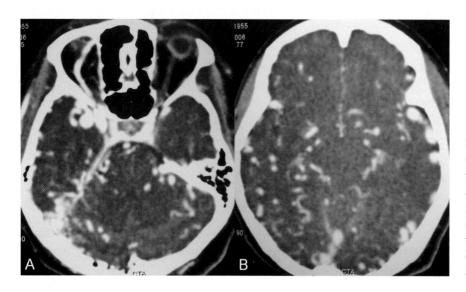

Fig. 26.1 Post-contrast CTA reveals **(A)** bulging of the right cavernous sinus and dilatation of the right superior ophthalmic vein. **(B)** Dilated vessels along the cortical surface of both cerebral hemispheres were also noted.

Radiologic Studies

CT/CTA

CT showed normal signal of the brain parenchyma. Post-contrast studies and CTA demonstrated prominently enhancing vessels within the cortical sulci of both cerebral hemispheres. Bulging of the right cavernous sinus and right superior ophthalmic vein was noted, suggesting the presence of a cavernous sinus dural arteriovenous fistula (DAVF) with cortical reflux (**Fig. 26.1**).

DSA

The study showed high-flow DAVFs along the right transverse sinus with multiple arterial feeders from branches of the middle meningeal arteries and occipital arteries bilaterally, the right meningohypophyseal trunk of the right internal carotid artery (ICA), and the posterior meningeal arteries from the vertebral arteries (VAs). Both antegrade and retrograde drainage of the shunt was noted through the patent right transverse and sigmoid sinuses to the jugular bulb, and reflux was noted into the superior sagittal sinus, occipital cortical veins, and deep venous system. The proximal left transverse sinus was occluded. Delayed drainage of the normal right cerebral hemisphere was observed through the right cavernous sinus and subsequently through the right superior ophthalmic vein. The left cerebral hemisphere drained through the left vein of Labbé into the left sigmoid sinus and left jugular bulb (**Fig. 26.2**). The late venous phase of the VA injection showed rerouting of the normal posterior fossa drainage toward the right cavernous sinus and left sigmoid sinus and through the perimedullary veins of the cervical spine.

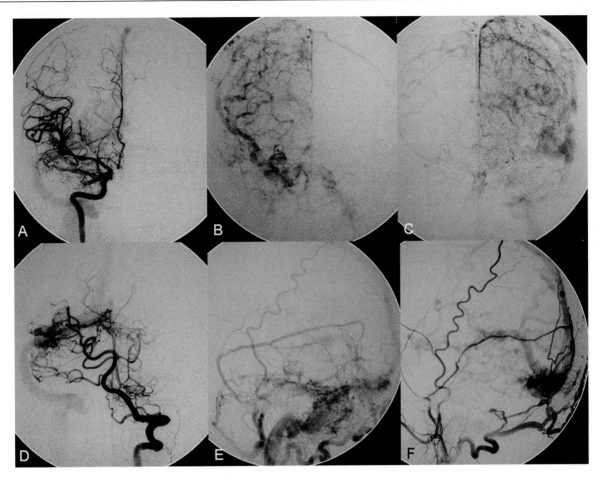

Fig. 26.2 DSA. Right ICA angiogram in AP view in **(A)** arterial and **(B)** late venous phase shows an AV shunt at the right transverse sinus supplied by the tentorial branch of the meningohypophyseal trunk. There is antegrade drainage of the shunt into the right sigmoid sinus and right jugular bulb, with retrograde drainage into the superior sagittal sinus. Left ICA angiogram in **(C)** AP view in late venous phase reveals normal drainage of the left cerebral hemisphere through the left vein of Labbé. Left VA angiogram in **(D)** AP view shows supply to the DAVF from the posterior meningeal arteries with pia-induced shunts from branches of the right posterior cerebral artery and right anterior inferior cerebellar artery, representing the high-flow nature of the lesion. Note the occlusion of the proximal left transverse sinus. **(E)** Right ECA and **(F)** left ECA angiograms show multiple arterial feeders to the DAVF, mainly from branches of the middle meningeal arteries and occipital arteries, bilaterally. There is retrograde drainage into the occipital cortical veins, straight sinus, and deep venous system.

Diagnosis

Aggressive DAVF of the left transverse sinus (Borden type 2)

Treatment

EQUIPMENT

- Standard 5F and 6F access (puncture needles, 5F and 6F vascular sheaths)
- Standard 5F and 6F multipurpose catheters (Guider Soft Tip; Boston Scientific, Natick, MA) with continuous flush and a 0.035-in hydrophilic guidewire (Terumo, Somerset, NJ)
- A 0.015-in over-the-wire microcatheter (Prowler 10; Cordis, Warren, NJ) with a 0.010-in hydrophilic guidewire (Agility 10; Cordis)

- A 0.021-in over-the-wire microcatheter (Prowler Plus; Cordis) with a 0.014-in micro-guidewire (Synchro 14; Boston Scientific)
- A 10% glucose solution
- Histoacryl/Lipiodol (1 mL/2 mL)
- Bare and fibered pushable platinum coils (Boston Scientific)
- Coil pusher (Boston Scientific)
- Contrast material

DESCRIPTION

Following diagnostic angiography, a 5F multipurpose catheter was advanced into the internal maxillary and occipital arteries bilaterally. To reduce the high flow of the shunt, transarterial embolization into the branches of the middle meningeal arteries and occipital arteries was performed bilaterally as close to the shunt zone as possible with glue at 50% concentration and an over-the-wire microcatheter. A 6F multipurpose catheter was then advanced from the femoral vein to the right internal jugular vein and placed at the right jugular bulb. After bilateral external carotid artery (ECA) injections, the shunt zone was interpreted to start from the torcular and extend all the way down to the level of the proximal right sigmoid sinus. A 0.021-in over-the-wire microcatheter was advanced over a micro-guidewire to the torcular region. Control runs via hand injection through the microcatheter were performed to verify the position. A large, bare, detachable platinum "framing" coil was selected to avoid distal migration of the pushable coils, followed by several large fibered coils and then smaller coils for dense packing. The microcatheter was progressively withdrawn toward the right sigmoid sinus with packing of the coils until the control run showed closure of the DAVF. The transvenous microcatheter and guiding catheter were removed, and a final control angiogram demonstrated obliteration of the DAVF (**Fig. 26.3**).

Discussion

Background

DAVFs involving the transverse and sigmoid sinuses most commonly present with pulsatile tinnitus, headaches, or intracranial hemorrhage. Exophthalmos and chemosis of the eye are unusual presentations that are more frequently seen with lesions located at the level of the cavernous sinus. The presence of these symptoms in a patient with a DAVF not located at the cavernous sinus suggests that the cavernous sinus is functioning as an alternative drainage pathway for either the shunt or the normal brain. Similar to the transarterial approach, transvenous management is technically challenging when the involved dural sinus is still patent and, more importantly, when it is functioning to drain the normal brain. It is often more difficult to preserve the dural sinus when a transvenous route is used, although small case series of patients in whom only one compartment of the dural sinus was involved have reported successful treatment of the involved compartment with transvenous coiling. In most cases, the entire dural sinus is involved; therefore, certain questions need to be answered before transvenous treatment with sacrifice of the dural sinus is considered: (1) Does the shunt require treatment? (2) How does the normal brain, including the cerebellum, drain? With DAVFs of the transverse and sigmoid sinuses, care must be taken concerning the entrance of the vein of Labbé and the inferior cerebellar vein into the sinus because both may play a major role in drainage of the temporo-occipital lobe and posterior fossa structures.

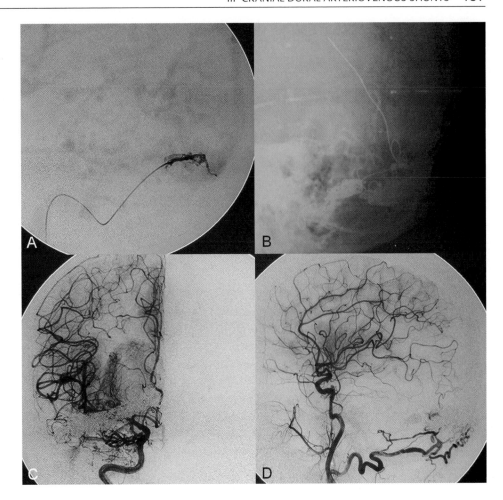

Fig. 26.3 (A) Hand injection through the microcatheter to verify the position within the right transverse sinus. **(B)** Skull radiography shows the coil meshwork. One coil migrated into the straight sinus and was not removed. Control right ICA angiogram in **(C)** AP view and left common carotid artery angiogram in **(D)** lateral view show closure of the DAVF.

Noninvasive Imaging Workup

CT/MRI

- Bulging of the cavernous sinus and dilatation of the superior ophthalmic vein are more commonly seen in cavernous sinus DAVFs but may be seen in cases in which the cavernous sinus functions as an alternative drainage pathway for the brain or shunt. If the dilated cortical veins are located diffusely along the surface of both hemispheres of the brain rather than localized along the sylvian fissure or cerebellar folia, then it is likely that the cavernous sinus is functioning as an alternative drainage route for the brain rather than being caused by a cavernous sinus DAVF.

CTA/MRA

- Early filling of the involved sinus and cortical venous reflux can both be seen on CTA and MRA; however, angiography is required for detailed evaluation of the arterial feeders and possible endovascular routes.

Invasive Imaging Workup

- Angiography is required in the pre-treatment evaluation of DAVFs; all potential feeders must be evaluated, including both ECAs, both ICAs, and both VAs.
- A delayed venous phase of both the ICAs and VAs is *necessary* for an evaluation of the brain and posterior fossa drainage.

Treatment Options

RADIOSURGERY

- Given the long time required for radiosurgery to become effective and the significant risk for symptoms during this period, radiosurgery is not recommended for the treatment of aggressive dural AV shunts.

SURGICAL TREATMENT

- Other surgical options that have been reported range from simple disconnection of the cortical venous reflux to sinus packing and resection or skeletonization of the diseased sinus segment.
- Preoperative proximal embolization with particles is useful to decrease surgical blood loss.

ENDOVASCULAR TREATMENT

- Embolization is the preferred treatment of DAVFs, as has been stated in previous cases.
- In DAVFs of the transverse and sigmoid sinuses, identification of the vein of Labbé and inferior cerebellar vein, which both drain into the transverse sinus, is necessary to avoid venous infarctions of the temporo-occipital lobe and posterior fossa. If both already have alternative pathways and/or are involved in the cortical venous reflux, then it can be assumed that the transverse sinus may be closed safely.
- Transarterial embolization immediately before the transvenous approach is recommended to diminish the flow in the sinus and allow the coils to be deposited safely.
- Identification of the exact extent of the dural sinus involved with disease is required. Treatment should start from the most distal segment. If the distal segment is incompletely treated and the proximal segment is closed, it is technically difficult to reposition the microcatheter through the treated segment.
- A large detachable framing coil should be used initially to avoid migration of the coil caused by flow.
- If a previously patent sinus is closed, bed rest for at least 24 hours following the procedure is advised to avoid migration of the coils.

Possible Complications

- Venous infarction and even death may occur if the dural sinus is draining healthy brain, including the cerebellum, and the dural sinus is inadvertently sacrificed despite this contraindication.
- Distal migration of the coils may occur during or after the procedure.

- Venous thrombosis may occur at the puncture site.
- Venous perforation may occur.

Published Literature on Treatment Options

Many case reports and case series have been reported concerning compartmentalization in DAVFs involving the dural sinuses; however, in most cases, the entire dural sinus wall is involved. In DAVFs with cortical venous reflux, a transvenous route is effective, with complete early occlusion rates of up to 80% and low complication rates. The combined use of a transarterial route to decrease flow in high-flow shunts may be helpful. Apart from platinum coils, permanent liquid materials (glue and Onyx) have also been used in transvenous embolization. However, caution must be exercised when the dural sinuses are still patent because of an increased risk for pulmonary emboli. In our practice, we occasionally inject glue within the coil meshwork to close the final residual shunt and induce thrombosis.

PEARLS AND PITFALLS

- In benign DAVFs of the dural sinuses, the results of CT and MRI are often negative, and CTA or MRA is necessary for the diagnosis.
- Benign DAVFs have a benign natural history and do not require treatment unless the patient cannot tolerate the symptoms (e.g., bruit).
- Venous drainage of the normal brain must be evaluated with late venous phases on angiography before a transvenous embolization is considered.
- Although the primary goal in treating aggressive DAVFs is to disconnect the shunt from the retrograde leptomeningeal veins of the brain, such precise targeting can hardly be achieved in DAVFs involving large segments of the dural sinus wall and with extensive upstream reflux into the various venous passages. Therefore, in these special circumstances, elimination of venous reflux is best accomplished with venous sacrifice of the abnormal sinus.

Further Reading

de Paula Lucas C, Prandini MN, Spelle L, Piotin M, Mounayer C, Moret J. Parallel transverse-sigmoid sinus harboring dural arteriovenous malformation. How to differentiate the pathological and normal sinus in order to treat and preserve patency and function. Acta Neurochir (Wien) 2010;152(3):523–527

Kirsch M, Liebig T, Kühne D, Henkes H. Endovascular management of dural arteriovenous fistulas of the transverse and sigmoid sinus in 150 patients. Neuroradiology 2009;51(7):477–483

Piske RL, Campos CM, Chaves JB, et al. Dural sinus compartment in dural arteriovenous shunts: a new angioarchitectural feature allowing superselective transvenous dural sinus occlusion treatment. AJNR Am J Neuroradiol 2005;26(7):1715–1722

CASE 27

Case Description

Clinical Presentation

A 59-year-old woman presents with the sudden onset of confusion and disorientation. Her past medical history is negative except for hypertension, treated with a β-blocker. Physical examination reveals no neurologic deficits. MRI and contrast-enhanced MRA are performed, followed by angiography.

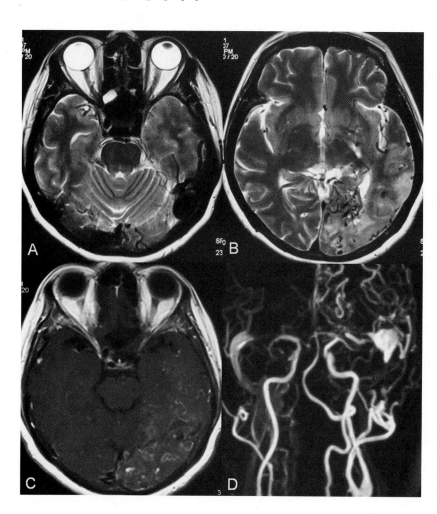

Fig. 27.1 MRI. **(A,B)** T2-weighted and **(C)** post-contrast T1-weighted images reveal venous congestion and multiple flow-void structures along the cortical sulci. **(D)** Contrast-enhanced MRA shows an AV shunt into a dilated venous structure at the left transverse sinus region.

Radiologic Studies

MRI/MRA

MRI showed hypersignal T2/FLAIR changes of edema in the left temporo-occipital lobe with ill-defined, mild contrast enhancement, consistent with venous congestion. Abnormal flow voids were noted along the adjacent cortical sulci of the left temporo-occipital lobe. MRA demonstrated an abnormal arteriovenous shunt into an ectatic venous structure at the left transverse sinus region (**Fig. 27.1**).

160

DSA

Injection of the left internal carotid artery (ICA) showed filling of an ectatic isolated left transverse sinus segment by the left meningohypophyseal trunk and a pseudophlebitic appearance of the cortical veins in the venous phase, suggestive of venous congestion. Small branches of the left occipital artery and meningeal branches of the left vertebral artery (VA) additionally fed the dural arteriovenous fistula (DAVF), which in turn showed evidence of cortical venous reflux. Thrombosis of the left transverse sinus proximal and distal to the lesion created the appearance of an isolated sinus segment ("trapped sinus"). Further reflux of the venous drainage from this sinus pouch into the left vein of Labbé and left occipital cortical veins was observed (**Fig. 27.2**).

Diagnosis

Aggressive DAVF of the left transverse sinus with an isolated "trapped" sinus (Borden type 2)

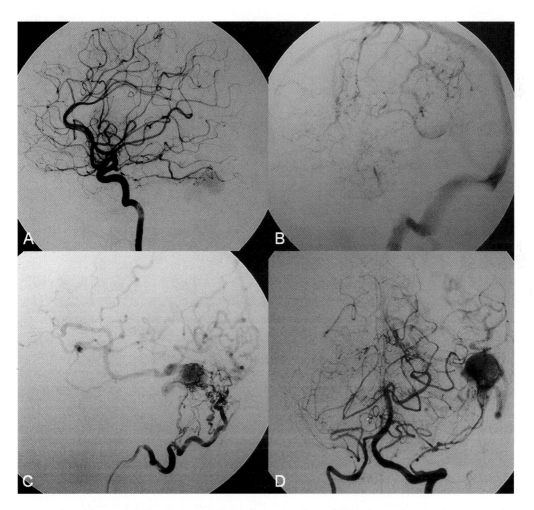

Fig. 27.2 DSA. Left ICA injection (lateral) in **(A)** arterial phase shows faint filling of an ectatic venous pouch at the left transverse sinus region by tentorial branches of the left meningohypophyseal trunk of the left ICA. Stagnation and poor filling of the cortical veins at the left temporo-occipital lobe is noted in **(B)** the late venous phase, indicating venous congestion. Left occipital angiogram in **(C)** lateral view and left vertebral angiogram in **(D)** AP view show tiny arterial feeders from both the occipital artery and left posterior meningeal artery.

Treatment

EQUIPMENT

- Standard 6F access (puncture needle, 6F vascular sheath)
- Standard 6F multipurpose catheter (Envoy; Cordis, Warren, NJ) with continuous flush and a 0.038-in hydrophilic guidewire (Terumo, Somerset, NJ)
- A 0.021-in over-the-wire microcatheter (Prowler Select Plus; Cordis) with a 0.014-in hydrophilic guidewire (Synchro 14; Boston Scientific, Natick MA)
- Contrast material
- Fibered pushable platinum coils (VortX 18; Boston Scientific)
- Coil pusher (Boston Scientific)

DESCRIPTION

Following diagnostic angiography, a 6F multipurpose catheter was advanced into the left internal jugular vein and placed at the left jugular bulb. To create a tract for the microcatheter, the 0.038-in guidewire was gently advanced with rotation under an arterial roadmap via a left VA injection into the thrombosed left sigmoid sinus and isolated left transverse sinus segment. Once the guidewire penetrated the isolated sinus, a blank roadmap was done. The guidewire was then withdrawn, and a microcatheter was quickly introduced over a micro-guidewire along the tract into the isolated sinus. Hand injection of contrast through the microcatheter was performed to confirm the position of the microcatheter. Multiple fibered platinum coils were then mechanically deployed to close the diseased sinus segment from the most proximal end (close to the torcular). Periodic control runs through the left VA were performed, and once closure of the DAVF was obtained, the microcatheter and venous catheter were removed. Final control angiogram of the left common carotid artery demonstrated complete obliteration of the DAVF (**Fig. 27.3**).

Discussion

Background

DAVFs with isolated sinuses are always malignant and classified as Borden type 2. Cortical venous reflux in these cases, associated with thrombosis of the dural sinus proximal and distal to the involved segment, redirects all the flow toward the cortical veins. The clinical presentation is aggressive, including intracranial hemorrhage and nonhemorrhagic neurologic symptoms in up to 40% of all cases. The transverse-sigmoid sinus is the most common location for a "trapped" sinus. In these cases, the involved sinus segment is never used for drainage of the normal brain and can therefore be occluded during treatment.

Noninvasive Imaging Workup

CT/CTA

- Intraparenchymal hemorrhage and subcortical calcification may be seen on unenhanced CT scans. Venous congestion may be seen as hypodensity on CT; however, it is better demonstrated by FLAIR sequences on MRI. Contrast-enhanced CT is required to show the dilated vessels along the cortical sulci.
- Both static and dynamic CTA can demonstrate an ectatic isolated sinus.

MRI/MRA

- Abnormal dilated vessels along the cortical sulci are best seen on T2-weighted images and post-gadolinium T1-weighted images.

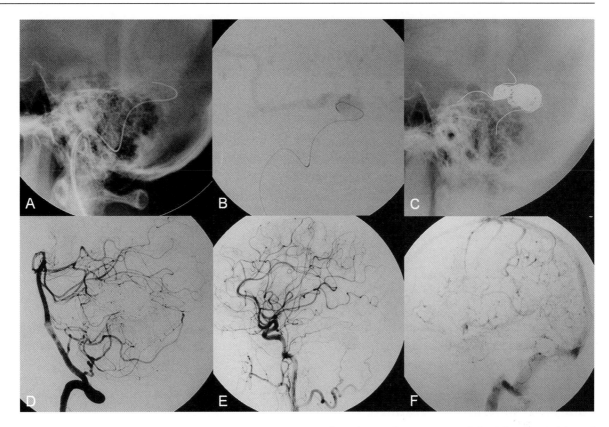

Fig. 27.3 (A) Plain radiography demonstrating the location of the guiding catheter and the 0.038-in guidewire. **(B)** Hand injection through the microcatheter confirms the position of the microcatheter within the isolated sinus. **(C)** Plain radiography after deployment of the fibered platinum coils and control angiograms of the left VA in **(D)** lateral view and of the left common carotid artery in lateral view in **(E)** late arterial and **(F)** late venous phases demonstrate complete closure of the fistula, with a decrease of the venous congestion at the left temporo-occipital lobe.

- Venous congestion and/or infarction are seen as hyperintensity on T2-weighted images and FLAIR. Focal enhancement of these areas may be a sign of chronic venous ischemia.
- Both static and dynamic MRA can demonstrate an ectatic isolated sinus.

Invasive Imaging Workup

- Angiography is always required in the pre-treatment evaluation of DAVFs, along with a careful analysis of how the normal brain drains and how the fistula is fed.

Treatment Options

SURGICAL TREATMENT

- If endovascular options alone fail to reach the fistulous site, a burr hole may facilitate the insertion of a microcatheter, followed by the deposition of embolic material in the isolated venous pouch.
- Other surgical options that have been reported range from simple disconnection of the cortical venous reflux to sinus packing and resection of the diseased sinus segment.
- Preoperative proximal embolization with particles is recommended to decrease surgical blood loss.

ENDOVASCULAR TREATMENT

- In cases with an isolated venous pouch, either transarterial embolization with liquid embolic agents or transvenous embolization with coils and/or liquid embolic agents may be used to occlude the diseased sinus segment. The choice depends on the angioarchitecture. If there is a large arterial feeder, the transarterial route is preferred. If not, a transvenous approach should be attempted. In our experience, it has been possible to reach the isolated segment through the thrombosed dural sinus in either antegrade or retrograde fashion in 70 to 80% of cases.
- Fibered coils are preferred because of their thrombogenicity; they may be used in conjunction with bare platinum coils.
- During a transvenous approach, care must be taken to occlude the segment that is most distal to the entry zone to avoid persistence of the DAVF.
- Periprocedural heparin is recommended if the procedure is anticipated to take longer than 30 minutes.

Possible Complications

- The risk for dural laceration and subdural or epidural hematoma is low, especially if the guidewire is advanced gently with a rotating movement. Care should be taken to remain inside the expected dural sinus and to avoid entering cortical veins.

Published Literature on Treatment Options

Since the first report of embolization of a DAVF with an isolated transverse-sigmoid sinus through a blind transvenous approach by Gobin et al in 1993, limited case series and case reports regarding this technique have been published. In our experience, the complication rate has been lower than 5%, the success rate between 70 and 80%, and the subsequent cure rate ~80 to 90%. These figures are in agreement with the opinion of most authors, who conclude that the "blind" transvenous approach is a safe and feasible alternative to surgery for the treatment of DAVFs with isolated dural sinuses.

PEARLS AND PITFALLS_____

- A DAVF with an isolated sinus is always aggressive and therefore must be treated and cured as soon as possible.
- The isolated sinus segment never functions as normal drainage of the brain and can be sacrificed during treatment.
- Endovascular treatment is the preferred method, and the choice of a transarterial versus a transvenous approach depends on the angioarchitecture of the DAVF.

Further Reading

Gobin YP, Houdart E, Rogopoulos A, Casasco A, Bailly AL, Merland JJ. Percutaneous transvenous embolization through the thrombosed sinus in transverse sinus dural fistula. AJNR Am J Neuroradiol 1993;14(5):1102–1105

Komiyama M, Ishiguro T, Matsusaka Y, Yasui T, Nishio A. Transfemoral, transvenous embolisation of dural arteriovenous fistula involving the isolated transverse-sigmoid sinus from the contralateral side. Acta Neurochir (Wien) 2002;144(10):1041–1046, discussion 1046

Naito I, Iwai T, Shimaguchi H, et al. Percutaneous transvenous embolisation through the occluded sinus for transverse-sigmoid dural arteriovenous fistulas with sinus occlusion. Neuroradiology 2001;43(8):672–676

Sugiu K, Tokunaga K, Nishida A, et al. Triple-catheter technique in the transvenous coil embolization of an isolated sinus dural arteriovenous fistula. Neurosurgery 2007; 61(3, Suppl)81–85, discussion 85

Wong GK, Poon WS, Yu SC, Zhu CX. Transvenous embolization for dural transverse sinus fistulas with occluded sigmoid sinus. Acta Neurochir (Wien) 2007;149(9):929–935, discussion 935–936

CASE 28

Case Description

Clinical Presentation

A 71-year-old woman presents with a history of left-sided pulsatile tinnitus for 8 months. Her history is otherwise unremarkable. A pulsatile bruit is detected overlying the left posterior auricular region on physical examination. MRI and 3D TOF MRA are performed, followed by angiography.

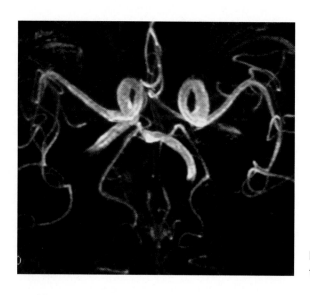

Fig. 28.1 3D TOF MRA suggests abnormal vessels along the left petrous angle.

Radiologic Studies

MRI/MRA

Results of detailed MRI of the internal carotid arteries (ICAs) were normal (not shown). No other causes of pulsatile tinnitus, such as high jugular bulbs, aberrant course of the ICAs, or a glomus tumor, were identified. The 3D TOF MRA study demonstrated abnormal vessels along the left petrous margin (**Fig. 28.1**).

DSA

Bilateral injections of the external carotid arteries (ECAs) showed an arteriovenous fistula surrounding the left jugular bulb, draining into the left condylar confluence, and fed mainly by the neuromeningeal branches of the ascending pharyngeal arteries. Feeding arteries through the clival branches of the left ICA and both vertebral arteries (VAs) were also noted. The right ICA was normal. Venous drainage was directed into the left internal jugular vein and vertebral venous plexus (**Fig. 28.2**). The natural history of the disease and risks for treatment were discussed with the patient, and she preferred to be treated because of the insomnia caused by the pulsatile tinnitus.

Diagnosis

Benign dural arteriovenous fistula (DAVF) of the condylar confluence (Borden type 1)

166

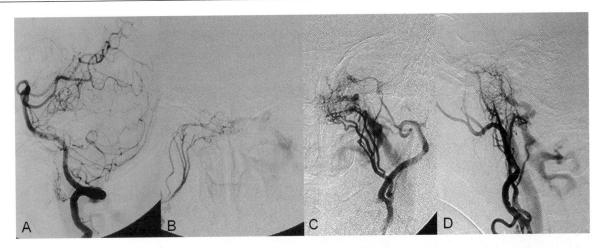

Fig. 28.2 DSA. Left vertebral angiogram in **(A)** lateral view, right ascending pharyngeal angiogram in **(B)** AP view, and left ascending pharyngeal angiogram in **(C)** AP and **(D)** lateral views demonstrate an AVF surrounding the left jugular bulb, draining into the left condylar confluence, and supplied by bilateral neuromeningeal branches of the ascending pharyngeal arteries. There is venous drainage into the internal jugular vein and vertebral venous plexus.

Treatment

EQUIPMENT

- Arterial 5F and venous 6F access (puncture needles, 5F and 6F vascular sheaths)
- Berenstein 5F catheter with continuous flush (Boston Scientific, Natick, MA)
- Standard 6F multipurpose catheter (Guider Soft Tip; Boston Scientific) with continuous flush and a 0.035-in hydrophilic guidewire (Terumo, Somerset, NJ)
- A 0.021-in over-the-wire microcatheter (Prowler Select Plus; Cordis, Warren, NJ) with a 0.014-in hydrophilic guidewire (Synchro14; Boston Scientific)
- Contrast material
- Fibered pushable platinum coils (VortX; Boston Scientific)
- Coil pusher (Boston Scientific)

DESCRIPTION

Following diagnostic angiography, a 6F multipurpose catheter was advanced into the left internal jugular vein and placed at the left jugular bulb (**Fig. 28.3**). A microcatheter was introduced over a guidewire into the left posterior condylar vein under a contralateral right ECA arterial roadmap (performed via the 5F arterial Berenstein catheter). Three fibered platinum coils were mechanically deployed, closing the left posterior condylar vein. Control runs through the contralateral right common carotid artery (CCA) showed closure of the DAVF. The microcatheter and venous catheter were removed, and control angiograms of the left CCA demonstrated complete obliteration of the DAVF.

Discussion

Background

DAVFs surrounding the jugular bulb have been classified differently by various authors in the literature. The most commonly used classification is based on the vein in which the DAVF occurs; they can therefore be separated into anterior condylar (hypoglossal), posterior condylar, and marginal sinus DAVFs. Separation of these three entities by angiography and cross-sectional imaging is often

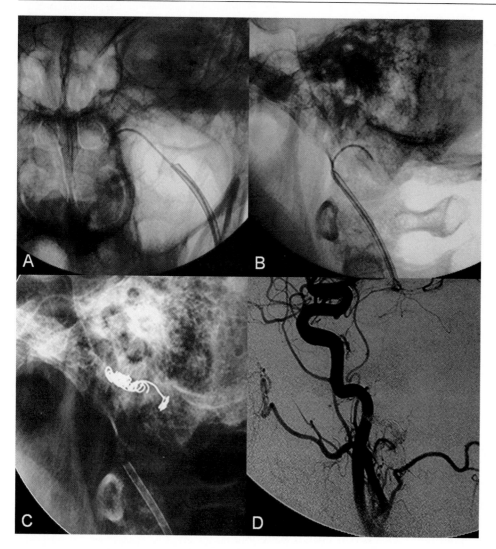

Fig. 28.3 Plain radiography in **(A)** AP and **(B)** lateral views demonstrating the location of the guiding catheter and guidewire. **(C)** Plain radiography in lateral view and **(D)** left CCA angiogram after embolization show the coil mesh and complete obliteration of the fistula.

difficult and may be unnecessary. They all have similar characteristics. Patients often present with symptoms of pulsatile tinnitus; arterial feeders consist of branches from the ascending pharyngeal artery, dural branches of the VA, and occasionally the occipital artery; and drainage is typically through the internal jugular vein or vertebral plexus. These DAVFs are rarely aggressive, and cortical venous reflux is present only if thrombosis of the venous outlet occurs, with intracranial rerouting of the venous drainage. Because they are often Borden type 1 or "benign" DAVFs, treatment may not be indicated, except when patients are unable to tolerate the tinnitus. Because of the high risk of transarterial embolization through the neuromeningeal trunk of the ascending pharyngeal artery, a transvenous route is preferred. The involved venous segment does not have a major role in drainage of the normal brain and therefore can be occluded safely during treatment.

Noninvasive Imaging Workup

PHYSICAL EXAMINATION

- A slight bruit may be present at the posterior auricular region.

CT/MRI

- The results of high-resolution CT and MRI to investigate pulsatile tinnitus are often negative.
- Both are used mainly to exclude other causes of pulsatile tinnitus; the most common of these are glomus tumor, aberrant ICA, and high jugular bulb.
- In some cases, dilated condylar veins may resemble a tumor at the hypoglossal canal or jugular foramen on post-contrast studies.

CTA/MRA

- The findings on static CTA and MRA may be subtle, with only mildly dilated abnormal vessels surrounding the jugular region.
- Early shunting into the jugular bulb and internal jugular vein can be identified with dynamic CTA and MRA.
- If cortical venous reflux does occur, abnormal vessels may be seen within the posterior fossa and/or upper cervical cord.

Invasive Imaging Workup

- As for other DAVFs, all potential feeders must be evaluated—in particular, the ascending pharyngeal arteries and VAs for DAVFs in this location.

Differential Diagnosis

- Major considerations are other causes of pulsatile tinnitus, including glomus tumor, aberrant ICA, and high jugular bulb.

Treatment Options

CONSERVATIVE OR MEDICAL MANAGEMENT

- If the DAVF is a Borden type 1, without any cortical venous reflux, then treatment may not be required.
- Spontaneous thrombosis can occur and result in closure of the fistula.
- In rare instances, thrombosis of a "benign" venous drainage route may cause rerouting of the drainage toward the cortical veins; therefore, follow-up dynamic imaging is necessary in these patients, especially if symptoms change.
- Disappearance of a bruit may point to either spontaneous occlusion or intracranial rerouting and should therefore prompt further angiographic workup.

ENDOVASCULAR TREATMENT

- Transvenous embolization is the first treatment option in DAVFs of the condylar confluence, and the shunt zone can easily be reached through the internal jugular vein and jugular bulb.

- Transarterial embolization with permanent liquid materials is reserved for cases without trans-venous access.

SURGICAL TREATMENT

- Surgical disconnection of the cortical/spinal venous reflux may be used when embolization fails to occlude the fistula.

Possible Complications

- In addition to standard angiographic complications at both the arterial and venous sites, com-pression of the hypoglossal nerve by the embolic material (often coils) can occur, which may be avoided by using softer coils or loose packing with thrombogenic fibered coils.

Published Literature on Treatment Options

Only a few case reports and small case series have documented the success of transvenous emboli-zation of DAVFs within this region because of their rarity and "benign" clinical course, which usu-ally does not require treatment. The major arterial feeder is often the ascending pharyngeal artery, and transarterial embolization of its neuromeningeal branch is associated with a high risk for lower cranial nerve palsy and stroke resulting from the anastomosis of this artery to both the ICA and VA. Complete cure is difficult to obtain with transarterial embolization alone and can be more eas-ily achieved with transvenous embolization. Surgical obliteration of the DAVF through a far-lateral transcondylar approach has been reported; however, surgery is often reserved for disconnection of cortical/spinal venous reflux in cases in which embolization has failed.

PEARLS AND PITFALLS _____

- DAVFs of the condylar confluence are often benign (Borden type 1) and commonly present with pulsatile tinnitus.
- Treatment is rarely indicated for benign DAVFs, and spontaneous thrombosis with subsequent closure of the fistula can occur in these patients; however, follow-up dynamic imaging is neces-sary to confirm the complete occlusion of the DAVF.
- The ascending pharyngeal artery is usually the main arterial feeder, so that the risk for lower cranial nerve palsy and stroke is high if transarterial embolization is performed.
- Transvenous embolization has a low risk for complications and high cure rates and therefore should be considered first for the treatment of DAVFs within this region.

Further Reading

Ernst R, Bulas R, Tomsick T, van Loveren H, Aziz KA. Three cases of dural arteriovenous fistula of the anterior condylar vein within the hypoglossal canal. AJNR Am J Neuroradiol 1999;20(10):2016–2020

Kiyosue H, Okahara M, Sagara Y, et al. Dural arteriovenous fistula involving the posterior condylar canal. AJNR Am J Neuroradiol 2007;28(8):1599–1601

Liu JK, Mahaney K, Barnwell SL, McMenomey SO, Delashaw JB Jr. Dural arteriovenous fistula of the anterior condylar confluence and hypoglossal canal mimicking a jugular foramen tumor. J Neurosurg 2008;109(2):335–340

Manabe S, Satoh K, Matsubara S, Satomi J, Hanaoka M, Nagahiro S. Characteristics, diagnosis and treatment of hypoglossal canal dural arteriovenous fistula: report of nine cases. Neuroradiology 2008;50(8):715–7211

McDougall CG, Halbach VV, Dowd CF, Higashida RT, Larsen DW, Hieshima GB. Dural arteriovenous fistulas of the marginal sinus. AJNR Am J Neuroradiol 1997;18(8):1565–1572

Satomi J, van Dijk JMC, Terbrugge KG, Willinsky RA, Wallace MC. Benign cranial dural arteriovenous fistulas: outcome of conservative management based on the natural history of the lesion. J Neurosurg 2002;97(4):767–770

CASE 29

Case Description

Clinical Presentation

A 64-year-old woman presents with a 6-month history of severe frontal headaches, blurred vision, and diplopia. She has an underlying history of diabetes mellitus, hypertension, and dyslipidemia (treated with glibenclamide, propranolol, enalapril, and simvastatin). Physical examination reveals mild chemosis and proptosis with ophthalmoplegia in the right eye. MRI of the orbits and 3D TOF MRA are performed, followed by angiography.

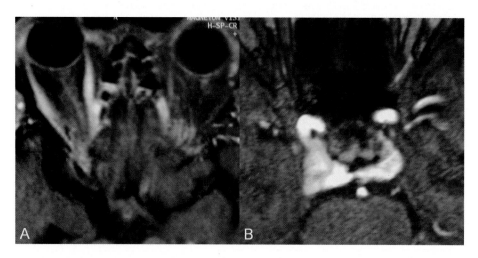

Fig. 29.1 **(A)** MRI T1-weighted image after gadolinium enhancement of the orbits. **(B)** 3D TOF MRA source image at the level of the cavernous sinuses.

Radiologic Studies

MRI/MRA

MRI of the orbits (**Fig. 29.1**) showed right exophthalmos with diffuse enlargement and diffuse homogeneous enhancement of the extraocular muscles. Bulging of the right cavernous sinus, seen on both T2 and 3D TOF MRA, was also observed. No definite dilated vessels were seen along the cortical sulci, and the signal intensity of the brain parenchyma was normal on the remaining sequences.

DSA

Bilateral injections of the internal carotid arteries (ICAs) showed an arteriovenous fistula at the posterior aspect of the right cavernous sinus, fed by meningohypophyseal branches from both ICAs. Supply from the right artery of the foramen rotundum from the distal internal maxillary artery was also noted. There was retrograde venous drainage via the right sphenoparietal sinus, and further drainage through the deep sylvian vein into the basal vein of Rosenthal and superficial sylvian vein into the frontal cortical veins (**Fig. 29.2**).

Diagnosis

Aggressive dural arteriovenous fistula (DAVF) of the right cavernous sinus (Borden type 2)

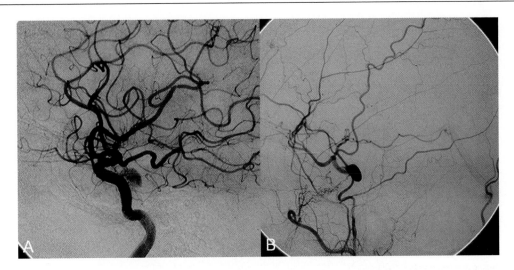

Fig. 29.2 DSA. **(A)** Right ICA angiogram in lateral view and **(B)** right ECA angiogram in lateral view show early filling of the posterior aspect of the right cavernous sinus, supplied by branches of the meningohypophyseal trunk of the right ICA and the right artery of the foramen rotundum from the distal internal maxillary artery. Cortical venous reflux into the frontal cortical veins and basal vein of Rosenthal through the superficial and deep sylvian veins is noted.

Treatment

EQUIPMENT

- Combined transvenous (6F) and transarterial (5F) access (puncture needles, 6F and 5F vascular sheaths)
- Standard 5F Berenstein catheter (Boston Scientific, Natick, MA) and 6F multipurpose catheter (Guider Soft Tip; Boston Scientific) with continuous flushes and a 0.038-in hydrophilic guidewire (Terumo, Somerset, NJ)
- A 0.021-in over-the-wire microcatheter (Prowler Select Plus; Cordis, Warren, NJ) with a 0.014-in hydrophilic guidewire (Synchro 14; Boston Scientific)
- Contrast material
- Pushable fibered platinum coils (VortX; Boston Scientific)
- Coil pusher (Boston Scientific)

DESCRIPTION

A 6F multipurpose catheter was advanced into the right internal jugular vein. The 0.0038-in guidewire was gently advanced with rotation under an arterial roadmap into the thrombosed right inferior petrosal vein. The catheter was then gently advanced into the proximal inferior petrosal vein for increased stability. The guidewire was further advanced superiorly toward the right cavernous sinus, creating a tract for the microcatheter. (Several channels leading to different compartments of the cavernous sinus are usually encountered, and multiple attempts may be necessary to find the correct compartment. Once the guidewire penetrates the involved cavernous sinus compartment, a blank roadmap is done. The guidewire is then withdrawn, and a microcatheter is quickly introduced over a micro-guidewire along the tract into the cavernous sinus compartment.) The position of the microcatheter was confirmed with hand injection of contrast. Multiple fibered platinum coils were then mechanically deployed, initially at the connection to the sphenoparietal sinus and deep sylvian vein to close the cortical venous reflux, then slowly backward toward the entry zone of the microcatheter. Periodic control runs through the right external carotid artery (ECA) were performed. After complete closure of the DAVF, the microcatheter and venous catheter were removed. A final control right ECA angiogram confirmed complete obliteration of the DAVF (**Fig. 29.3**).

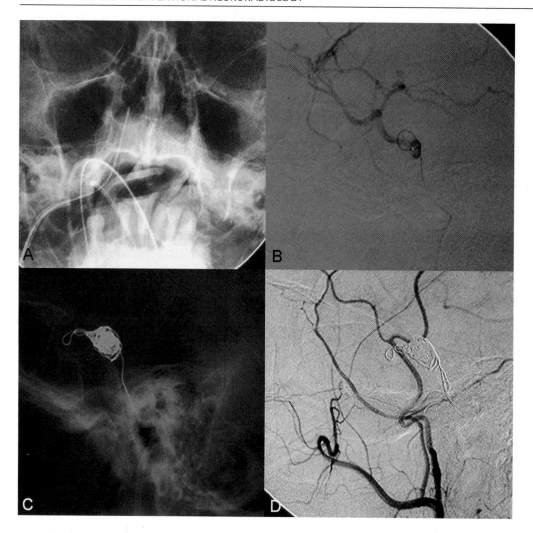

Fig. 29.3 (A) Plain radiography in AP view reveals the location of the guiding catheter and guidewire. **(B)** Microcatheter injection verifies the position within the correct compartment of the cavernous sinus. **(C)** Plain radiography in lateral view and **(D)** right ECA angiogram after embolization demonstrate the coil mesh and confirm complete obliteration of the DAVF.

Discussion

Background

DAVFs of the cavernous sinus are also known as an indirect type of carotid-cavernous fistulae. Their arterial supply can be from the meningeal branches of the ECA, ICA, or both. The presenting symptoms depend on the pattern of venous drainage. Drainage anteriorly into the superior and inferior ophthalmic veins most commonly causes ocular symptoms of chemosis, proptosis, and ophthalmoplegia. Posterior drainage through the inferior petrosal vein may cause pulsatile tinnitus, and venous infarctions or hemorrhage may rarely result from cortical venous reflux through the sphenoparietal sinus into the superficial and deep sylvian veins and the superior petrosal vein into the posterior fossa veins. Although the ocular symptoms are considered to be "benign," long-standing increased intraocular pressure may lead to secondary glaucoma and subsequent loss of vision. Cavernous sinus DAVFs of the benign type are usually managed conservatively. Endovascular treatment is the preferred option for malignant lesions with cortical venous reflux. Because the cavernous sinus usually does not have any major role in drainage of the brain in a normal adult, transarterial or transvenous obliteration of the affected portion of the sinus can be performed for cure.

Noninvasive Imaging Workup

PHYSICAL EXAMINATION

- Chemosis, proptosis, and ophthalmoplegia are usually present.
- A bruit is rarely encountered; when present, it classically indicates a high-flow shunt, and if the patient has a history of trauma, it raises suspicion for a direct (traumatic) carotid-cavernous fistula, as discussed in Case 42.

CT/MRI

- Bulging of the cavernous sinus with dilatation of the superior ophthalmic vein is best visualized as flow voids on T2-weighted images and on contrast-enhanced CT scans.
- Asymmetric dilatation of the sphenoparietal sinus, just inferior to the temporal pole, may suggest cortical venous reflux; however, angiography is still the gold standard for the evaluation of cortical venous reflux.
- The exact site of the lesion cannot be evaluated with CT and MRI because blood may shunt from side to side through intercavernous anastomoses.

CTA/MRA

- Static CTA and MRA are of limited value in the evaluation of cavernous sinus DAVFs and are used only to confirm the diagnosis.
- Dynamic CTA and MRA may be able to evaluate the location of the lesion and detect cortical venous reflux.

Invasive Imaging Workup

- The major venous drainage is directed toward four compartments: anteriorly, connecting to the superior and inferior ophthalmic veins; laterally, to the sphenoparietal sinus and medial temporal vein; posteriorly, connecting to the superior and inferior petrosal veins; and medially, toward the other side via intercavernous anastomoses.

Differential Diagnosis

- Orbital lesions, such as thyroid ophthalmopathy and orbital pseudotumor, can present with exophthalmos; however, they are not associated with bulging of the cavernous sinus or dilatation of the superior ophthalmic vein.
- Thrombosis of the cavernous sinus typically appears as a filling defect on contrast-enhanced studies with the clot shown as a high T1 signal within the cavernous sinus.
- Direct carotid-cavernous fistulae (see Cases 42 and 43) are direct high-flow shunts between the ICA and cavernous sinus and are usually traumatic in origin. A loud bruit overlying both the orbit and the posterior auricular region suggests this diagnosis.

Treatment Options

CONSERVATIVE OR MEDICAL MANAGEMENT

- Spontaneous thrombosis with subsequent closure occurs in ~15 to 50% of DAVFs; therefore, benign (Borden type 1) cavernous sinus DAVFs without increased ocular pressure or with medically manageable increased ocular pressure (glaucoma) may very well be managed conservatively.
- Dynamic imaging is indicated for follow-up and to document complete closure in these cases because thrombosis of the benign venous drainage routes may lead to cortical or spinal venous reflux in ~3 to 4%.

- External ocular compression of the angular vein with or without external carotid compression has been reported to facilitate spontaneous thrombosis; however, this can be used only in cases with drainage through the superior ophthalmic vein without cortical venous reflux. This must be documented by DSA while ocular compression is applied. The maneuver further increases the intraocular pressure, so it should be employed with caution in patients who present with secondary glaucoma.

SURGICAL TREATMENT

- The sphenoparietal sinus may be surgically disconnected to manage supratentorial cortical venous reflux.
- Surgical packing of the cavernous sinus has been reported in cases in which all other options have failed.

ENDOVASCULAR TREATMENT

- If there is good arterial access through a large arterial feeder, transarterial embolization with permanent liquid material, aiming to partially fill the cavernous sinus, is our first choice because of the shorter procedure time. Caution must be exercised to avoid the orbital and cavernous anastomoses between the ECA and ICA within this region. Transvenous embolization is preferred if multiple small feeders are present within the wall of the cavernous sinuses, with a low likelihood of complete occlusion via the arterial route.
- Various transvenous routes have been reported. Our general practice is to choose (1) a visualized route, (2) the straightest/shortest route, and (3) a route on the same side as the lesion. The inferior petrosal venous approach, even if not visualized, is generally the easiest. The second choice is via the superior ophthalmic vein from the angular and facial vein through the external jugular vein.
- DAVFs involving the cavernous sinuses bilaterally are relatively common. They are usually connected through intercavernous anastomoses and can be treated from a unilateral transvenous approach.
- Both direct puncture of the cavernous sinus through the orbit and open surgery have been reported but should be carried out only in experienced hands and only if the other options fail.
- Exophthalmos and ophthalmoplegia may temporarily worsen after complete treatment because of progressive thrombosis of the ophthalmic veins; they can be managed with steroids in most cases, and anticoagulation treatment is rarely required.

Possible Complications

- Temporary worsening of exophthalmos and ophthalmoplegia can usually be managed with steroids.

Published Literature on Treatment Options

In the large series of 141 patients who had cavernous sinus DAVFs treated with transvenous embolization reported by Kirsch et al in 2006, the initial cure rate was 81%, with long-term follow-up cure rates of up to 94.5%. The overall complication rate (including asymptomatic emboli and venous perforation) was ~8%, without any permanent neurologic sequelae. These results are similar to those in previously reported smaller series and our own experience, indicating that the transvenous route is an effective and relatively safe treatment modality. Transarterial embolization for cavernous sinus DAVFs is often made challenging by the presence of numerous tiny arterial feeders from both the ICA and ECA. Because complete occlusion of the involved cavernous sinus compartment is required for cure, proximal occlusion of the arterial feeder is insufficient, and particle embolization is no longer acceptable. It also carries a higher risk for complications because of the anastomoses between the ECA and ICA in this territory.

PEARLS AND PITFALLS

- CT/MRI and static CTA/MRA are *not* sufficient for an exact evaluation of the side of the cavernous DAVF and the presence of cortical venous reflux.
- Transvenous embolization for cavernous sinus DAVFs is safer and more effective than transarterial embolization.
- The inferior petrosal vein, whether or not visualized, is the preferred access route. Placement of the guiding catheter into the proximal inferior petrosal vein helps to improve the stability of the microcatheter and can be done safely with gentle rotation.

Further Reading

Agid R, Willinsky RA, Haw C, Souza MP, Vanek IJ, terBrugge KG. Targeted compartmental embolization of cavernous sinus dural arteriovenous fistulae using transfemoral medial and lateral facial vein approaches. Neuroradiology 2004;46(2):156–160

Benndorf G, Bender A, Lehmann R, Lanksch W. Transvenous occlusion of dural cavernous sinus fistulas through the thrombosed inferior petrosal sinus: report of four cases and review of the literature. Surg Neurol 2000;54(1):42–54

Kim DJ, Kim DI, Suh SH, et al. Results of transvenous embolization of cavernous dural arteriovenous fistula: a single-center experience with emphasis on complications and management. AJNR Am J Neuroradiol 2006;27(10):2078–2082

Kirsch M, Henkes H, Liebig T, et al. Endovascular management of dural carotid-cavernous sinus fistulas in 141 patients. Neuroradiology 2006;48(7):486–490

Preechawat P, Narmkerd P, Jiarakongmun P, Poonyathalang A, Pongpech SM. Dural carotid cavernous sinus fistula: ocular characteristics, endovascular management and clinical outcome. J Med Assoc Thai 2008;91(6):852–858

White JB, Layton KF, Evans AJ, et al. Transorbital puncture for the treatment of cavernous sinus dural arteriovenous fistulas. AJNR Am J Neuroradiol 2007;28(7):1415–1417

CASE 30

Case Description

Clinical Presentation

A 54-year-old man with an underlying history of diabetes mellitus and hypertension, both managed with medication, presents with a 6-month history of behavioral change and memory loss. Physical examination shows cognitive deficits without any motor or sensory impairment. MRI and angiography are performed.

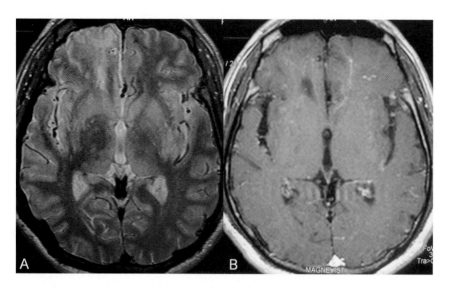

Fig. 30.1 MRI. **(A)** T2-weighted image and **(B)** post-gadolinium T1-weighted image.

Radiologic Studies

MRI

The MRI study showed hyperintense T2 signal changes in the right frontal lobe with minimal enhancement in both frontal lobes following the administration of gadolinium. Small tubular flow voids were also observed along the cortical surface of both frontal regions and the left temporo-occipital region. The remainder of the brain parenchyma was normal (**Fig. 30.1**).

DSA

The study showed multiple dural arteriovenous fistulae (DAVFs) along the anterior and middle segments of the superior sagittal sinus and at the left transverse sinus. These were associated with thrombosis of the anterior superior sagittal sinus and left transverse sinus. The anterior superior sagittal sinus DAVF received supply from the anterior branches of the middle meningeal arteries (MMAs) bilaterally and the right anterior falcine artery from the right ophthalmic artery, with retrograde reflux into the frontal cortical veins bilaterally. There was supply from the MMAs bilaterally and indirectly from the superficial temporal arteries bilaterally to the middle superior sagittal sinus DAVF, which drained into the parasagittal cortical veins. Supply to the left transverse sinus DAVF was via branches of the left MMA, left occipital artery, and left posterior meningeal artery from the left vertebral artery, with reflux of the venous drainage into the left vein of uncus and further drainage into the left basal vein of Rosenthal. There was a delayed venous phase with stagnation of contrast at the level of the frontal lobes on both internal carotid artery (ICA) injections **(Fig. 30.2)**.

Diagnosis

Multiple aggressive DAVFs at the level of the superior sagittal sinus and left transverse sinus (Borden type 2)

Treatment

EQUIPMENT

- Standard 5F access (puncture needle, 5F vascular sheath)
- Standard 5F multipurpose catheter (Guider Soft Tip; Boston Scientific, Natick, MA) with continuous flush and a 0.035-in hydrophilic guidewire (Terumo, Somerset, NJ)

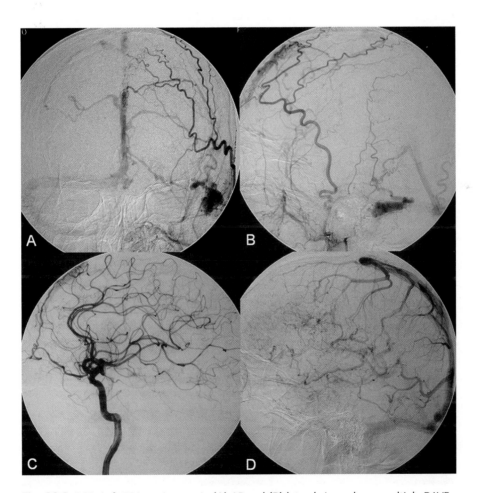

Fig. 30.2 DSA. Left ECA angiogram in **(A)** AP and **(B)** lateral views shows multiple DAVFs. **(C)** Right ICA angiogram, lateral view in arterial phase, reveals additional supply to the anterior superior sagittal sinus DAVF from the anterior falcine artery. Contrast stagnation with delayed filling of the frontal cortical veins is seen in **(D)** the late venous phase with associated thrombosis of the anterior superior sagittal sinus.

- A 0.015-in over-the-wire microcatheter (Prowler 10; Cordis, Warren, NJ) with a 0.010-in hydrophilic guidewire (Agility 10; Cordis)
- A 10% glucose solution
- Histoacryl/Lipiodol (1 mL/2 mL)
- Contrast material

DESCRIPTION

We decided to embolize the anterior superior sagittal sinus DAVF first because of the evidence of venous congestion within the frontal lobes. A 5F multipurpose catheter was advanced into left internal maxillary artery, after which an over-the-wire microcatheter was introduced over a micro-guidewire into the anterior branch of the left MMA and placed as close to the shunt zone as possible. A control run via hand injection through the microcatheter verified the position, and a glucose solution was used to flush the microcatheter. Then we injected a mixture of 50% glue in an attempt to fill the venous segment. The procedure was repeated for the DAVF at the left transverse sinus through the petrosquamous branch of the left MMA, with glue filling the venous pouch. The 5F multipurpose catheter was next moved to the right internal maxillary artery, and the middle superior sagittal sinus DAVF was embolized with a mixture of 50% glue through the anterior branch of the right MMA. The glue partially filled the middle superior sagittal sinus venous segment, and the final control angiogram of the right external carotid artery (ECA) still showed minimal shunting, which underwent progressive thrombosis and was completely obliterated on the 2-month follow-up angiogram (**Fig. 30.3**).

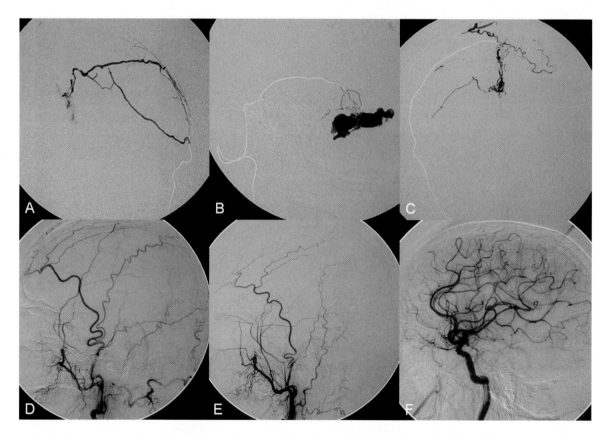

Fig. 30.3 Final glue casts within the anterior branch of the left MMA. **(A)** AP view, petrosquamous branch of the left MMA; **(B)** lateral view and anterior branch of the right MMA; **(C)** AP view. There was partial filling with glue in both the **(A)** anterior and **(C)** middle superior sagittal sinus venous segments. **(C)** Note the retrograde filling into superficial temporal artery feeders bilaterally. Follow-up angiograms at 2 months of the **(D)** right ECA, **(E)** left ECA, and **(F)** right ICA. Angiograms in lateral view demonstrate complete closure of the multiple fistulae.

Discussion

Background

Multiple DAVFs are rare, with an incidence reported in previous literature ranging from 7 to 10%. As reported by Geibprasert et al, they are usually seen in regions adjacent to the dorsal epidural group of dural AV shunts, which includes mainly the superior sagittal sinus, torcular, and transverse sinuses. Although the etiology of DAVFs is still unknown, this observation may suggest a role of venous hypertension and/or venous thrombosis in the formation of such DAVFs. In our experience, the rate of hemorrhagic presentation in patients with multiple DAVFs has been three times higher than the rate of hemorrhagic presentation in patients with a single DAVF. This is likely a consequence of the higher rate of cortical venous reflux, which was present in more than 80% of the patients with multiple DAVFs in the report of van Dijk et al.

Noninvasive Imaging Workup

CT/MRI

- When DAVFs without cortical venous reflux are located at the superior sagittal sinus or the transverse and sigmoid sinuses, CT and MRI often yield false-negative results.
- Structural imaging is usually not sufficient to diagnose multiple dural AV shunts.

CTA/MRA

- Early filling of the involved sinus and cortical venous reflux can both be seen CTA and MRA; however, angiography is required for a detailed evaluation of the arterial feeders and possible endovascular routes, and for visualization of the multiple shunting zones.

Invasive Imaging Workup

- The rather high incidence of multiple DAVFs and their considerably worse prognosis is another reason why the evaluation of these lesions always requires full six-vessel angiography. The reporting physician should be aware of the possibility of multiple fistulae and specifically search for them.

Treatment Options

SURGICAL TREATMENT

- Because it is rare for two shunts to be disconnected via the same approach, multiple shunts are a clear indication for endovascular treatments. The surgical options do not differ from those presented in previous cases.
- Preoperative proximal embolization with particles can decrease surgical blood loss.

ENDOVASCULAR TREATMENT

- For the endovascular treatment of multiple DAVFs, the same rules described in previous cases apply.
- Classically, the shunt with the highest flow is treated first.
- All shunts should be treated in one session to avoid hemodynamic changes in one compartment, which may increase the risk for hemorrhage in another compartment.
- The treatment of all shunts is mandatory if the outflow routes of all shunts are the same and treatment of the first shunt has occluded the ouflow of the shunts not yet treated.

Possible Complications

- The hemodynamic alterations that result from embolizing one shunt may increase the risk for changing the outflow pattern of a second shunt. Therefore, the treatment of all shunts with cortical venous reflux in the same session is recommended.
- If both malignant and benign shunts are present, the malignant ones must be treated, whereas the benign ones may be followed conservatively.

Published Literature on Treatment Options

As for all DAVFs, curative treatment is indicated if cortical venous reflux (Borden types 2 and 3) is present. In patients who have multiple DAVFs, the ones with cortical venous reflux should be treated first; the benign lesions without cortical venous reflux can be followed closely with imaging studies. The choice of endovascular approach depends on the angioarchitecture, and combined treatment modalities may be necessary to cure multiple aggressive DAVFs.

PEARLS AND PITFALLS _____

- Multiple DAVFs are rare but occur in ~8% of patients with DAVFs. They tend to be located along the superior sagittal and transverse dural sinuses.
- They are associated with a higher risk for cortical venous reflux and therefore a higher risk for hemorrhage and neurologic deficits.
- The lesions with cortical venous reflux must be treated first; lesions without cortical venous reflux may be followed closely with imaging studies.

Further Reading

Barnwell SL, Halbach VV, Dowd CF, Higashida RT, Hieshima GB, Wilson CB. Multiple dural arteriovenous fistulas of the cranium and spine. AJNR Am J Neuroradiol 1991;12(3):441–445

Geibprasert S, Pereira V, Krings T, et al. Dural arteriovenous shunts: a new classification of craniospinal epidural venous anatomical bases and clinical correlations. Stroke 2008;39(10):2783–2794

van Dijk JM, TerBrugge KG, Willinsky RA, Wallace MC. Multiplicity of dural arteriovenous fistulas. J Neurosurg 2002;96(1):76–78

CASE 31

Case Description

Clinical Presentation

A 27-year-old man presents with severe hemorrhage after extraction of a loose left lower molar tooth. He was previously healthy and was not on any medication. CT and MRI are performed, followed by angiography.

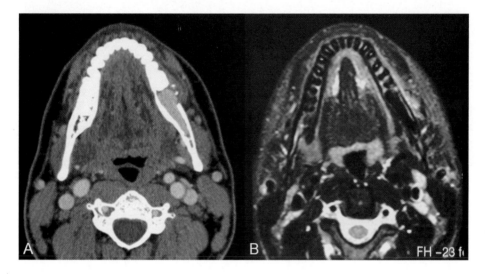

Fig. 31.1 **(A)** Post-contrast CT scan and **(B)** T2-weighted MRI.

Radiologic Studies

CT/MRI

Post-contrast CT scan showed an osteolytic lesion at the left side of the mandible with evidence of cortical disruption. There was intense homogeneous enhancement of this lesion, which had an elongated appearance and extended along the mandible. A T2-weighted MR sequence demonstrated the left mandibular lesion as a flow-void structure, consistent with a vascular lesion (**Fig. 31.1**).

DSA

Angiography of the left internal maxillary artery (IMA) and left facial artery (FA) demonstrated a high-flow arteriovenous shunt within the mandible. There was supply from two converging arteries—the inferior alveolar artery from the IMA and the mental artery from the FA—with drainage into an ectatic venous compartment within the left mandible before further drainage into the external jugular vein (**Fig. 31.2 A,B**).

Diagnosis

Mandibular arteriovenous fistulous malformation

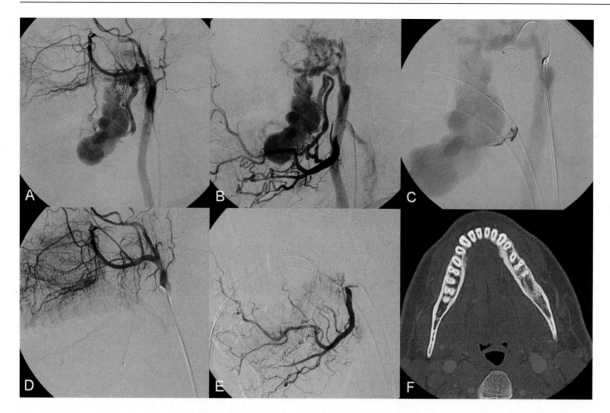

Fig. 31.2 DSA. **(A)** Left IMA and **(B)** left FA angiograms in lateral views. **(C)** Hand injection through the microcatheter wedged within the left inferior alveolar artery in lateral view before glue injection. **(D)** Follow-up left IMA and **(E)** left FA angiograms at 2 months show complete closure of the fistula. **(F)** Axial CT scan of the mandible in bone window at 1 year after embolization reveals remodeling of the mandibular bone.

Treatment

EQUIPMENT

- Standard 5F Access (puncture Needle, 5F vascular sheath)
- Standard 5F multipurpose catheter (Envoy; Cordis, Warren, NJ) with continuous flush and a 0.035-in hydrophilic guidewire (Terumo, Somerset, NJ)
- A 0.012-in flow-related microcatheter (Magic 1.2; Balt International, Montmorency, France) with a 0.008-in hydrophilic guidewire (Mirage; ev3, Plymouth, MN)
- A 10% glucose solution
- Histoacryl/Lipiodol (1 mL/2 mL)
- Contrast material

DESCRIPTION

Following diagnostic angiography, a 5F multipurpose catheter was advanced into the left IMA. A flow-directed microcatheter was introduced over a micro-guidewire into the inferior alveolar branch of the IMA in a wedged position as close to the fistula as possible. Control runs via hand injection through the microcatheter verified the position of the microcatheter. The microcatheter was then flushed with a glucose solution, after which glue at 50% concentration was injected to close the fistulous point under a blank roadmap; this resulted immediately in total obliteration of the fistula (**Fig. 31.2C–E**). The microcatheter was removed, and control angiography confirmed the complete closure. Follow-up angiography at 3 months revealed no recurrence of the fistula. A follow-up CT scan at 1 year after the procedure demonstrated remodeling of the mandibular bone (**Fig. 31.2F**).

Discussion

Background

Intraosseous mandibular arteriovenous malformations (AVMs) and fistulae are rare entities that must be recognized because they may present with life-threatening hemorrhage after tooth extraction or biopsy. These lesions are typically encountered in children and adolescents. Most patients have a history of recurrent minor episodes of bleeding while brushing their teeth. Other, unusual presenting symptoms include facial swelling, changes in skin and mucosal color, bruit, and dental loosening.

Noninvasive Imaging Workup

CT/MRI

- The high-flow characteristics of facial and scalp AVMs are seen as enhancing tubular structures on post-contrast CT scans or as flow voids on T2-weighted MR sequences.
- Bone resorption is a result of the high-flow nature of these lesions, which can be identified as well-defined osteolytic lesions on bone window CT images.
- MRI will show tubular flow voids within the bone.

CTA/MRA

- Dilated arterial feeders and early filling of the venous segment within the bone may be seen on CTA and MRA.

Invasive Imaging Workup

- Angiography is often done before embolization in an emergency setting.
- Although the major feeders are from the external carotid artery (i.e., branches of the IMA and FA), the intracranial circulation, especially the vertebral arteries in the case of mandibular AVMs, should also be injected to exclude associated intracranial AVMs in the setting of a cerebrofacial arteriovenous metameric syndrome (CAMS).
- A nidus-type lesion with multiple arterial feeders is more often encountered than a fistula-type lesion.

Treatment Options

SURGICAL TREATMENT

- In the past, surgery was the treatment of choice for mandibular AVMs; currently, it is still performed when a cure cannot be obtained with endovascular treatment.
- Two techniques can be employed: transmandibular curettage and bone resection with transplantation.
- Surgical ligation of the external carotid artery is ineffective because of the recruitment of collateral feeders and is never indicated because it precludes further endovascular treatment.

ENDOVASCULAR TREATMENT

- Embolization is the preferred treatment choice in an emergency setting to arrest the acute bleeding that occurs.
- Transarterial embolization with liquid material should aim at closing the fistulous point in fistula-type lesions and at filling the venous segment in nidus-type lesions.
- Transarterial embolization with particles alone will result in incomplete occlusion, recurrence, and rebleeding and is therefore not recommended.

- Proximal arterial occlusion will lead to the recruitment of other vessels to fill the AVM and is contraindicated because these smaller vessels will be more difficult to catheterize.
- If transarterial embolization is unable to completely occlude the venous segment within the mandible, another endovascular approach can be proposed, such as transvenous embolization with coils or direct percutaneous/transosseous puncture into the venous segment to deliver the embolic material.
- If a surgical procedure is planned for definitive treatment of a facial/mandibular AVM, preoperative embolization may help to decrease surgical blood loss. In this instance, the major feeders are typically embolized with liquid material, followed by particle embolization of the remaining, smaller arterial feeders.

Possible Complications

- Pulmonary emboli may develop.
- Stroke and cranial nerve palsies due to extracranial-intracranial anastomoses and embolization of arteries that supply the cranial nerves are extremely rare.
- Local infection and a reaction to the embolic material may occur. Occasionally, a foreign body granuloma may develop, and surgical removal of the embolic material may be required.

Published Literature on Treatment Options

Because mandibular AVMs are rare, only small case series and case reports are found in the literature. In contrast to our presented case, a fistulous lesion, most mandibular AVMs are of the nidus type; therefore, transarterial glue embolization may not result in complete cure if the glue fails to fill the venous segment sufficiently. Many authors prefer direct puncture through the bone to deliver the embolic material, usually glue, into the mandibular venous segment. There have been several case reports of transvenous approaches to the mandibular vein; however, many authors feel that although this is a good alternative treatment, it is often time-consuming and may require a large number of platinum coils, which may not be suitable if the patient is actively bleeding.

PEARLS AND PITFALLS

- Mandibular AVMs can present with life-threatening bleeding following tooth extraction or biopsy and require emergent embolization.
- Occasionally, they may be a part of a cerebrofacial arteriovenous metameric syndrome (CAMS); therefore, vascular studies of the intracranial circulation are indicated.
- Sufficient filling of the intraosseous venous segment is usually needed to cure these lesions, which may be achieved by a transarterial, transvenous, or direct puncture route.

Further Reading

Kiyosue H, Mori H, Hori Y, Okahara M, Kawano K, Mizuki H. Treatment of mandibular arteriovenous malformation by transvenous embolization: A case report. Head Neck 1999;21(6):574–577

Persky MS, Yoo HJ, Berenstein A. Management of vascular malformations of the mandible and maxilla. Laryngoscope 2003;113(11):1885–1892

Rodesch G, Soupre V, Vazquez MP, Alvarez H, Lasjaunias P. Arteriovenous malformations of the dental arcades. The place of endovascular therapy: results in 12 cases are presented. J Craniomaxillofac Surg 1998;26(5):306–313

CASE 32

Case Description

Clinical Presentation

A 22-year-old woman presents with progressive enlargement of a soft pulsatile mass at the vertex that she has had since the age of 12 years. Physical examination reveals a compressible scalp mass at the midline parietal region. The mass is pulsatile, with a thrill on palpation. Outside CT reveals a vascular lesion, and the patient is referred to us for further angiographic evaluation.

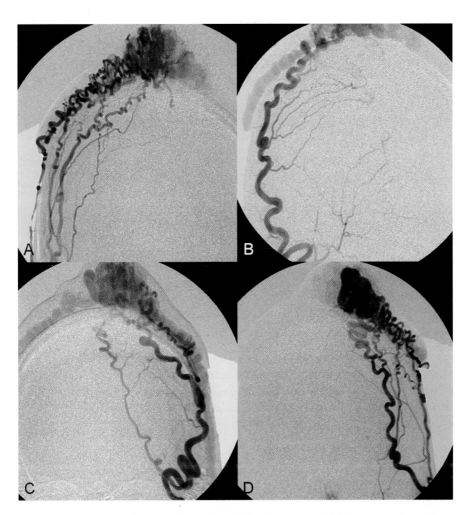

Fig. 32.1 DSA. **(A)** Right internal maxillary, **(B)** right occipital, **(C)** left internal maxillary, and **(D)** left occipital angiograms.

187

Radiologic Studies

DSA

Angiograms of the internal maxillary arteries and the occipital arteries revealed a scalp arteriovenous malformation (AVM) at the high parietal region with multiple arterial feeders from subcutaneous branches of the superficial temporal and occipital arteries bilaterally. There was drainage into large ectatic venous pouches that corresponded to the pulsatile mass on physical examination before further drainage into scalp veins bilaterally (**Fig. 32.1**).

Diagnosis

Scalp AVM

Treatment

EQUIPMENT

- Standard 5F access (puncture needle, 5F vascular sheath)
- Standard 5F multipurpose catheter (Envoy; Cordis, Warren, NJ) with continuous flush and a 0.035-in hydrophilic guidewire (Terumo, Somerset, NJ)
- A 0.012-in flow-related microcatheter (Magic 1.2; Balt International, Montmorency, France) with a 0.008-in hydrophilic guidewire (Mirage; ev3, Plymouth, MN)
- A 21-gauge BD Angiocath (B Braun, Melsungen, Germany) with a connection tube
- A 10% glucose solution
- Histoacryl/Lipiodol (1 mL/3 mL, 1 mL/1 mL)
- Contrast material

DESCRIPTION

The procedure was done under general anesthesia. The skin of the scalp overlying the pulsatile mass was prepared before the procedure. Following diagnostic angiography, a 5F multipurpose catheter was advanced into the right occipital artery. A flow-related microcatheter was introduced over a micro-guidewire into the subcutaneous branch of the occipital artery. Attempts were made to place the microcatheter as close to the AVM as possible; however, this was technically difficult because of multiple kinks in the subcutaneous artery. A hand injection through the microcatheter verified its position. The microcatheter was then flushed with glucose solution, followed by the injection of glue at 25% concentration under a blank roadmap, which resulted in proximal occlusion of the occipital artery branch. The glue did not penetrate the venous pouch. The microcatheter was removed, and the procedure was repeated for the subcutaneous branches of the left superficial temporal and left occipital arteries, with similar results. Because proximal ligation would lead to subsequent reopening of the AVM, direct puncture of the venous pouch was done with a 21-gauge Angiocath, followed by hand injection of contrast to verify the position and venous outflow. The Angiocath was then flushed with glucose solution, and glue at 50% concentration was injected under a blank roadmap. Manual compression of the venous outflow was used to prevent glue migration. The direct puncture was repeated one more time and resulted in complete obliteration of the venous pouch and scalp AVM. The needle was removed, and a control angiogram of the external carotid arteries revealed complete closure of the scalp AVM (**Fig. 32.2**).

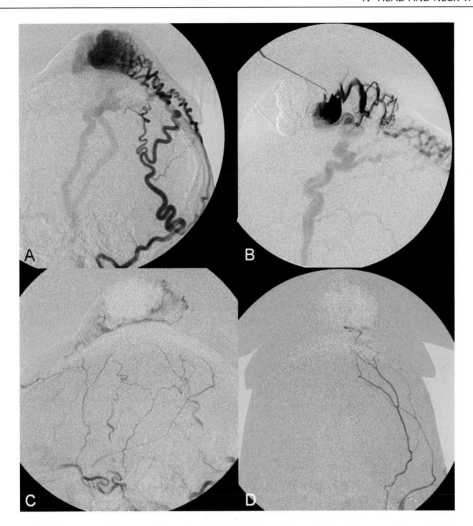

Fig. 32.2 DSA. Left occipital angiogram in **(A)** lateral view before the procedure and **(B)** hand injection via a 21-gauge needle into the venous pouch demonstrate the connection between the venous pouch and the scalp veins. Left external carotid artery angiogram in **(C)** lateral and **(D)** AP views after transarterial embolization and direct puncture reveals complete obliteration of the scalp AVM.

Discussion

Background

Scalp AVMs are abnormal AV communications localized within the subcutaneous fatty layer of the scalp. Although we use the term *malformation* to describe these lesions because of the multiplicity of arterial feeders, the AV connections are typically of the fistulous type, without an intervening capillary bed. These lesions have been referred to in the literature as *cirsoid aneurysm, aneurysma serpentinum, aneurysma racemosum,* and *plexiform angioma.* They are characterized by an AV shunt, the absence of an intervening capillary bed, and dilated, tortuous draining veins that often cause a cosmetic deformity and may occasionally bleed. The etiology of these lesions is still poorly understood; however, it is generally accepted that they can be either congenital or traumatic in origin. It is estimated that ~30% or more of these lesions are related to blunt, nonpenetrating trauma, with delayed occurrence of the shunt. Iatrogenic fistulae after hair transplantation have also been described in the literature. Most of the patients present with progressive scalp swelling. Rapid enlargement may occur during puberty, menstruation, and pregnancy. Large lesions may be associated with scalp necrosis and secondary malignant changes.

Noninvasive Imaging Workup

CT/MRI

- High-flow scalp AVMs are seen as enhancing tubular structures on post-contrast CT scan or as flow voids on T2-weighted MR sequences.

CTA/MRA

- Dilated arterial feeders and early filling of the ectatic venous pouches can be seen on CTA and MRA.

Invasive Imaging Workup

- Angiography is necessary for planning the treatment of scalp AVMs.
- The major arterial feeders are the subcutaneous arteries from the superficial temporal, occipital, and posterior auricular arteries. Occasional collaterals from the meningeal arteries may be seen, but this is unusual.
- The venous drainage pattern must be evaluated, in particular to detect intracranial connections and variations, such as a sinus pericranii.

Treatment Options

SURGICAL TREATMENT

- Surgical resection is an excellent treatment choice for scalp AVMs and typically yields good cosmetic results. Presurgical embolization and the use of skin expanders in preparation for surgical resection of the AVM are required, especially for large lesions.
- In some cases, although the lesion has already been cured with endovascular treatment, surgical removal of the embolic material may be necessary.
- Ligation of the proximal arterial feeders is no longer performed because of the recruitment of collateral feeders, which complicates future treatment.
- Some large, high-flow AVMs involving the facial region are very difficult to manage, even with multimodality treatment, and may eventually result in a disastrous outcome.

ENDOVASCULAR TREATMENT

- With the increased use of direct puncture in recent years, the role of endovascular techniques as a definitive treatment for scalp AVMs has increased.
- The aim of treatment is closure of the dilated venous pouch(es) in which the arterial feeders converge.
- Transarterial embolization alone usually cannot cure these lesions because of the tortuosity of the subcutaneous branches and difficulties encountered in navigating the microcatheter sufficiently distally to deposit embolic material in the venous pouch.
- Direct percutaneous puncture of the venous pouch has been described. Because of the high-flow nature of scalp AVMs, it may be difficult to control the injection of embolic material into the venous pouch; therefore, various techniques to compress the venous outflow ("cookie cutter" technique) with the use of more concentrated glue (40–50%) have been described.
- Transarterial embolization may be used before direct puncture to help control the injection of embolic material.
- Particles are not routinely used except for embolization before direct puncture or a surgical procedure.

Possible Complications

- Glue migration may result in pulmonary emboli or intracranial venous thrombosis in cases with a connection between the scalp and intracranial venous system.
- Skin necrosis or hair loss may result from the extensive occlusion of normal subcutaneous arteries during transarterial embolization.
- Local infection and reaction to the embolic material may occur.
- Persistent cosmetic problems may be caused by a cast of liquid embolic material underneath the skin.

Published Literature on Treatment Options

In a surgical series of 21 patients reported by Fisher-Jeffes et al, six patients had post-surgical complications of skin necrosis, bleeding, and wound sepsis, and in four patients, the lesion recurred. Since Barnwell et al described the use of direct puncture for the treatment of three patients with curative results, this technique has evolved, and other authors have developed techniques to compress the venous outflow and better control the injection of glue into the venous pouch. These developments have increased the cure rates for endovascular treatment to 70 to 100% and decreased the risk for complications of glue migration. However, because a large amount of glue may be necessary for large lesions, many authors still support the use of combined treatment with the post-surgical removal of disfiguring and hard glue casts. There have been some reports in the literature of the use of sclerosing agents, such as alcohol and sodium tetradecyl sulfate; however, we discourage these techniques because the high-flow nature of scalp AVMs makes it difficult or impossible to retain the sclerosing agents in the lesion, with a concomitant high risk for systemic toxicity.

PEARLS AND PITFALLS _____

- Scalp AVMs are high-flow fistulous communications within the subcutaneous layer and therefore typically recruit arterial supply from multiple subcutaneous branches.
- The aim of the endovascular treatment of scalp AVMs is to occlude the proximal venous segment/pouch, which can be accomplished by direct puncture.
- Compression of the venous outflow during glue injection helps to prevent glue migration ("cookie cutter" technique).

Further Reading

Barnwell SL, Halbach VV, Dowd CF, Higashida RT, Hieshima GB. Endovascular treatment of scalp and artereovenous fistulas. Radiology 1989;173:533–539

Fisher-Jeffes ND, Domingo Z, Madden M, DeVilliers JC. Arteriovenous malformations of the scalp. Neurosurgery 1995;36:656–660

Han MH, Seong SO, Kim HD, Chang KH, Yeon KM, Han MC. Craniofacial arteriovenous malformation: preoperative embolization with direct puncture and injection of n-butyl cyanoacrylate. Radiology 1999;211(3):661–666

Nagasaka S, Fukushima T, Goto K, Ohjimi H, Iwabuchi S, Maehara F. Treatment of scalp arteriovenous malformation. Neurosurgery 1996;38(4):671–677, discussion 677

Ryu CW, Whang SM, Suh DC, et al. Percutaneous direct puncture glue embolization of high-flow craniofacial arteriovenous lesions: a new circular ring compression device with a beveled edge. AJNR Am J Neuroradiol 2007;28(3):528–530

CASE 33

Case Description

Clinical Presentation

A 46-year-old man presents with a bluish, soft, nonpulsating mass lesion at the right side of his tongue. The lesion has slowly expanded over more than 10 years. It occasionally bleeds and increases in size when he is bending forward or lying down. MRI of the face and tongue is performed.

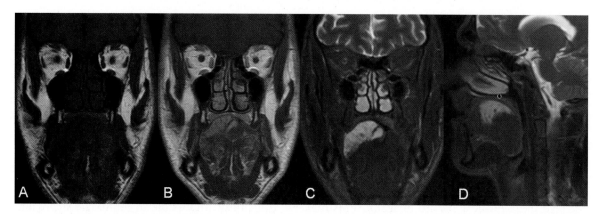

Fig. 33.1 MRI. T1-weighted images **(A)** before gadolinium and **(B)** after gadolinium in coronal view and T2-weighted images in **(C)** coronal and **(D)** sagittal views.

Radiologic Studies

MRI

MRI showed an isosignal T1 and a hypersignal T2 lesion, in comparison with muscle, at the right side of the tongue. Post-gadolinium studies showed moderate enhancement, corresponding to a venous malformation (**Fig. 33.1**).

Diagnosis

Venous malformation (VM) of the right side of the tongue

Treatment

EQUIPMENT

- 22-Gauge BD Angiocaths (B Braun, Melsungen, Germany)
- Low-osmolarity, water-soluble iodinated contrast material
- Bleomycin (1 mg/mL) to a maximum dose of 15 mg

DESCRIPTION

Percutaneous sclerotherapy was performed under fluoroscopic guidance, sterile conditions, and general anesthesia. 22-Gauge Angiocaths were percutaneously inserted into the VM until the return of blood was observed. Phlebography with a small amount (1–2 mL) of contrast material confirmed the position of the needle within the VM and assessed venous drainage. Three milliliters of bleomycin was injected into the VM under simultaneous subtracted fluoroscopy. When the injected material entered the malformation, it replaced the previously injected contrast material, pushing it into the periphery and into the draining veins of the VM, and it appeared as negative contrast (white) on simultaneous fluoroscopic subtraction (negative subtraction technique). The procedure was performed three times, each time with different puncture needles and at different puncture sites, for a total dose of 9 mg of bleomycin during the session. Two additional percutaneous sclerotherapy sessions were performed at 2-month intervals. Follow-up MRI at 1 year showed a reduced size of the VM with clinical improvement (**Fig. 33.2**).

Discussion

Background

VMs are congenital, slow-flow vascular lesions consisting of dysmorphic vascular channels lined by flattened endothelium. Although present at birth, they may appear clinically at any point during life and often have a history of slow, progressive enlargement. Clinical presentations range from a faint blue patch on the skin to a soft, compressible, nonpulsatile mass. Lesions in the oral cavity may lead to dysphagia, difficulties with speech or swallowing, orthodontic concerns, and airway obstruction.

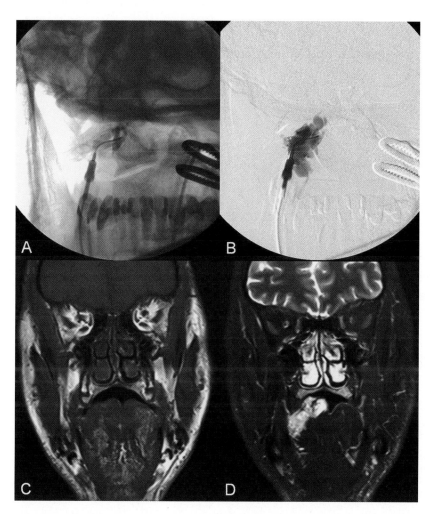

Fig. 33.2 Phlebography. **(A)** Nonsubtracted and **(B)** subtracted images before the injection of bleomycin. MRI. **(C)** T1-weighted and **(D)** T2-weighted images at 1-year follow-up after three sessions of treatment show decreased size of the lesion.

Noninvasive Imaging Workup

PHYSICAL EXAMINATION

- A bluish mass lesion is soft, nonpulsatile, and compressible.
- The lesion changes in size with a change in position and during the Valsalva maneuver.

CT/MRI

- The lesion is seen as isodense to slightly hyperdense on unenhanced CT. It is isointense to hypointense on T1-weighted and hyperintense on T2-weighted MR images in comparison with muscle. Post-contrast studies show enhancement, which is used to differentiate VMs from lymphatic malformations.
- Round calcifications representing phleboliths may be seen.

CTA/MRA

- No abnormal arterial feeders or enlargement is seen on static CTA/MRA and during the arterial phase of dynamic studies.
- Filling of the ectatic venous pouches may be seen during the late venous phase of dynamic CTA/MRA.

Invasive Imaging Workup

- Angiography is usually not required and is performed only when the diagnosis is uncertain or a mixed type of vascular malformation is suspected.

Treatment Options

PERCUTANEOUS SCLEROTHERAPY

- Many sclerotherapeutic agents are available. Alcohol is the most commonly used, and in recent years, experience with bleomycin has increased.
- Bleomycin is diluted to a concentration of 1 mg/mL, with dosage regimens as follows:
  - In children younger than 1 year of age, the maximum dose is 0.5 to 1 mg/kg per session.
  - In children older than 1 year of age and in adults, the maximum dose is 15 mg per session.
- If on phlebography the venous pouches drain into risky areas, such as the cavernous sinus, blockage with external compression or transvenous coiling can be done before the sclerotic agent is injected, although in our experience bleomycin is much less dangerous than alcohol.

SURGICAL TREATMENT

- Surgical resection has been used mainly in the past. It is now used only when other options have failed, to improve cosmetic results, or when a life-threatening condition, such as a mass effect on airways, is present.

Possible Complications

- Skin discoloration, which may be aggravated by the use of adhesive tape surrounding the region
- Cellulitis/ulceration
- Nausea and vomiting
- Flulike symptoms
- Partial temporary hair loss

Published Literature on Treatment Options

Bleomycin is a cytotoxic antitumoral antibiotic with a known side effect of vascular endothelial destruction. It was first reported for the treatment of cystic hygromas. In 2004, Muir et al reported the prospective treatment of 95 patients with hemangiomas and congenital vascular malformations, 31 of which were VMs; the response rate in this subset was 84%. Temporary, minor complications occurred in 8.4%, which included superficial ulceration, cellulitis, flulike symptoms, and transient hair loss. None of the patients had toxic hematologic effects or showed signs of pulmonary involvement (fibrosis, hypertension). In a large series of 260 patients with VMs treated with pingyangmycin, a bleomycin analog, Zhao et al reported a subjective rating of "good" or "excellent" by 89% of the patients. Only one patient experienced ulceration at the injection site, which resulted in subsequent scarring. Bleomycin is therefore considered to be a safe and effective treatment, with an extremely low profile of adverse side effects. Concerns have been raised regarding the potential development of pulmonary fibrosis, which is the major complication seen in cancer patients treated with systemic bleomycin. To date, no cases of pulmonary fibrosis have been reported in the literature after its use as a sclerotherapy agent. This is likely because when used for sclerotherapy, it does not enter the bloodstream, as it does in patients to whom it is administered systemically. There is no consensus regarding what sclerosing agent should be used. In the matched-pair analysis of Spence et al that compared alcohol and bleomycin treatments, alcohol had a slightly higher success rate than bleomycin (100% vs. 88.2%), and the average number of treatment sessions required was significantly lower in patients treated with alcohol than in those treated with bleomycin (1.9 vs. 3.4), indicating that bleomycin is a less potent agent. On the other hand, the most striking difference between the two sclerosant agents was in the rates of adverse events and complications. Among patients treated with alcohol, 50% experienced unwanted sequelae, as opposed to none of the patients treated with bleomycin in the matched pairs. In particular, the risk for swelling, pain, and skin necrosis is reduced when bleomycin is used. Bleomycin is therefore in our opinion the sclerosant agent of choice, especially in vulnerable areas such as the periorbital region, lips, tongue, and parapharyngeal spaces, locations where alcohol would typically not be used.

PEARLS AND PITFALLS _____

- The characteristic imaging findings of VMs include phleboliths, high signal on T2, enhancement, and an absence of abnormally enlarged arterial feeders on angiography.
- Alcohol is the most commonly used sclerotic agent for the treatment of VMs; however, bleomycin offers the benefit of less swelling and pain with similar results.
- Lesions in certain locations, such as the tongue, lips, and periorbital regions, are best treated with bleomycin.

Further Reading

Muir T, Kirsten M, Fourie P, Dippenaar N, Ionescu GO. Intralesional bleomycin injection (IBI) treatment for haemangiomas and congenital vascular malformations. Pediatr Surg Int 2004;19(12):766–773

Spence J, Krings T, Terbrugge K, daCosta LB, Agid R. Percutaneous treatment of facial venous malformations: a matched comparison of alcohol and bleomycin sclerotherapy. Head Neck April 29, 2010. [Epub ahead of print]

Zhao JH, Zhang WF, Zhao YF. Sclerotherapy of oral and facial venous malformations with use of pingyangmycin and/or sodium morrhuate. Int J Oral Maxillofac Surg 2004;33(5):463–466

CASE 34

Case Description

Clinical Presentation

A 52-year-old woman presents with swelling of the right side of her face that has been slowly progressing for several years and that fluctuates in size during changes of position. MRI and contrast-enhanced MRA are performed, followed by angiography.

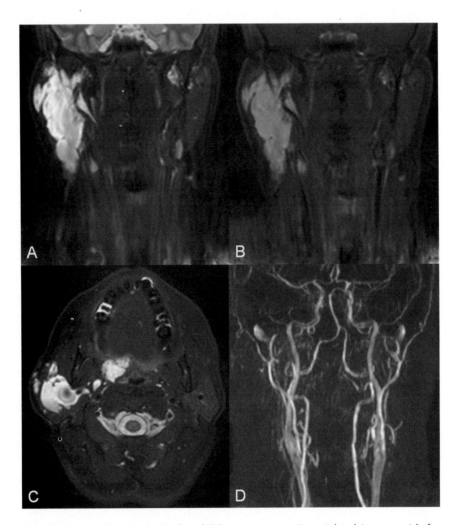

Fig. 34.1 MRI. **(A)** T2-weighted and **(B)** post-contrast T1-weighted images with fat saturation in coronal view. **(C)** Axial T2-weighted image with fat saturation and **(D)** contrast-enhanced MRA show a large hypersignal T2 lesion at the right side of the face, also involving the parotid space, with intense enhancement. Note the lack of any arterial supply, corresponding to a VM.

Radiologic Studies

MRI/MRA

MRI showed a large hypersignal T2 lesion at the right side of the face and parotid space, with intense enhancement on a post-gadolinium study. A few small, round, markedly hyposignal T2 structures were observed within the lesion, compatible with phleboliths. No enlarged arterial supply was identified on contrast-enhanced MRA. These findings corresponded to the diagnosis of a venous malformation (**Fig. 34.1**).

Diagnosis

Venous malformation (VM) of the right side of the face and parotid space

Treatment

EQUIPMENT

- 22-Gauge BD Angiocaths (B Braun, Melsungen, Germany)
- Low-osmolarity, water-soluble iodinated contrast material
- 100% Ethyl alcohol

DESCRIPTION

Percutaneous sclerotherapy was performed under fluoroscopic guidance, sterile conditions, and general anesthesia. 22-Gauge Angiocaths were percutaneously inserted into the VM until the return of blood was observed. Phlebography with a small amount (1–2 mL) of contrast material confirmed the position of the needle within the VM and assessed venous drainage. Three to four milliliters of pure alcohol was injected into the VM under simultaneous subtracted fluoroscopy with the negative subtraction technique described in Case 33. When the alcohol entered the malformation, it replaced the previously injected contrast material, pushing it into the periphery and into the draining veins of the VM, and it appeared as negative contrast (white) on simultaneous fluoroscopic subtraction (**Fig. 34.2**). A total of five injections were done with different puncture needles and with different needle positions for a total dose of 15 mL of pure alcohol. Follow-up MRI at 9 months showed a reduced size of the VM with decreased facial asymmetry.

Discussion

Background

VMs are commonly encountered within the head and neck region. Typical symptoms include swelling, pain, ulceration, and bleeding, although most patients are asymptomatic or have only cosmetic concerns. These lesions tend to involve multiple anatomic spaces and may encase neuromuscular structures, making surgical treatment difficult with a high risk for complications. In recent years, sclerotherapy has played an increasing role, either as a single-modality treatment or as part of a combined-modality treatment, used preoperatively to reduce the size of a lesion or postoperatively in case of incomplete resection or recurrence.

Noninvasive Imaging Workup

PHYSICAL EXAMINATION

- A soft, nonpulsatile, compressible mass changes in size with a change in position and during the Valsalva maneuver.

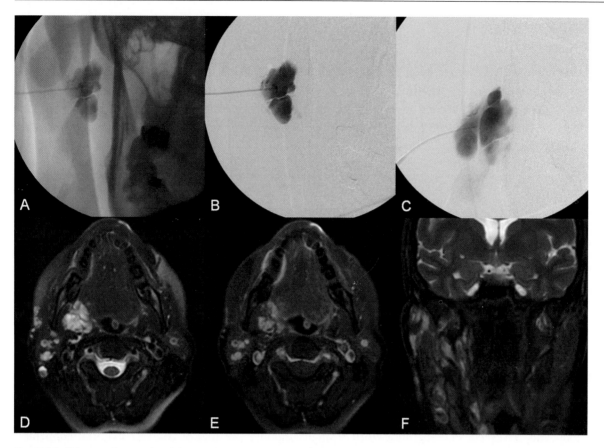

Fig. 34.2 **(A)** Nonsubtracted and **(B,C)** subtracted images of the phlebogram before the injection of alcohol in two different punctures demonstrate filling of the venous pouch with contrast without any dangerous venous drainage. MRI. **(D)** T2-weighted and **(E)** T1-weighted post-gadolinium images in axial view and **(F)** T2-weighted image in coronal view at 9-month follow-up show decreased size of the superficial component of the lesion.

- The bluish discoloration may not be seen if the lesion is located entirely within the subcutaneous or deeper layers.
- Depending on its location, a lesion may impede speech and swallowing and obstruct the upper airway, although most lesions are asymptomatic.

CT/MRI

- The lesion is isodense to slightly hyperdense on unenhanced CT. It is isointense to hypointense on T1-weighted and hyperintense on T2-weighted MR images in comparison with muscle.
- The lesion is usually infiltrative and may involve multiple anatomic spaces.
- Post-contrast studies show enhancement, which is used to differentiate VMs from lymphatic malformations.
- Round calcifications representing phleboliths may be seen; they appear as signal voids on MRI.

Invasive Imaging Workup

- Angiography is usually not required and is performed only when the diagnosis is uncertain.

Treatment Options

PERCUTANEOUS SCLEROTHERAPY

- Ethyl alcohol is the most commonly used sclerotherapeutic agent.
- The maximum dose of ethyl alcohol is 1 mL/kg per session.
- In superficial lesions with a high risk for ulceration, a more diluted concentration (0.66 mg/mL) may be used.
- If on phlebography the venous pouches drain into risky areas, such as the cavernous sinus, blockage by external compression or transvenous coiling must be done before the sclerotic agent is injected.
- Preoperative antibiotic management is recommended (cephazolin 100 mg/kg up to 2 g) immediately before the procedure.
- Steroids may be used following the procedure if excessive swelling occurs.

SURGICAL TREATMENT

- Historically, VMs have been treated surgically, although in recent years, percutaneous sclerotherapy has been used more often, either as a preoperative support to reduce lesion size, as a postoperative complement, or as a single approach.

Possible Complications

- Local tissue injury (e.g., skin blistering, necrosis, ulceration, and peripheral nerve palsies)
- Infection and inflammation of the area (i.e., thrombophlebitis and cellulitis)
- Pulmonary thromboembolism from thrombus dislodgement of the sclerosed VM
- Systemic intoxication, especially in patients who receive large doses of ethanol
- Swelling and pain

Published Literature on Treatment Options

The efficacy of alcohol as a sclerotherapeutic agent ranges from 75 to 100% in previous literature. In the largest series, of 87 patients reported by Lee et al, which included lesions in all locations, the rate of overall clinical improvement was 95.4%, with complications occurring in 47 of a total of 397 sessions (12.4% of sessions, 27.9% of patients). Most complications were minor and transient, although more serious sequelae developed in 11 patients, including 5 cases of peripheral nerve palsy (2 permanent), 5 cases of deep vein thrombosis (1 with pulmonary embolism), and 1 case of calf muscle fibrosis. Of the 40 patients with craniofacial VMs reported by Berenguer et al in 1999, 30 (75%) were cured or had marked improvement of their lesions following alcohol sclerotherapy. Again, a high rate of local complications was observed, although most were temporary: skin blistering in 20 patients (50%), deep ulceration in 5 patients (13%), and nerve injury in 3 patients (7.5%). Permanent nerve injury secondary to treatment developed in 1 patient (2.5%).

In patients with facial VMs, absolute indications for treatment are obstruction of the upper airways and impeded speech or swallowing; relative indications for treatment are swelling, pain, and recurrent hemorrhage, as well as cosmetic concerns. Alcohol sclerotherapy temporarily worsens swelling, which must be taken into account when lesions are close to the upper airways or tongue and may require a temporary tracheostomy. In these situations, bleomycin treatment or partial surgical resection should be strongly considered. The aim of treatment is symptom palliation and size reduction, and sclerotherapy sessions can be repeated until either the patient feels that the residual symptoms are tolerable or the clinician feels that there is no further role for treatment.

PEARLS AND PITFALLS

- Ethyl alcohol is an effective sclerotherapeutic agent for the treatment of VMs; however, it is associated with a high rate of temporary local complications and post-procedural swelling and pain.
- Dangerous venous drainage of the venous pouches, such as those in the cavernous sinus, must be avoided. Blockage with external compression or transvenous coiling before injection of the sclerotic agent can be used. Bleomycin should be strongly considered as an alternative agent in these circumstances.

Further Reading

Agid R, Burvin R, Gomori JM. Sclerotherapy for venous malformations using a "negative subtraction" technique. Neuroradiology 2006;48(2):127–129

Berenguer B, Burrows PE, Zurakowski D, Mulliken JB. Sclerotherapy of craniofacial venous malformations: complications and results. Plast Reconstr Surg 1999;104(1):1–11, discussion 12–15

Lee BB, Do YS, Byun HS, Choo IW, Kim DI, Huh SH. Advanced management of venous malformation with ethanol sclerotherapy: mid-term results. J Vasc Surg 2003;37(3):533–538

CASE 35

Case Description

Clinical Presentation

A 9-month-old girl presents with the history of a left cheek mass since the age of 1 month that shows rapid enlargement despite treatment with oral prednisolone and V-beam laser. Physical examination reveals a soft-tissue mass at the left cheek with mild overlying discoloration. The parents are advised concerning the natural history of the lesion and insist on partial treatment. MRI is performed, followed by angiography and partial trans-arterial particle embolization within the same session.

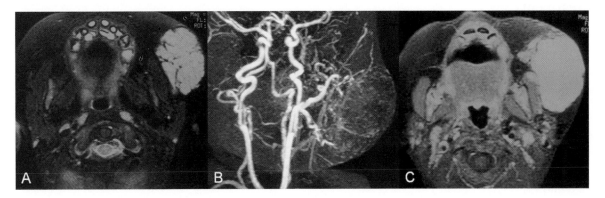

Fig. 35.1 MRI. **(A)** T2-weighted and **(B)** post-contrast T1-weighted images with fat saturation. **(C)** Post-contrast MRA in oblique view.

Radiologic Studies

MRI/MRA

MRI showed a hyposignal T1/hypersignal T2 well-defined lobulated mass lesion at the subcutaneous layer of the left cheek with intense enhancement on a post-contrast study. Static MRA revealed enlargement of multiple branches of the left external carotid artery supplying the mass lesion. These findings were consistent with the proliferative phase of a hemangioma (**Fig. 35.1**).

DSA

Injections of the left facial and internal maxillary arteries demonstrated a multilobulated capillary tumor blush at the level of the left cheek. Enlargement of multiple branches of the left facial, left transverse facial, and left internal maxillary arteries supplying the lesion was also observed (**Fig. 35.2**).

Diagnosis

Facial hemangioma of the left cheek

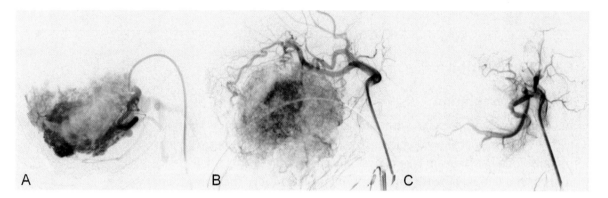

Fig. 35.2 DSA. **(A)** Left facial and **(B)** left internal maxillary angiograms in lateral view. **(C)** Angiogram of the left internal maxillary artery after particle embolization shows obliteration of the supply to the tumor.

Treatment

EQUIPMENT

- Standard 4F access (puncture needle, 4F vascular sheath)
- Standard 4F multipurpose catheter (Cordis, Warren, NJ) with continuous flush and a 0.035-in hydrophilic guidewire (Terumo, Somerset, NJ)
- A 0.015-in over-the-wire microcatheter (Prowler 10; Cordis) with a 0.010-in hydrophilic guidewire (Agility 10; Cordis)
- Polyvinyl alcohol particles (Ivalon), 300 to 500 μm
- Contrast material

DESCRIPTION

Following diagnostic angiography, a 4F multipurpose catheter was advanced into the proximal left facial artery. An over-the-wire microcatheter was introduced over a micro-guidewire into the distal branches. A mixture of 300- to 500-μm polyvinyl alcohol particles and contrast media was injected slowly under a blank roadmap until stagnation of the distal branches was observed. The microcatheter was removed, the 4F multipurpose catheter was advanced into the proximal left internal maxillary artery, and the microcatheter was placed into the distal internal maxillary artery and transverse facial artery, followed by particle embolization with the same technique used to close the remaining arterial supply to the lesion. The microcatheter was removed, and the final control run showed obliteration of the supply to the hemangioma (**Fig. 35.2C**).

Discussion

Background

Hemangiomas are the most common tumors of infancy and can be seen in up to 10 to 12% of all children younger than 1 year of age. In 1982, Mulliken and Glowacki were the first to characterize hemangiomas as a separate entity from vascular malformations. Histologically, a hemangioma is a true neoplasm, in which an increased turnover of endothelial cells, mast cells, fibroblasts, and macrophages enables its capability for proliferation. After birth, hemangiomas typically grow rapidly; this proliferative phase may last up to 18 months. The growth rate then stabilizes, and lesions enlarge only with growth of the child for some time before entering a spontaneous involutional phase, which may last until the child is 10 to 12 years of age (50% of all cases spontaneously involute by 5 years, 70% at 7 years, and up to 80–90% by 12 years). Areas of necrosis and ulceration can complicate this stage; however, scarring is rare, and the overlying skin will appear normal in up to 50% of cases. The remaining 50% may have residual discoloration of the skin ranging from telangiectases to a fatty fibrous replacement with scarring. Only ~20% of all hemangiomas are associated with problems that may require treatment. These include cardiac failure (in very large lesions), coagulation disorders, palpebral occlusion (blindness), cartilage necrosis (in lesions located at the tip of the nose), orbital deformity, oral mass effect, impaired mandibular growth, subglottic location, and steroid resistance, dependence, or intolerance. The general rule for treatment is that the resulting scar should always be smaller than the sequelae of spontaneous involution.

Noninvasive Imaging Workup

HISTORY AND PHYSICAL EXAMINATION

- A history of rapid postnatal growth followed by stabilization and involution is often helpful for the diagnosis.
- Superficial hemangiomas are characteristically red and raised, with a strawberry-like appearance. The lesions are warm and soft, and they may be pulsatile. Deeper lesions may be difficult to diagnose because of a bluish discoloration due to the dilated draining veins; however, a pale halo surrounding the lesion may be seen, which helps in the diagnosis.

ULTRASOUND WITH DOPPLER IMAGING

- A hemangioma is seen as a solid mass lesion with increased vascularity on flow imaging. A high flow rate with decreased arterial resistance and increased venous velocity, indicating the presence of micro-shunting, will be apparent on Doppler assessment.

CT/CTA

- CT and CTA are not routinely used in the evaluation of hemangiomas so as to avoid radiation exposure.

MRI/MRA

- Hemangiomas are isointense to hypointense on T1-weighted images and moderately hyperintense on T2-weighted images.
- Intense homogeneous enhancement is seen in the proliferative phase, which may become heterogeneous during involution.
- Enlargement of the feeding arteries can be demonstrated on MRA.

Invasive Imaging Workup

- Angiography is not required for the diagnosis of a hemangioma and is performed only at the time of embolization.
- Dilatation of the arterial feeders and a dense capillary tumor blush are often detected, with dilatation of the adjacent veins. Rapid venous filling, indicating arteriovenous shunting, may also be present, although no fistulae exist.

Treatment Options

PHARMACOLOGIC TREATMENT

- Systemic corticosteroids are usually considered as the first-line treatment for hemangiomas. They are effective mainly in the early, active, proliferating phase, usually within the first 6 to 8 months of life. The recommended dose of prednisolone is 2 to 3 mg/kg of body weight per day for 4 to 6 weeks, followed by tapering of the dose over 2 to 3 months, although some authors have reported higher response rates with high doses of up to 5 mg/kg of body weight.

- The use of interferon alfa-2a is controversial. Although successful treatment has been reported, significant side effects, including irreversible neurotoxicity, have occurred. Therefore, this treatment is typically reserved for cases of severe, bilateral, vision-threatening lesions that fail to respond to steroid treatment.
- Vincristine and actinomycin are chemotherapeutic agents used only in cases of Kasabach-Merritt syndrome with consumptive coagulopathy that do not respond to other forms of treatment.

LASER TREATMENT

- Many forms of medical lasers have been used for the treatment of hemangiomas. The results are likely to be best with lesions in superficial locations, whereas the deeper ones are associated with a higher rate of complications. Subglottic hemangiomas have been reported to respond well to endoscopic diode laser treatment.

SURGICAL TREATMENT

- Surgical resection and reconstruction may be required for large hemangiomas and those with extensive ulceration and necrosis.
- Preoperative proximal embolization with particles may have a role to decrease surgical blood loss.

ENDOVASCULAR TREATMENT

- Arterial embolization with particles or permanent liquid agents (N-butyl-cyanoacrylate) is aimed at producing ischemia and necrosis within the tumor and is indicated for the treatment of those hemangiomas that have failed to respond to pharmacologic treatment and that will have permanent sequelae if left untreated (location at tip of the nose or orbit; large, life-threatening hemangiomas). Obliteration of at least 70% of the arterial supply is often required for a significant clinical response, and the result may be transient, so that multiple procedures are required.
- In certain cases, partial transarterial embolization with particles may be used to induce the involutional phase for cosmetic reasons.
- The intralesional injection of bleomycin, with doses similar to those used in venous malformations, has been reported with promising results.
- The intralesional injection of alcohol or glue has also been reported; however, these agents are reserved for those cases that have failed all other treatment options.

Possible Complications

- Volume and contrast material overload is often a technical challenge in children. Multiple sessions may be necessary.
- Superficial ulceration may occur, especially if Gelfoam powder is used, as a consequence of skin necrosis. Treatment with local antiseptics or antibiotics may be needed.
- Stroke or cranial nerve palsies may develop because of the patency of extracranial-to-intracranial anastomoses in children.
- Fever of noninfectious origin is associated with necrosis of large lesions and may persist for 2 to 3 weeks.

Published Literature on Treatment Options

The treatment of hemangiomas varies depending on the institution and the location of the hemangioma. It is generally accepted that not all hemangiomas require treatment, and corticosteroids, either systemic or intralesional, are often the first treatment of choice. The rate of response to steroids varies from 30 to 93%. Laser treatment has the best results in superficially located lesions, particularly those with a subglottic location. Transarterial embolization is rarely indicated and is reserved for cases with life-threatening bleeding, consumptive coagulopathy, or cardiac failure in which other treatment options have failed.

PEARLS AND PITFALLS _____

- Hemangiomas are true neoplasms and can be differentiated from vascular malformations by their ability to proliferate and grow.
- Hemangiomas involute spontaneously in up to 80 to 90% of all patients by the age of 12 years; therefore, treatment in most cases is unnecessary.
- The indications for treatment of a hemangioma include the following: cardiac failure, coagulation disorder, palpebral occlusion, orbital deformity, location at the tip of the nose (because of cartilage necrosis), oral mass effect, impaired mandibular growth, and subglottic location.
- Pharmacologic treatment with corticosteroids is the first choice for complicated hemangiomas; other treatment modalities, including transarterial embolization, are reserved for those rare cases that fail this option.

Further Reading

Argenta LC, David LR, Sanger C, Park C. Advances in hemangioma evaluation and treatment. J Craniofac Surg 2006;17(4):748–755

Lasjaunias P, Berenstein A, terBrugge K. Surgical Neuroangiography. Vol 3: Clinical and Interventional Aspects in Children. 2nd ed. New York, NY: Springer-Verlag; 2006

Mulliken JB, Young AE. Vascular Birthmarks: Hemangiomas and Malformations. Philadelphia: WB Saunders Company; 1988

Song JK, Niimi Y, Berenstein A. Endovascular treatment of hemangiomas. Neuroimaging Clin N Am 2007;17(2):165–173

CASE 36

Case Description

Clinical Presentation

A 50-year-old woman has a history of headaches for nearly a year. One month before admission, she developed numbness of the right side of her face with ataxia. Physical examination shows decreased sensation in the territory of cranial nerve V, mild right-sided facial weakness, and ataxia. No motor weakness is present. MRI is performed, followed by angiography with preoperative embolization.

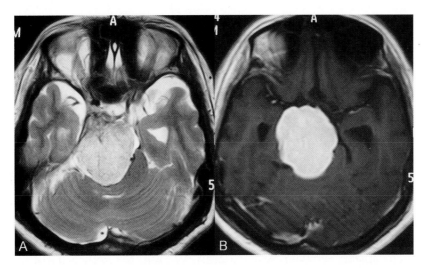

Fig. 36.1 MRI. **(A)** T2-weighted and **(B)** post-gadolinium T1-weighted images.

Radiologic Studies

MRI

MRI revealed a well-defined extra-axial mass lesion at the right petroclival region with hypointense T1/hyperintense T2 signal and intense homogeneous enhancement on a post-contrast study. The lesion caused a significant mass effect on the right side of the pons and midbrain (**Fig. 36.1**). A linear, enhancing dural tail was observed along the clivus. The findings were consistent with the diagnosis of a petroclival meningioma.

DSA

The study demonstrated a hypervascular tumor blush, supplied predominantly by branches of the right meningohypophyseal trunk from the right internal carotid artery (ICA) and meningeal branches from the right neuromeningeal trunk of the right ascending pharyngeal artery (**Fig. 36.2 A,B**). Minimal supply from branches of the left meningohypophyseal trunk and left ascending pharyngeal artery was also observed.

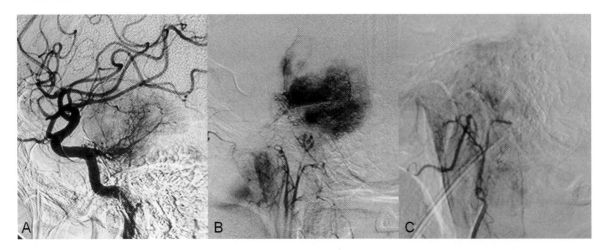

Fig. 36.2 DSA. **(A)** Right ICA and **(B)** right ascending pharyngeal artery angiograms in lateral view demonstrate a hypervascular tumor blush. **(C)** Angiogram of the right ascending pharyngeal artery after particle embolization shows obliteration of the supply to the tumor.

Diagnosis

Right petroclival meningioma

Treatment

EQUIPMENT

- Standard 5F access (puncture needle, 5F vascular sheath)
- Standard 5F multipurpose catheter (Guider Soft Tip; Boston Scientific, Natick, MA) with continuous flush and a 0.035-in hydrophilic guidewire (Terumo, Somerset, NJ)
- A 0.018-in over-the-wire microcatheter (Prowler Select; Cordis, Warren, NJ) with a 0.014-in hydrophilic guidewire (Agility 14; Cordis)
- Polyvinyl alcohol particles (Ivalon), 300 to 500 μm
- Contrast material

DESCRIPTION

Following diagnostic angiography, a 5F multipurpose catheter was advanced into the proximal right external carotid artery (ECA). An over-the-wire microcatheter was introduced over a micro-guidewire into the neuromeningeal trunk of the right ascending pharyngeal artery. A mixture of 300- to 500-μm polyvinyl alcohol particles with contrast media was injected slowly under a blank roadmap until stagnation of the distal branches was observed. The microcatheter was removed, and the 5F multipurpose catheter was advanced into the proximal left ECA. The microcatheter was then placed into the left ascending pharyngeal artery, followed by particle embolization with the same technique. The microcatheter was removed, and the final control run showed obliteration of the external carotid supply to the tumor (**Fig. 36.2C**). Attempts to catheterize the meningohypophyseal trunks from the ICAs failed to reach a safe position for particle or glue embolization. The patient underwent surgical removal of the tumor within 24 hours after the procedure without any complications.

Discussion

Background

Meningiomas are extra-axial tumors arising from arachnoid cells of the meninges, which originate from the neural crest. They account for ~13 to 20% of all primary intracranial tumors and can be found at any location along the arachnoid membrane, most commonly along the cerebral convexity. The peak incidence is at 45 years of age, with a strong female predominance. Malignant lesions are very rare, but metastases may occur by seeding via the cerebrospinal fluid. Extraneural metastases to the lungs, liver, and lymph nodes may also occur. Because most meningiomas are benign and curable tumors, complete surgical resection remains the treatment of choice.

Noninvasive Imaging Workup

CT

- More than 50% of meningiomas are hyperdense on unenhanced CT scans, and calcification can be seen in ~14%. Hypodensity surrounding the tumor is likely related to brain edema. Hyperostosis of the adjacent bone can also be seen on bone window.
- Marked homogeneous enhancement with well-defined borders is typically seen on post-contrast CT.
- Heterogeneous enhancement and tumor necrosis are unusual and suggest a more aggressive lesion.

MRI

- Meningiomas are often homogeneously isointense to the brain parenchyma on T1-weighted sequences and hyperintense on T2-weighted sequences. Areas of flow void may be seen on T2-weighted images, which may represent the highly vascular nature of these lesions and/or calcifications.
- Contrast enhancement is necessary to determine the relationship of a meningioma to adjacent major cerebral arteries and veins.

CTA/MRA

- The use of both CTA and dynamic MRA to determine the vascularity of meningiomas before pre-operative embolization has been reported.
- Enlargement of the feeding arteries, typically from the middle meningeal artery for convexity lesions, can be demonstrated.

Invasive Imaging Workup

- Angiography is usually not required for the diagnosis of a meningioma and is performed in most instances at the time of embolization.
- The major arterial feeders to the center and dural base of a meningioma are typically from dural branches. In larger tumors, recruitment of pial supply from the anterior cerebral artery, middle cerebral artery, posterior cerebral artery, or cerebellar arteries to peripheral parts of the tumor may be seen.
- Intraventricular meningiomas are supplied by the choroidal arteries.

Treatment Options

RADIOSURGERY

- Radiosurgery has been increasingly used in recent years for meningiomas of the skull base. In small lesions, radiosurgery may be applied as a single modality or as an adjunctive treatment for residual tumor after surgical resection.
- In our experience, the aim of radiosurgery is mainly to control tumor growth and recurrence. The size of the tumor usually does not significantly decrease after radiosurgery.

SURGICAL TREATMENT

- Complete surgical resection is the best available treatment.
- Various surgical methods have been used, depending on the location.

ENDOVASCULAR TREATMENT

- Preoperative embolization can help reduce the vascularity of the tumor and therefore decrease blood loss and facilitate complete removal of the tumor during surgery.
- As in the presurgical management of arteriovenous malformations, embolization can be performed to occlude those feeding arteries that will be difficult to reach at surgery. It can also be used to devascularize the tumor bed and induce shrinkage and necrosis, thereby facilitating removal at surgery. The superselectivity required and the embolic material chosen will be different in these two circumstances.
- Delay of surgery for up to 3 weeks after embolization to allow time for maximum tumor necrosis, which softens the tumor and facilitates complete removal, has been reported.
- Although some studies have preferred the use of smaller particles (i.e., 45–150 μm) for maximum tumor necrosis, in our experience, particles of 300 to 500 μm are safer to avoid penetration through the skull base and intratumoral anastomoses with subsequent emboli and ischemic stroke. However, if larger particles are used, as in our case, the optimal surgical timing is within 24 hours.
- The use of permanent liquid embolic agents (i.e., glue and Onyx) has been reported for the preoperative embolization of meningiomas; in our opinion, both should be used with caution because of their ability to penetrate the above-mentioned anastomoses.
- The dural branches arising from the ECAs, usually the middle meningeal artery, are embolized first. The tip of the microcatheter should ideally be placed within or adjacent to the tumor bed. If a good, far-distal position within the arterial feeders from the dural branches of the ICA or vertebral artery (VA) can be obtained, these will subsequently be embolized. In cases of aggressive lesions, recurrent tumors, or young patients, the pial supply may also be embolized to improve the chance for complete resection.
- Swelling of a tumor after embolization may occur very rarely, usually within 48 to 72 hours of the procedure, and may be treated with steroids. This type of complication does not appear to occur when the tumor bed is satisfactorily embolized but may reflect incomplete embolization when there is dual supply from both pial and dural vasculature.

Possible Complications

- Hemorrhage may be intratumoral or may be epidural, subdural, or subarachnoidal when it is due to arterial perforation.

- Stroke or cranial nerve palsies may result from distal embolization through the skull base and intratumoral anastomotic channels.
- Swelling of the tumor may occur after embolization.

Published Literature on Treatment Options

Many studies in previous literature have shown benefits of the preoperative embolization of meningiomas, especially larger ones, to help reduce blood loss during surgery, time required for surgical resection, and length of hospital stay. Blood loss is significantly reduced if the tumor is devascularized more than 90%. In the past, it was generally accepted that the optimal timing for surgery after embolization to reduce the blood loss was within 24 hours; however, this concept has changed in the past years. Several authors have used permanent liquid embolic agents (glue and Onyx), which makes it possible to delay surgery until maximum tumor necrosis and softening occur. This phenomenon also occurs with the use of smaller particles, which penetrate and occlude the capillary bed of the tumor; when these embolic agents are used, the optimal interval between embolization and surgery for tumor softening is 7 to 9 days. The complication rates for the preoperative embolization of meningiomas vary among institutions but are generally accepted to be between 5 and 7%. A significant risk factor for complications is the use of smaller particles or liquid embolic agents. The use of a temporary balloon has been advocated to reduce the chance of stroke during the embolization of branches of the ICAs and VAs.

The balloon can be positioned across the origin of the feeding dural vessel after it has been superselectively catheterized. The balloon is inflated while the embolization is performed via the microcatheter with either particles or liquids. Another method is to position the balloon distal to the tumor-feeding dural branch and inflate the balloon while embolization is performed in the main parent vessel ((ICA, VA) through a microcatheter positioned immediately adjacent to the origin of the tumor-feeding dural branch. Flow into the dural branch must be significant for the embolic material to reach this vessel while the balloon is inflated for distal protection. Once flow to the tumor has greatly diminished, the parent vessel is "cleaned" with repeated injections of saline and either removal of the mixture of blood and saline or intentional flushing of the column down to the external carotid system. The balloon system is then deflated and removed. Obviously, anticoagulation is necessary under these circumstances

PEARLS AND PITFALLS _____

- Most meningiomas are benign tumors, and therefore complete surgical resection is the best treatment modality.
- The major arterial supply to the central tumor and dural attachment is through the meningeal arteries, which in most cases originate from the ECA and can be embolized with a low risk for complications.
- Smaller particles are associated with a higher risk for complications, and liquid embolic agents (e.g., glue and Onyx) should be used carefully because of their ability to penetrate through the skull base and intratumoral anastomoses.
- As in the embolization of arteriovenous malformations, the tip of the microcatheter should ideally be placed as close as possible to the tumor bed. At that point, liquid material or small particles can be gently injected for deeper penetration of the tumor.

Further Reading

Dowd CF, Halbach VV, Higashida RT. Meningiomas: the role of preoperative angiography and embolization. Neurosurg Focus 2003;15(1):E10

Engelhard HH. Progress in the diagnosis and treatment of patients with meningiomas. Part I: diagnostic imaging, preoperative embolization. Surg Neurol 2001;55(2):89–101

Lasjaunias P, Berenstein A, terBrugge K. Surgical Neuroangiography. Vol 2: Clinical and Endovascular Treatment Aspects in Adults. 2nd ed. New York, NY: Springer-Verlag; 2004

Tymianski M, Willinsky RA, Tator CH, Mikulis D, TerBrugge KG, Markson L. Embolization with temporary balloon occlusion of the internal carotid artery and in vivo proton spectroscopy improves radical removal of petrous-tentorial meningioma. Neurosurgery 1994;35(5):974–977, discussion 977

CASE 37

Case Description

Clinical Presentation

An 18-year-old man presents with a history of recurrent episodes of epistaxis for 3 months and progressive stuffiness of the right nostril. His neurologic examination is normal. CT is performed, followed by angiography with preoperative embolization.

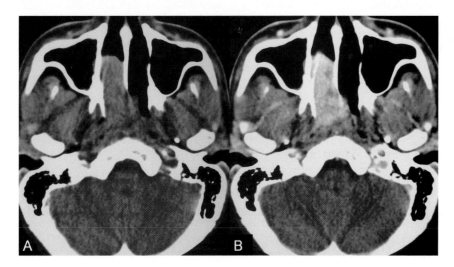

Fig. 37.1 (A) Unenhanced and **(B)** post-contrast axial CT scans at the level of the nasopharynx.

Radiologic Studies

CT

CT showed a slightly hyperdense mass at the right posterior nasal cavity involving the nasal septum and extending into the nasopharynx. Marked, slightly heterogeneous enhancement was seen on a post-contrast study (**Fig. 37.1**). Given the age and sex of the patient, these findings led to the diagnosis of a juvenile angiofibroma.

DSA

The study revealed a hypervascular tumor blush, supplied predominantly by branches of the right internal maxillary artery and ascending palatine artery from the right facial artery (**Fig. 37.2 A,B**). Minimal supply from the mandibular artery of the right internal carotid artery (ICA) through the foramen lacerum was also observed.

Diagnosis

Right-sided juvenile angiofibroma

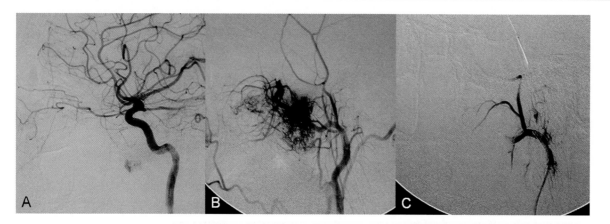

Fig. 37.2 DSA. **(A)** Right ICA and **(B)** right internal maxillary artery angiograms in lateral view. **(C)** Post-particle embolization angiogram of the right internal maxillary artery shows obliteration of the supply to the tumor.

Treatment

EQUIPMENT

- Standard 5F access (puncture needle, 5F vascular sheath)
- Standard 5F multipurpose catheter (Guider Soft Tip; Boston Scientific, Natick, MA) with continuous flush and a 0.035-in hydrophilic guidewire (Terumo, Somerset, NJ)
- A 0.021-in over-the-wire microcatheter (Prowler Select Plus; Cordis, Warren, NJ) with a 0.014-in hydrophilic guidewire (Agility 14; Cordis)
- Polyvinyl alcohol particles (Ivalon), 355 to 500 μm
- Contrast material

DESCRIPTION

Following diagnostic angiography, a 5F multipurpose catheter was advanced into the proximal right external carotid artery. An over-the-wire microcatheter was introduced over a micro-guidewire into the distal internal maxillary artery beyond the origin of the middle meningeal artery. A mixture of 355- to 500-μm polyvinyl alcohol particles with contrast media was injected slowly under a blank roadmap until stagnation of the distal branches was observed. The microcatheter was then advanced into the right ascending palatine artery of the right facial artery, followed by particle embolization with the same technique. The microcatheter was removed, and the final control run showed obliteration of the external carotid supply to the tumor (**Fig. 37.2C**). The patient underwent further surgical removal of the tumor within 24 hours after the procedure without any complications.

Discussion

Background

Juvenile angiofibromas are relatively uncommon tumors of vascular origin that are histologically benign but locally invasive. They account for ~0.5% of all head and neck tumors, typically developing in male adolescents. The peak age is ~14 to 17 years. The clinical symptoms of a juvenile angiofibroma are related directly to its size and extension. The most common are nasal obstruction and epistaxis. The tumor typically originates in the posterior nasal cavity and usually extends to the pterygopalatine fossa. Occasionally, it may arise from the nasal septum. The classification system of Fisch is often employed for staging juvenile angiofibromas; stages I and II tumors are still localized to the nasal cavity, nasopharynx, and pterygopalatine fossa, whereas stages III and IV tumors involve the infratemporal fossa, orbit, and skull base. Complete surgical resection is the best treatment choice; however, local recurrence may be seen in up to 35% of cases. Malignant transformation is extremely rare and in most cases reported in the literature is secondary to radiation therapy.

Noninvasive Imaging Workup

CT

- An intense, rather homogeneously enhancing soft-tissue mass can be identified on unenhanced and post-contrast CT scans. Extension through the pterygopalatine fossa with subsequent expansion is a common finding.
- Bone windows are useful to detect small areas of bone erosion by the tumor.

MRI

- Juvenile angiofibromas usually have an intermediate signal on T1-weighted sequences, compared with the high signal of fat and low signal of muscle, and they have a high signal on T2-weighted sequences. Small flow voids may also be seen on T2-weighted sequences, which are related to the vascularity of the tumor.
- Intense contrast enhancement can be visualized on post-gadolinium T1-weighted sequences, and coronal and sagittal views are necessary for the evaluation of intracranial extension and skull base involvement.

CTA/MRA

- CTA and MRA are not routinely used for the evaluation of juvenile angiofibromas.
- Enlargement of the internal maxillary arteries, which are the major feeding arteries, may be seen. In stages III and IV with skull base involvement, narrowing of the ICAs due to encasement by the tumor may be visualized.

Invasive Imaging Workup

- Angiography is not required for the diagnosis of a juvenile angiofibroma and is performed only before embolization.
- The extracranial portion of the tumor is supplied mainly by branches of the internal maxillary artery, the accessory meningeal artery, the ascending pharyngeal artery, and intrapetrous and intracavernous branches of the ICA, which extend extracranially through the neural foramina.
- Tumors with orbital and skull base extension may recruit additional supply from the ethmoidal branches of the ophthalmic artery and intracranial branches of the intracavernous ICA.

Treatment Options

RADIOSURGERY

- Although the use of radiation alone for the treatment of advanced juvenile angiofibromas (stages III and IV) has been reported, we still believe that radiosurgery should be reserved for cases with residual tumor after surgery because of the possibility of secondary malignant transformation, secondary tumor formation, and other late complications related to radiation.

SURGICAL TREATMENT

- Complete surgical resection is the best available treatment.

- In general, for stages I and II tumors, endoscopic surgery is usually sufficient, and preoperative embolization may not be necessary. A multimodality approach is usually employed for stages III and IV tumors, in which preoperative embolization is followed by radical surgery and possible radiosurgery for residual intracavernous tumor.

ENDOVASCULAR TREATMENT

- Preoperative embolization can help reduce the vascularity of the tumor and therefore decrease blood loss and facilitate complete removal of the tumor during surgery.
- The supplying vessels from the external carotid artery, including the internal maxillary artery, accessory meningeal artery, ascending palatine artery from the facial artery, and ascending pharyngeal arteries, are the major targets of preoperative embolization.
- Particles are the preferred embolic material, and the particle size should be larger than 150 to 200 μm to avoid penetration through the skull base and intratumoral anastomoses. Studies have also shown that because of the presence of micro-arteriovenous shunts within the tumoral bed, the use of smaller particles may result in the formation of pulmonary emboli. In our experience, we usually use 355- to 500-μm polyvinyl alcohol particles for tumor devascularization, followed by Gelfoam strip or tube particles to close the proximal feeding artery.
- The optimal time for surgery is within 24 hours after embolization.
- Percutaneous puncture and direct embolization with liquid agents such as glue or Onyx have been reported for juvenile angiofibromas that are supplied mainly by branches of the ICA; however, experience with this technique is necessary because it carries a significantly higher risk for embolic complications to the brain caused by retrograde penetration of the embolic material through tumoral anastomoses into the ICA.
- In cases with extensive involvement of the skull base, sacrifice of the ICA after a balloon occlusion test may facilitate complete removal of the tumor.

Possible Complications

- Stroke, cranial nerve palsies, or blindness may result from distal embolization through the skull base and intratumoral anastomotic channels.

Published Literature on Treatment Options

Preoperative embolization is currently generally accepted as the standard management of juvenile angiofibromas, particularly large tumors with skull base extension (Fisch stages III and IV). In smaller tumors (stages I and II), several studies have shown that preoperative embolization helps to decrease blood loss during endoscopic surgery, the duration of packing, and length of hospital stay. Although several reports have been published about the direct percutaneous puncture and intratumoral embolization of juvenile angiofibromas, this technique requires significant operator experience to avoid the potentially devastating complications of ICA stroke.

PEARLS AND PITFALLS

- Juvenile angiofibromas are benign, locally aggressive vascular tumors that occur predominantly in male adolescents.
- Complete surgical resection is the best treatment modality and can be facilitated by preoperative embolization, especially in patients with large lesions.

- Smaller particles are associated with a higher risk for complications because of their ability to penetrate through the skull base and intratumoral anastomoses, causing stroke or cranial nerve palsy, and through intratumoral micro-arteriovenous shunts, causing pulmonary emboli.

Further Reading

Andrade NA, Pinto JA, Nóbrega MdeO, Aguiar JE, Aguiar TF, Vinhaes ES. Exclusively endoscopic surgery for juvenile nasopharyngeal angiofibroma. Otolaryngol Head Neck Surg 2007;137(3):492–496

Casasco A, Houdart E, Biondi A, et al. Major complications of percutaneous embolization of skull-base tumors. AJNR Am J Neuroradiol 1999;20(1):179–181

Valavanis A, Christoforidis G. Applications of interventional neuroradiology in the head and neck. Semin Roentgenol 2000;35(1):72–83

CASE 38

Case Description

Clinical Presentation

A 42-year-old man feels a slowly growing mass in his neck below the angle of the mandible. On examination, a nontender mass is palpated in the carotid space that is mobile in the lateral plane but immobile in the craniocaudal plane. There are no signs of pain or dysphagia, and the patient does not experience syncope. Contrast-enhanced MRI is performed.

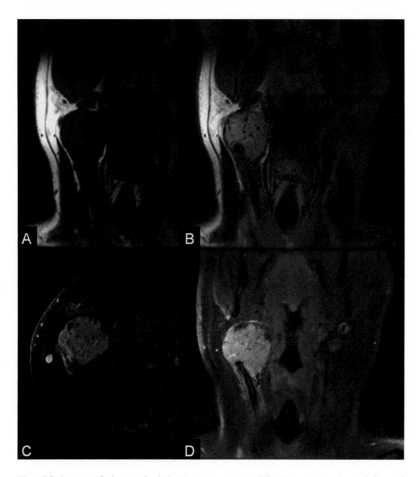

Fig. 38.1 MRI of the neck. **(A)** T1 pre-contrast, **(B)** T1 post-contrast, **(C)** axial fat-suppressed T2, and **(D)** coronal T1 post-contrast fat-suppressed sequences demonstrate an intensely enhancing T2-hyperintense lesion with intralesional flow voids at the carotid bifurcation. This lesion separates the ECA and ICA.

Radiologic Studies

MRI

MRI demonstrated a densely enhancing T2-hyperintense lesion in direct proximity to the right neurovascular bundle with intratumoral flow voids and separation of the external and internal carotid arteries (**Fig. 38.1**). No other tumors were visible.

218

Diagnosis

Carotid body tumor

Treatment

EQUIPMENT

- Standard 6F access (puncture needle, 6F vascular sheath)
- Multipurpose 6F catheter (Envoy; Cordis, Warren, NJ) with continuous flush and a 0.035-in hydrophilic guidewire (Terumo, Somerset, NJ)
- Straight microcatheter (Prowler Plus; Cordis) with a 0.014-in guidewire (Synchro 14; Boston Scientific, Natick, MA)
- Contour polyvinyl alcohol particles, 255 to 350 μm (Boston Scientific)
- Contrast material

DESCRIPTION

Presurgical embolization was requested. Both common carotid arteries (CCAs) and the ipsilateral vertebral artery (VA) were injected to rule out multiplicity. Angiography demonstrated the classic displacement of the internal carotid artery (ICA) versus the external carotid artery (ECA), a sign favoring a carotid body tumor (**Fig. 38.2**). A microcatheter was advanced into the ascending pharyngeal artery, superior laryngeal artery, and facial artery as well as the lingual, inferior laryngeal, and ascending cervical arteries (**Fig. 38.3**). In the former three vessels, a tumor blush was visualized, and particle embolization was performed under negative roadmap conditions with one vial of Contour 255- to 350-μm polyvinyl alcohol particles dissolved in a 50:50 mixture of contrast and saline. Controls were performed via the microcatheter after flushing with saline; particle injection was stopped after visualization of the collateral supply to the arteries supplying the brain. The final control demonstrated nearly complete obliteration of the vascular supply to the tumor, with a residual tiny blush arising from recurrent vasa vasorum of the ICA; these were not further embolized (**Fig. 38.4**).

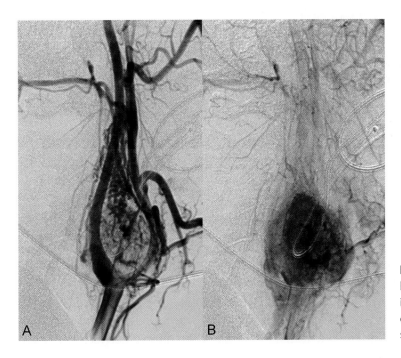

Fig. 38.2 DSA. Right CCA angiogram, lateral view in **(A)** arterial and **(B)** capillary phases demonstrates a hypervascular tumor at the carotid bifurcation separating the ECA and ICA.

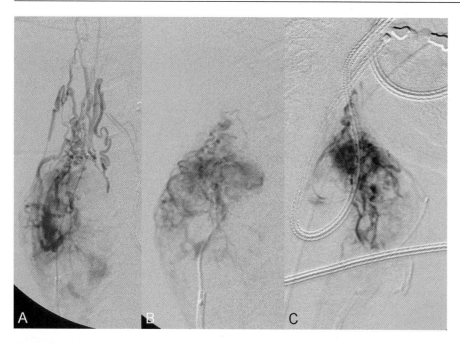

Fig. 38.3 Superselective injections into **(A)** the ascending pharyngeal artery, **(B)** the superior laryngeal artery, and **(C)** the facial artery reveal the arterial supply to the multiple compartments of the tumor.

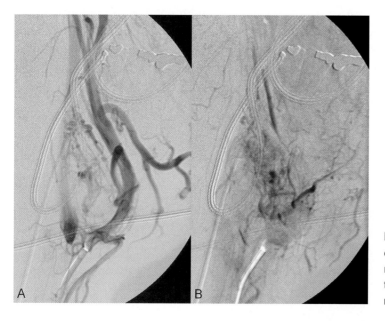

Fig. 38.4 DSA. Right CCA angiogram in lateral view after embolization in **(A)** arterial and **(B)** capillary phases shows nearly total obliteration of the vascular supply to the tumor and minimal residual supply from the vasa vasorum of the ICA.

Discussion

Background

Paragangliomas are slowly growing lesions that arise from nests of chemoreceptor tissue (paraganglia) in various parts of the body. Tumors can be distinguished in four main locations in the head and neck region: the carotid body tumor at the carotid bifurcation, the glomus vagale tumor along the nasopharyngeal and oropharyngeal neurovascular bundle, the glomus jugulare, and the glomus tympanicum (see Case 39). Carotid body tumors are equally distributed between the sexes.

Paragangliomas are multicentric in 5 to 10% of sporadic cases and in 30 to 40% of familial cases; their occurrence may be metachronous. Paragangliomas affect the carotid body in 90% of familial cases (vs. 35% of sporadic cases); in addition, patients are affected at a younger age (40 vs. 55 years), and malignant transformation is more frequent. On histologic examination, carotid body tumors have a highly vascular stroma containing sinusoidal spaces that separate the tumor cells from the bloodstream. Because of the presence of anastomoses between the sinusoids and veins, rapid venous filling during angiography is often noted. These slowly growing benign neoplasms do not regress spontaneously, and all paragangliomas can eventually become malignant or aggressive, so that radical surgery is indicated. The indication is further supported by the fact that only 10% of patients are alive 20 years after the discovery of a paraganglioma.

Noninvasive Imaging Workup

CLINICAL FINDINGS

- The clinical findings are classically related to a mass effect. Carotid body tumors become symptomatic because of endocrine activity in only 1 to 5% of cases. However, because secretory paragangliomas are associated with higher morbidity and mortality rates and because preoperative and intraoperative treatment with α-adrenergic receptor blockers may be required, these patients must be identified.
- Patients who have paragangliomas with endocrine activity experience palpitations, tachycardia, headaches, and repetitive hypertensive crises. Laboratory findings include increased levels of catecholamines in the blood and of normetanephrine and homovanillic acid in the urine.
- Carotid body tumors are nontender masses on examination that are mobile in the lateral plane. They may cause dysphagia and can occasionally transmit the carotid pulse or present with a bruit.
- Extension into the parapharyngeal space, cranial nerve involvement (superior laryngeal nerve leading to hoarseness, descending branch of cranial nerve XII leading to hemiatrophy of the tongue), Horner's syndrome, and stroke from ICA invasion are all rarely seen.

IMAGING FINDINGS

- In patients with carotid body tumors, Doppler and duplex ultrasound show a tumor mass separating the ICA and ECA. The major vessels feeding the tumor can encircle the mass, with smaller vessels extending into the tumor.
- CT demonstrates a densely enhancing mass in the neurovascular bundle. The ECA and ICA are stretched around the mass, which is centered within the carotid bifurcation.
- MRI demonstrates the so-called salt-and-pepper pattern of a well-circumscribed, encapsulated mass. On T2-weighted sequences, serpiginous and punctate flow voids within the mass look like pepper, whereas on T1-weighted sequences, subacute hemorrhage within the tumor looks like salt (methemoglobin on T1-weighted images). Extension into tissue and secondary tumor locations may be seen. Post-contrast, fat-suppressed T1-weighted sequences depict the tumor best.

Invasive Imaging Workup

- The ascending pharyngeal artery always contributes to the supply of a paraganglioma.
- The angiographic protocol should also include arteries supplying the brain (ipsilateral VA and ICA) to demonstrate potentially dangerous anastomotic sites.
- ECA branches (in addition to the ascending pharyngeal artery) that may contribute to the arterial supply of cervical paragangliomas are the facial, lingual, superior and inferior laryngeal, and ascending cervical arteries. In addition, supply via dilated vasa vasorum may be present.

Differential Diagnosis

- A meticulous evaluation of noninvasive images will help to exclude branchial cleft cysts, neurogenic tumors, aneurysm, or dolichocarotid sinus based on the classic findings of hypervascularity and a mass lesion that typically distends the ECA and ICA.

- A glomus vagale tumor can occur at any point along the course of the vagus nerve. Clinically, involvement of the lower cranial nerves (IX–XII) is more often seen. Angiographic images do not show distension of the ICA and ECA but rather anterior and medial displacement of the ICA and compression of the internal jugular vein (**Fig. 38.5**).

Treatment Options

SURGICAL TREATMENT

- Given the extreme vascularity of these tumors, endovascular therapy is typically requested before radical surgical excision.

ENDOVASCULAR TREATMENT

- Endovascular techniques play an adjunctive role in surgical management. The goal of embolization is shrinkage of tumor vascularity to decrease intraoperative blood loss.

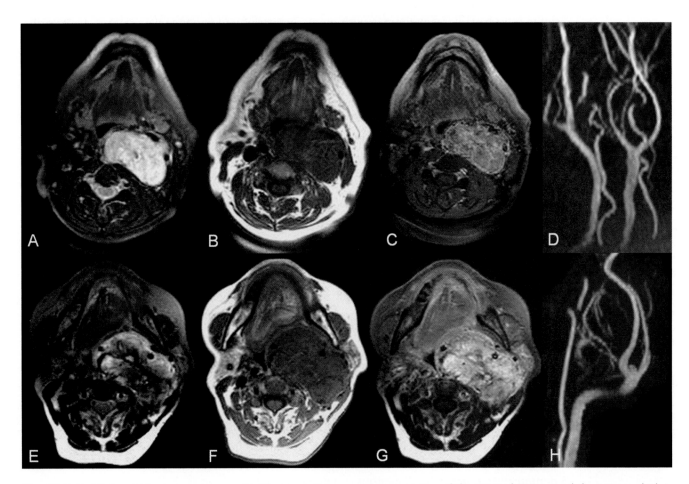

Fig. 38.5 (A–D) Carotid body tumor versus **(E–H)** glomus jugulare tumor. **(A,E)** MRI. T2-weighted, **(B,F)** T1-weighted, **(B,F)** pre-contrast, and **(C,G)** post-contrast sequences. Although the signal characteristics of the tumor matrix are similar, **(D,F)** MRA demonstrates separation of the ICA and ECA around the tumor, which is classic for carotid body tumor, whereas anterior and medial displacement of the ICA and ECA and compression of the jugular vein are typical of a glomus jugulare tumor.

- Embolization with polyvinyl alcohol particles and direct puncture and embolization with liquid materials are potential treatment options.
- Because capillaries within the tumor are 200 μm in diameter, 250- to 350-μm polyvinyl alcohol particles are used in our practice. Particle sizes below 150 μm are not recommended because they may induce skin necrosis, interfere with subsequent wound healing, occlude supply to the cranial nerves, or penetrate via anastomoses into the ICA or VA territories.
- The delay between embolization and surgery is 2 days to 2 weeks, sufficient time for embolization-related edema to decrease but not enough time for recanalization to occur.
- Particles are prepared in a diluted suspension and injected via a microcatheter as microboluses. The process is monitored with negative fluoroscopy.
- The pattern of flow is monitored throughout the procedure to avoid opening anastomoses.

Possible Complications

- Fever and pain may occur following particle embolization.
- Cranial nerve palsy and stroke may occur if dangerous anastomoses and supply to the cranial nerves are ignored.
- Skin or muscle necrosis or delayed wound healing may occur if a particle size that is too small is chosen.

Published Literature on Treatment Options

Whether or not a carotid body tumor is difficult to resect depends on its relation to the surrounding vessels. Adherence to the ICA or ECA or encasement of an artery will lead to a higher incidence of cerebrovascular complications and permanent cranial nerve impairment; the rates are in the range of 5% for cerebrovascular complications and 20% for permanent cranial nerve impairment if the tumor encases the carotid arteries. The surgical resection of paragangliomas can be complicated by profuse bleeding due to the extreme vascularity of these lesions. Preoperative embolization can reduce intraoperative blood loss significantly, especially in the case of vagal and jugulotympanic paragangliomas. For tumors in these locations, an occlusion test is also recommended to assess the possibility of sacrificing the ICA during radical surgery. Optimal therapy requires a multidisciplinary approach and is therefore likely to differ from center to center. Preoperative embolization is considered a safe adjuvant to surgery and is therefore widely employed.

PEARLS AND PITFALLS

- Multicentricity is seen in 10% of sporadic cases and in 30 to 40% of familial cases.
- The average age of patients with a paraganglioma is 55 years; in younger patients, the tumors tend to grow more rapidly, and they are more likely to involve cranial nerves and exhibit endocrine activity.
- In locations (high altitudes) where chronic hypoxia is endemic, these tumors occur 10 times more frequently.
- The ascending pharyngeal artery is the vessel that supplies each and every paraganglioma.

Further Reading

Geibprasert S, Pongpech S, Armstrong D, Krings T. Dangerous extracranial-intracranial anastomoses and supply to the cranial nerves: vessels the neurointerventionalist needs to know. AJNR Am J Neuroradiol 2009;30(8):1459–1468

Kasper GC, Welling RE, Wladis AR, et al. A multidisciplinary approach to carotid paragangliomas. Vasc Endovascular Surg 2006;40(6):467–474

Knight TT Jr, Gonzalez JA, Rary JM, Rush DS. Current concepts for the surgical management of carotid body tumor. Am J Surg 2006;191(1):104–110

Valavanis A, Christoforidis G. Applications of interventional neuroradiology in the head and neck. Semin Roentgenol 2000;35(1):72–83

van den Berg R. Imaging and management of head and neck paragangliomas. Eur Radiol 2005;15(7):1310–1318

CASE 39

Case Description

Clinical Presentation

A 53-year-old woman presented in 1992 with a left-sided glomus tympanicum tumor. She underwent embolization and surgical resection at that time. Seventeen years later, she presents with significant recurrence, and a translabyrinthine removal of the tumor is planned. She is referred to our service for preoperative embolization of this hypervascular lesion.

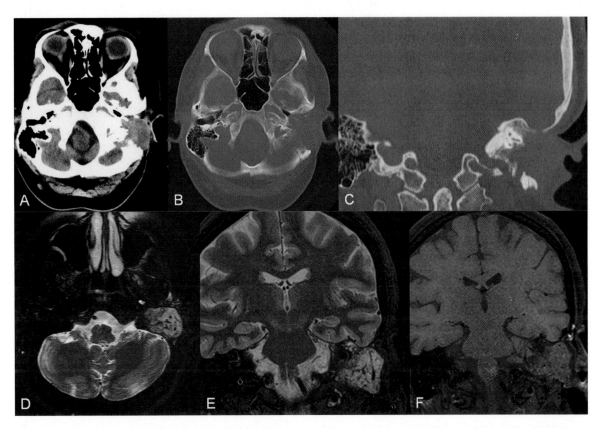

Fig. 39.1 **(A)** Unenhanced axial CT and bone windows in **(B)** axial and **(C)** coronal reformats show extension into the left petrous pyramid with bone destruction and erosion of the carotid canal. **(D)** Axial and **(E)** coronal T2-weighted and **(F)** coronal T1-weighted pre-contrast fat-suppressed MR sequences demonstrate extensive tumor within the left temporal bone with a classic "salt and pepper" pattern, corresponding to a glomus tumor.

Radiologic Studies

CT AND MRI

CT and MRI demonstrated an erosive tumor of the temporal bone with the classic "salt and pepper" pattern of a glomus tumor (**Fig. 39.1**). There was extension into the petrous pyramid with extensive erosion of the vertical section of the carotid canal but no evidence of erosion of the horizontal portion of the carotid canal (Fisch grade C2).

225

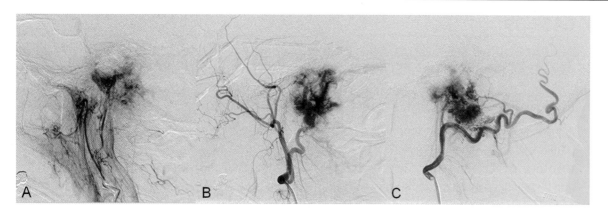

Fig. 39.2 Selective DSA of **(A)** the ascending pharyngeal artery, **(B)** the posterior auricular artery, and **(C)** the occipital artery in lateral view demonstrates the vascular supply of three different tumor compartments before embolization.

DSA

On angiography, the vertebral artery (VA) and right common carotid artery (CCA) appeared normal; however, extensive right-sided external carotid artery (ECA) supply to the tumor was demonstrated (**Fig. 39.2**).

Diagnosis

Recurrent temporal paraganglioma

Treatment

EQUIPMENT

- Standard 6F access (puncture needle, 6F vascular sheath)
- Multipurpose 6F catheter (Envoy; Cordis, Warren, NJ) with continuous flush and a 0.035-in hydro-philic guidewire (Terumo, Somerset, NJ)
- Straight microcatheter (Prowler Plus; Cordis) with a 0.014-in guidewire (Synchro 14; Boston Scientific, Natick, MA)
- Contour polyvinyl alcohol particles, 255 to 350 μm (Boston Scientific)
- Gelfoam pledgets
- Fibered coils (VortX; Boston Scientific) with a coil pusher (Boston Scientific)
- Contrast material

DESCRIPTION

First, the occipital artery was selected; here, multiple small vessels were seen to arise from the artery proximal to the anastomosis with the VA. In addition, larger feeders were present distal to the anastomosis. Distal embolization was performed with polyvinyl alcohol particles (250–355 μm) until stasis was achieved. The microcatheter was withdrawn to the level of the anastomosis between the occipital artery and VA. Here, three fibered coils were placed to occlude the vertebral anastomosis in an effort to protect it from subsequent embolization. The catheter was further withdrawn into the proximal occipital artery, where additional embolization of the tumor with polyvinyl alcohol particles could now be done safely, until stagnation was observed (**Fig. 39.3**). A Gelfoam pledget was placed in the occipital trunk. The posterior auricular artery was embolized in a similar fashion following control angiography to exclude any anastomoses to the brain or arteries supplying the

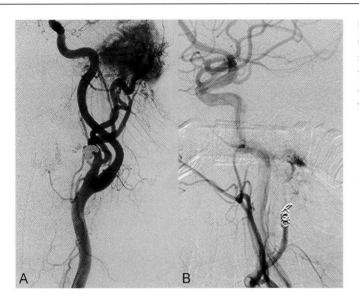

Fig. 39.3 Left CCA angiograms in lateral view **(A)** before and **(B)** after embolization demonstrate an 85% reduction in tumor vascularization. Note the coils deployed within the occipital artery to prevent the particles from entering the vertebral anastomosis.

cranial nerves (in particular, the facial nerve arcade). Finally, the ascending pharyngeal artery was catheterized, and embolization was performed with repeated control runs to exclude any opening of potential anastomoses to the VA or carotid artery. After significant reduction of the tumor supply, we found both the anastomosis to the VA and, via the clival branch, an anastomosis to the internal carotid artery (ICA). There was still some residual feeding to the tumor; however, we felt that further particle embolization, given the significant risk for reflux into these anastomoses, was not warranted. The patient awoke without neurologic deficits and proceeded to surgery the next day.

Discussion

Background

Paragangliomas constitute 0.6% of all head and neck tumors, but they are the second most common neoplasm of the temporal bone (following neurogenic tumors) and the most common neoplasm of the middle ear. Paragangliomas with a temporal bone origin account for 50% of all paragangliomas and have a female preponderance. General considerations regarding paragangliomas were presented in Case 38; the discussion in this case focuses on glomus tympanicum and glomus jugulare paragangliomas. These temporal paragangliomas arise from paraganglionic tissue along the tympanic branch of the glossopharyngeal nerve (Jacobson's nerve) and the auricular branch of the vagus nerve (Arnold's nerve), which together with the vagus nerve will form the jugular ganglion. The tumors can arise anywhere along these nerves, and their point of origin and route of spread determine their names. Glomus tympanicum tumors abut the cochlear promontory of the medial wall of the middle ear cavity, leaving the inferior walls of the middle ear cavity intact. Glomus jugulotympanicum tumors originate in the jugular foramen and then invade the middle ear; thus, their location is superolateral to the jugular foramen and below the middle ear cavity. Classically, the bony floor of the middle ear cavity is invaded and the jugular spine is eroded. Glomus jugulare tumors arise from the adventitia of the jugular vein and present as a mass in the jugular foramen. Their pattern of spread follows the path of least resistance (mastoid air cell tract, vascular channel, eustachian tube, neural foramen), and they are associated with a moth-eaten pattern of destruction of the temporal bone. Dehiscence of the inferior wall of the tympanic cavity indicates involvement of the mesotympanum and ossicles, whereas involvement of the bony labyrinth is associated with medial spread from middle ear locations.

Noninvasive Imaging Workup

CLINICAL FINDINGS

- Patients with a tympanic paraganglioma experience unilateral pulsatile tinnitus, and a vascular retrotympanic mass is visible on inspection. The tinnitus is subjective and early (because of promontory bone conduction), and it worsens during effort, the Valsalva maneuver, or cervical vascular compression. Involvement of the facial nerve is present in one-third of patients in the early phase, with spontaneous regression, and is believed to be due to transient arterial steal. Late clinical findings are disappearance of the tinnitus (because of cochlear destruction) with conductive and perceptive hearing loss, otorrhagia, and involvement of the lower cranial nerves due to late extension to the jugular bulb.
- Patients with jugular paragangliomas have jugular foramen syndromes. These include lower cranial nerve palsy (Vernet syndrome: cranial nerves IX, X, and XI; Collet-Sicard syndrome: Vernet syndrome plus cranial nerve XII); hypoglossal neuralgia; retro-auricular pain; and intermittent pulsatile or nonpulsatile tinnitus due to turbulent flow in the jugular vein.

IMAGING FINDINGS

- For patients with temporal paragangliomas, imaging must define the Fisch and Valavanis grade because this will determine treatment strategies.
  - A: tympanic cavity only
  - B: extension into mastoid cells
  - C: extension into petrous pyramid; C1: minimal erosion of the vertical section of the carotid canal; C2: extensive erosion; C3: C2 plus erosion of the horizontal portion of the carotid canal; C4: tumor reaching the foramen lacerum and cavernous sinus
  - Type D: intracranial and intradural extension; D1: < 2 cm, D2: > 2 cm
- CT and MRI demonstrate a densely enhancing, globular soft-tissue mass, the location and extent of which determine its name and grade.

Invasive Imaging Workup

- Angiographic workup must include global CCA, ICA, and ECA runs; both ascending pharyngeal arteries; and the ipsilateral VA (including venous phases for the evaluation of jugular vein occlusion). Supply may arise from the extradural branches of the vertebral artery at C1 through C3, and intradurally from the ipsilateral anterior and posterior inferior cerebellar arteries and the posterior auricular artery.
- Superselective injection of all arteries supplying the paraganglioma will demonstrate whether a "mono"-compartmental or "multi"-compartmental paraganglioma is present. Monocompartmental paragangliomas are found in 15% of cases and can be completely embolized through a single feeder.

Differential Diagnosis

- Vascular variations that must be differentiated from a temporal paraganglioma are a prominent jugular bulb and an intratympanic "aberrant" course of the ICA.
- Tumors that may mimic temporal paragangliomas are tympanic granulomas, neurogenic tumors, meningiomas, metastases, and hemangiomas.

Treatment Options

ENDOVASCULAR TREATMENT

- The extent of the arterial supply can be deduced in part from the extent and location of the lesion. Contributions from the petrosal branch of the middle meningeal artery, clival branches of the ICA, or meningeal branches of the VA can be anticipated if intracranial extradural involvement is present. Intradural involvement implies additional supply from the anterior or posterior inferior cerebellar artery.
- During embolization, careful attention must be paid to anastomoses with arteries supplying the brain.
- Occlusion of the ICA may have to be considered in cases of extensive destruction of the horizontal portion of the carotid canal (Fisch grade C3) or tumor within the foramen lacerum (Fisch grade C4).
- Particle embolization is followed by proximal Gelfoam embolization and is used for presurgical embolization.
- For palliative embolization without subsequent surgery, liquid agents may have to be used.

Possible Complications

See also Case 38.

- Embolization of the ascending pharyngeal artery with liquid agents may lead to lower cranial nerve palsy and is therefore not recommended.

Published Literature on Treatment Options

Treatment options for paragangliomas include microsurgical resection, radiation therapy, and embolization, or any combination of these modalities. In many centers, radical surgical removal is the treatment of choice and is indicated when the tumor is still small and resection is associated with a relative low risk. Size and extent, location, and multicentricity are important factors that determine the possibility of resecting a tumor with acceptable morbidity. Adjuvant endovascular treatments can decrease surgical risks; the preoperative embolization of paragangliomas larger than 3 cm reduces operative bleeding and shortens the duration of surgery.

Stereotactic radiosurgery has been proposed as an alternative treatment for tumors that cannot be resected. In the majority of cases reported, stabilization of tumor growth or even reduction of tumor size was noted; however, long-term follow-up is not yet available. Compared with surgical case series, there seems to be a lower rate of treatment-related morbidity but a higher rate of tumor recurrence.

Embolization alone can control tumor growth, with regression of symptoms following aggressive embolization, and this strategy may be employed as a palliative treatment. In addition to transarterial embolization, direct puncture embolization can be considered for the palliative management of paragangliomas of the head and neck.

PEARLS AND PITFALLS

- Although temporal paragangliomas are rare, they are the second most common neoplasm of the temporal bone and the most common neoplasm of the middle ear.
- Direct puncture for the treatment of a paraganglioma with a liquid embolic agent may lead to reflux into brain-supplying arteries that are not necessarily evident and seen during the direct micro-injections. A complete angiographic workup before direct puncture is therefore warranted.

Further Reading

Abud DG, Mounayer C, Benndorf G, Piotin M, Spelle L, Moret J. Intratumoral injection of cyanoacrylate glue in head and neck paragangliomas. AJNR Am J Neuroradiol 2004;25(9):1457–1462

Al-Mefty O, Teixeira A. Complex tumors of the glomus jugulare: criteria, treatment, and outcome. J Neurosurg 2002;97(6):1356–1366

Geibprasert S, Pongpech S, Armstrong D, Krings T. Dangerous extracranial-intracranial anastomoses and supply to the cranial nerves: vessels the neurointerventionalist needs to know. AJNR Am J Neuroradiol 2009;30(8):1459–1468

Gottfried ON, Liu JK, Couldwell WT. Comparison of radiosurgery and conventional surgery for the treatment of glomus jugulare tumors. Neurosurg Focus 2004;17(2):E4

Moret J, Lasjaunias P, Théron J. Vascular compartments and territories of tympano-jugular glomic tumors. J Belge Radiol 1980;63(2-3):321–337

Valavanis A, Christoforidis G. Applications of interventional neuroradiology in the head and neck. Semin Roentgenol 2000;35(1):72–83

Valavanis A, Fisch U. The contribution of computed tomography to the management of glomus tumors of the temporal bone. Rev Laryngol Otol Rhinol (Bord) 1983;104(5):411–415

van den Berg R. Imaging and management of head and neck paragangliomas. Eur Radiol 2005;15(7):1310–1318

CASE 40

Case Description

Clinical Presentation

A 50-year-old man with underlying von Hippel-Lindau disease presents with progressive weakness and numbness of the legs. He previously underwent surgical resection of a cervical hemangioblastoma. MRI is performed and surgical resection of lesions at T6 and T10-T11 is scheduled, to be preceded by spinal angiography and preoperative embolization.

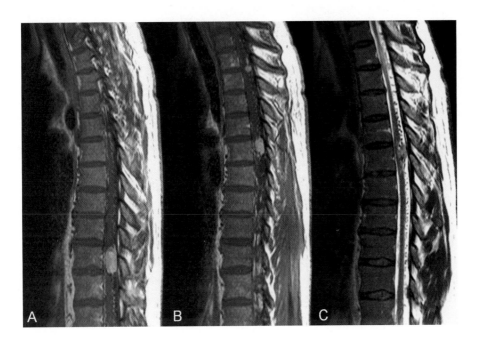

Fig. 40.1 MRI. **(A,B)** Post-gadolinium T1-weighted and **(C)** T2-weighted images.

Radiologic Studies

MRI

MRI demonstrated multiple, intensely enhancing, hyperintense T2 signal nodules located predominantly at the dorsal surface of the cord at the thoracic level. The largest lesions were located at T6 and T10-T11, with surrounding multiple flow voids suggestive of increased vascularity (**Fig. 40.1**). Mildly hyperintense T2 signal change of the cord was observed at the T2-T3 and T6 levels. These findings were consistent with multiple spinal hemangioblastomas.

DSA

Spinal angiography was performed under general anesthesia with a 4F Cobra II catheter. Injection of the right T8 segmental artery revealed a large radiculomedullary artery contributing to the anterior spinal artery, which had a small ascending and a large descending limb. In addition, a large posterior spinal artery arising from the radiculopial artery from this segmental artery supplied a large, prominent tumor blush at the upper margin of the T6 vertebral body, slightly to the right of midline. A tiny tumor blush was also noted at the upper T8 vertebral body level (**Fig. 40.2**). Additional injections of

231

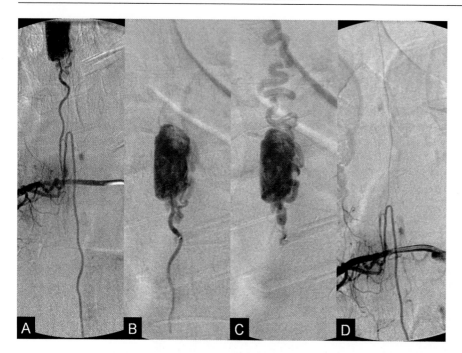

Fig. 40.2 DSA. **(A)** Right T8 segmental artery injection. Selective injections within the radiculopial artery in **(B)** late arterial and **(C)** venous phase demonstrate tumor blush and prominent veins draining the tumor. **(D)** Post-embolization injection of the right T8 segmental artery shows devascularization of the tumor with preservation of the radiculo-medullary artery and anterior spinal artery.

the left T12 segmental artery demonstrated a small to moderately sized but tortuous posterior spinal artery, which ascended and supplied a blush at the posterior aspect of the tumor at the T10-T11 level, and the right L1 segmental artery showed a large posterior spinal artery supplying several small tumor nodules, mostly around the right side of the cord at the T12 and L1 levels (not shown).

Diagnosis

Multiple spinal hemangioblastomas

Treatment

EQUIPMENT

- Standard 4F access (puncture needle, 4F vascular sheath)
- Standard 4F Cobra (Cook Medical, Bloomington, IN) and 4F multipurpose (Cook Medical) catheters with continuous flush and a 0.035-in hydrophilic guidewire (Terumo, Somerset, NJ)
- A 0.012-in flow-directed microcatheter (Magic; Balt International, Montmorency, France) with a 0.008-in guidewire (Mirage; ev3, Plymouth, MN)
- A 10% glucose solution
- Histoacryl/Lipiodol (16%)
- Contrast material

DESCRIPTION

Following diagnostic angiography, the patient was fully heparinized, and the 4F Cobra catheter was exchanged for a 4F multipurpose catheter, with the tip placed well into the right T8 segmental artery. With roadmap technique, the flow-directed microcatheter was advanced into the radiculopial artery, which supplied the dense tumor blush at T6. Superselective injection confirmed that this artery almost exclusively supplied the large tumor, with no additional significant cord-supplying branches seen. The tip of the microcatheter was advanced as close as possible to the tumor. A 16% mixture of Histoacryl and Lipiodol was prepared and injected via the posterior spinal artery into the tumor. Some penetration of the tumor was achieved, as well as an arterial ligation of the distal posterior spinal artery that supplied the tumor. The microcatheter was removed, and a post-embolization diagnostic run in the right T8 segmental artery through the guiding catheter showed devascularization of the tumor with preservation of the radiculomedullary artery and anterior spinal artery (**Fig. 40.2D**). There was stagnation of the radiculopial artery, which was occluded at the level of the glue embolization. The guiding catheter was then withdrawn. The supply to the tumor at the T10-T11 level was too tortuous to be catheterized safely. The patient awoke without neurological deficit and was operated upon two days later with no significant perioperative blood loss.

Discussion

Background

Spinal hemangioblastomas are rare benign vascular tumors that account for 1 to 7% of all spinal tumors. Approximately two-thirds of cases are sporadic, and the remaining one-third are associated with von Hippel-Lindau disease. The lesions are single in 80% of cases; the thoracic spine is the most common location, followed by the cervical spine. The tumors are more commonly located dorsal to the cord. Complete surgical removal is the treatment of choice for symptomatic hemangioblastomas, with preoperative embolization reserved for extensive and hypervascular lesions. Preoperative embolization for cerebellar hemangioblastomas can be very helpful before the surgical removal of large, hypervascular tumors but can be associated with a high rate of post-procedural ischemia, hemorrhage, and mortality.

Von Hippel-Lindau disease is a rare, autosomal-dominant, multisystem disorder characterized by the development of multiple benign and malignant tumors. The condition is associated with inactivation of the tumor suppressor gene located on chromosome 3p25.5. Currently, the most common causes of death in patients with von Hippel-Lindau disease are renal cell carcinoma and neurologic complications of cerebellar hemangioblastomas. The diagnosis can be made based on the presence of (1) more than one central nervous system hemangioblastoma, (2) one central nervous system hemangioblastoma with visceral manifestations of von Hippel-Lindau disease, or (3) any manifestation in a patient with a known family history.

Noninvasive Imaging Workup

CT

- CT is not routinely used for the investigation of spinal hemangioblastomas.
- A cerebellar hemangioblastoma is typically seen as a partly cystic, partly nodular mass in the cerebellar hemisphere or vermis with a slightly hyperdense mural nodule that enhances intensely on the post-contrast study. The cyst and its walls usually do not show any enhancement.

MRI

- Spinal hemangioblastomas are solid in ~25% of cases, whereas the remainder usually have mixed solid and cystic components. The solid component always shows intense enhancement with occasional intralesional hemorrhage. The tumors are typically located superficially on the dorsal surface of the cord and may be associated with a syrinx in up to 60 to 70% of cases. Intratumoral flow voids and prominent posterior draining veins are often detected, especially in large lesions.

Surrounding edema within the cord can also be seen. In some rare cases, extensive edema involving a large area of the spinal cord is noted in patients with multiple hemangioblastomas, producing venous hypertension similar to that occurring in spinal dural arteriovenous fistulae.

- MRI findings for cerebellar hemangioblastomas are similar to the CT findings, with varying cystic components and a solid nodule. Occasionally, subtle hemorrhage within the lesion may be detected on MRI.

CTA/MRA

- CTA and MRA are not routinely used for the evaluation of spinal hemangioblastomas because of the small size of the feeding arteries.
- Enlarged arterial feeders may be seen supplying large mural nodules in cerebellar hemangioblastomas.

Invasive Imaging Workup

- Dilated arteries, a prominent tumor blush, and enlarged draining veins on spinal angiography are characteristic of spinal hemangioblastomas. Given their dorsal location, the major supply to the tumors is usually from the radiculopial arteries but may occasionally be through vasa corona branches from the anterior spinal artery.
- The angiographic findings are similar for cerebellar hemangioblastomas. Angiography may help detect the smaller lesions that are often associated with von Hippel-Lindau disease.

Treatment Options

RADIOSURGERY

- There have been several reports of radiosurgery or radiotherapy for the treatment of spinal hemangioblastomas related to von Hippel-Lindau disease; however, in our opinion, surgical removal remains the best treatment option if it is possible.

SURGICAL TREATMENT

- Complete surgical resection is the best treatment modality for spinal hemangioblastomas.

ENDOVASCULAR TREATMENT

- The preoperative embolization of spinal hemangioblastomas is technically challenging because of their small size and the tortuosity of the feeding arteries.
- In our institution, embolization is done only if the supply is from a radiculopial artery (posterior spinal artery-axis). If the supply is from the anterior spinal artery-axis, the risk for embolization is too high and outweighs the benefits.
- We tend to use permanent liquid agents (glue) for embolization because of the small size of the feeding arteries.
- Periprocedural heparin is recommended.
- The preoperative embolization of cerebellar hemangioblastomas is recommended only for those lesions that are large and hypervascular. Because these tumors are fed by branches that also supply the healthy surrounding brain, extreme care must be taken to deposit the embolic material within the tumor, and reflux is obviously to be avoided. Therefore, the tip of the microcatheter must be as close as possible to the tumor bed, and the liquid embolic agent must be injected very gently, avoiding any reflux. Inadvertent embolization of healthy posterior fossa vessels will be associated with post-procedural ischemia or hemorrhage, potentially causing significant morbidity, delay of surgery, or even death.

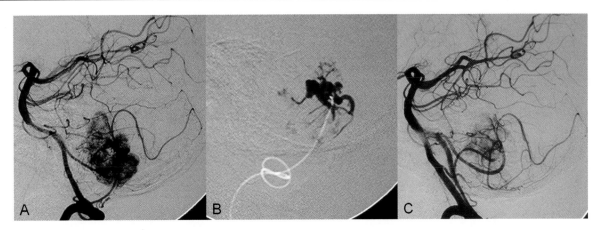

Fig. 40.3 DSA in a 56-year-old man with a cerebellar hemangioblastoma. Right vertebral artery angiograms in lateral view **(A)** before, **(B)** during, and **(C)** after embolization demonstrating a tumor blush supplied mainly by branches of the right posterior inferior cerebellar artery, which has an extradural origin. Note that the glue case only minimally penetrates the intratumoral bed and mainly closes the feeding arteries (ligation embolization).

Possible Complications

- Spinal ischemia may result from reflux of the embolic material into the normal cord supply.

Published Literature on Treatment Options

The treatment for symptomatic spinal hemangioblastomas is surgical removal. Preoperative embolization has been recommended for large and hypervascular lesions; in most smaller spinal lesions, it is not necessary. Preoperative embolization for hemangioblastomas within the cerebellum remains controversial. In a small series of five patients reported by Eskridge et al in 1996, preoperative particle embolization helped reduce blood loss during surgery, but worsening of hydrocephalus developed in one patient because of tumor swelling. In a series of three patients, Cornelius et al reported that intratumoral hemorrhage developed in all patients after the procedure, and they subsequently died. The authors suspected that the particles that they had used (100–300 μm in size) penetrated the capillary bed, causing intratumoral venous obstruction and hemorrhage. In our experience, we have successfully treated several cerebellar hemangioblastomas with glue embolization, without any complications (**Fig. 40.3**). Particles larger than 300 μm may also be used safely with the same goal. It is worthwhile to note that only complete embolization helps to reduce complications and morbidity during surgery; therefore, the risk of partial embolization must be weighed against its questionable benefits for surgery.

PEARLS AND PITFALLS

- The presence of multiple central nervous system hemangioblastomas suggests von Hippel-Lindau disease.
- Surgery is the best treatment modality for central nervous system hemangioblastomas, and the benefits of preoperative embolization are still controversial. Risk and benefits should be evaluated based on the experience of each institution.
- The preoperative embolization of spinal hemangioblastomas can be done relatively safely through the radiculopial arteries.

Further Reading

Cornelius JF, Saint-Maurice JP, Bresson D, George B, Houdart E. Hemorrhage after particle embolization of hemangioblastomas: comparison of outcomes in spinal and cerebellar lesions. J Neurosurg 2007;106(6):994–998

Eskridge JM, McAuliffe W, Harris B, Kim DK, Scott J, Winn HR. Preoperative endovascular embolization of craniospinal hemangioblastomas. AJNR Am J Neuroradiol 1996;17(3):525–531

Tampieri D, Leblanc R, TerBrugge K. Preoperative embolization of brain and spinal hemangioblastomas. Neurosurgery 1993;33(3):502–505, discussion 505

CASE 41

Case Description

Clinical Presentation

A 49-year-old man with a history of renal cell carcinoma is admitted to our hospital with low back pain, numbness in the groin, incontinence, and lower extremity muscle weakness and paresthesias that have been slowly progressive over the past week. Examination reveals local pain around the upper lumbar spine, reduced lower extremity reflexes, and loss of anal tone. MRI is performed to elucidate the nature of the cauda equina syndrome, followed by CT.

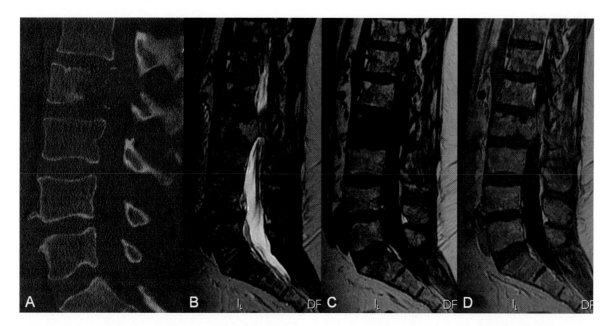

Fig. 41.1 **(A)** Sagittal CT reconstruction in bone window. **(B)** Sagittal T2-weighted and T1-weighted **(C)** pre-contrast and **(D)** post-contrast MR sequences of the lumbar spine demonstrate pathologic fracture of the L2 vertebral body with bone destruction and an associated mass lesion. Extension into the epidural sac is causing moderate spinal stenosis and nerve root compression.

Radiologic Studies

MRI AND CT

MRI demonstrated a destructive and strongly enhancing bony lesion at the L2 vertebral body. The lesion occupied the right posterior aspect and extended through the pedicle to the right transverse process and lamina of L2. Extension into the epidural space surrounding the epidural sac anteriorly and onto the right lateral aspect was causing moderate spinal stenosis with compression of the nerve roots of the cauda equina. The involved vertebral body was collapsed (**Fig. 41.1**). CT confirmed the mass and demonstrated its destructive nature.

Diagnosis

Spinal vertebral renal cell metastasis with vertebral body collapse and cauda equina syndrome

Treatment

EQUIPMENT

- Standard 5F access (puncture needle, 5F vascular sheath)
- 5F Cobra C2 glide catheter (Cook Medical, Bloomington, IN) with continuous flush and a 0.035-in hydrophilic guidewire (Terumo, Somerset, NJ)
- Straight microcatheter (Fast Tracker 18; Boston Scientific, Natick, MA) with a 0.014-in guidewire (Synchro 14; Boston Scientific)
- Contour polyvinyl alcohol particles, 355 to 500 μm (Boston Scientific)
- Contrast material

DESCRIPTION

Bilateral diagnostic spinal angiography was performed from T9 to L3. Supply to the anterior spinal artery was seen from the left T11 segmental artery, and supply to the posterolateral spinal artery was seen from the right T11 level. A marked tumor blush was visible after injection into the right L2 and L1 segmental arteries. No supply to the spinal cord was visualized from either level. Under roadmap guidance, the microcatheter was advanced into the segmental arteries at L1 and L2. Particle embolization was performed under negative roadmap conditions with two vials of 355- to 500-μm Contour polyvinyl alcohol particles dissolved in a 50:50 mixture of contrast and saline. Controls were performed after removal of the microcatheter in each pedicle at regular intervals to verify the result of embolization and to demonstrate that no spinal cord supply was visible following embolization of the tumor. Controls demonstrated nearly complete obliteration of the vascular supply to the vertebral metastasis (**Fig. 41.2**).

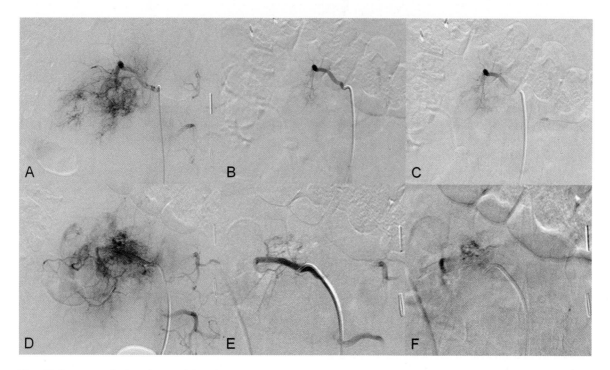

Fig. 41.2 DSA. Right **(A–C)** L1 and **(D–F)** L2 segmental artery angiograms **(A,D)** before and after embolization in **(B,E)** early arterial and **(C,F)** capillary phases reveal nearly complete obliteration of the vascular supply to the hypervascular vertebral metastasis.

Discussion

Background

Tumors metastasize to the spine in 30 to 70% of cases; common primary cancers are breast, lung, prostate, and renal cell carcinomas. Depending on the primary lesion, the vertebrae affected by metastatic disease will demonstrate extensive vascularity, with renal cell and thyroid carcinoma metastases the most vascular. Surgical resection of these hypervascular spinal metastases may lead to life-threatening loss of blood intraoperatively. The amount of blood lost depends on the degree of hypervascularity, the size and extent of the lesion, and the complexity and duration of surgery. Preoperative embolization to devascularize the tumor is therefore carried out in most centers.

Noninvasive Imaging Workup

CLINICAL FINDINGS

- The most common presenting symptom is back pain, which is often localized to the affected vertebral body. Pathologic fractures may occur. Neurologic deficits can result from spinal cord compression; nerve root compression due to neuroforaminal narrowing can also be seen.
- If symptomatic spinal cord compression is present, recovery from neurologic deficits is unlikely unless decompression is accomplished within 24 to 48 hours after the onset of symptoms.

IMAGING FINDINGS

- Plain films have the lowest sensitivity and may be used in the acute context to evaluate whether pathologic fractures are present.
- CT is able to differentiate lytic from sclerotic metastases, the latter suggesting prostate cancer, carcinoid, or sarcoma as the primary tumor.
- MRI is the method of choice to evaluate the metastatic spine. It has the highest sensitivity and can demonstrate associated soft-tissue expansion of the tumor as well as the degree of spinal cord compression.

Invasive Imaging Workup

- Angiography will demonstrate the origin of the feeding arteries, the degree of hypervascularity, and the origin of the spinal cord arterial supply. In most instances, embolization is performed in the same session as the diagnostic angiography
- For lesions of the cervical spine, injections into the vertebral arteries, thyrocervical trunk, costocervical trunk, and external carotid arteries are mandatory.
- For lesions of the thoracic and lumbar spine, the segmental arteries within at least two levels above and two levels below the tumor site should be visualized.
- For lower lumbar and sacral lesions, the lumbar arteries, medial sacral arteries, and internal iliac arteries must be visualized.

Differential Diagnosis

- Hemangiomas demonstrate a vertically striated pattern on plain films (corresponding to the "polka-dot" pattern seen on CT), and they have a higher signal on T1- and T2-weighted sequences. They may be expansile, and if neurologic symptoms occur, therapy may be warranted, including vertebroplasty, surgical removal, and palliative or curative embolization.

- Aneurysmal bone cysts are benign vascular lesions that present with pain and appear as expansile lytic lesions with a thin, intact cortical rim on CT. MRI will demonstrate a lobular lesion with septa and blood-fluid levels. The therapy of choice is surgical excision and reconstruction, preceded by endovascular embolization.
- Osteoblastomas arise from the posterior elements; they are lytic lesions with a reactive sclerotic margin and have a central density.
- Chordomas arise from notochordal remnants and are often found in the sacrum and the clivus. They are lytic lesions with intralesional calcifications and an associated soft-tissue mass.
- Primary malignant lesions of the spine are osteosarcoma, chondrosarcoma, and Ewing sarcoma. They are destructive lytic lesions with associated soft-tissue masses and a heterogeneous appearance on MRI. The role of the interventionalist in the management of these lesions is to perform percutaneous biopsies.

Treatment Options

SURGICAL TREATMENT

- The embolization of vertebral tumors is useful as an adjunct to surgery because it can minimize blood loss. Embolization also may decrease the surgical operating time and reduce complications by improving visualization in the operative field.

ENDOVASCULAR TREATMENT

- If the supply to the spinal cord is seen to be from the same segmental artery as the tumor supply, embolization carries a high risk for neurologic deficits.
- Embolization with polyvinyl alcohol particles is the method of choice to treat hypervascular metastases before surgery.
- The choice of particle size is based on the number of shunts within the tumor and the size of the vessels to be embolized. The smallest particles may induce skin necrosis and interfere with wound healing; therefore, we do not recommend particles smaller than 150 μm. Particles larger than 500 μm will not penetrate distally and may cause clotting in the microcatheter, and are therefore not recommended either.
- The particles are prepared in a diluted suspension and injected via a microcatheter as microboluses. The procedure is monitored with negative fluoroscopy.
- The pattern of flow is monitored throughout the procedure to avoid opening anastomoses.

Possible Complications

- In hypervascular lesions, the spinal cord supply may not be visible during the first angiography because visible contrast is shunted into the lesion; therefore, control runs may be necessary. If this is not done, neurologic deficits may ensue.
- Skin or muscle necrosis or delayed wound healing may occur if a particle size that is too small is chosen.

Published Literature on Treatment Options

Most authors agree that preoperative embolization significantly decreases perioperative blood loss, makes surgery easier, facilitates radical removal, and improves surgical results. The reduction in blood loss is estimated to be on the order of 30 to 50%; however, data from a "control" group are missing. Radical surgery should not be attempted in patients who have extensive metastases of renal cell carcinoma without prior embolization. However, preoperative embolization does not preclude extreme perioperative blood loss, and tumor size, radical versus palliative surgery, and technical complexity have been found to be strongly correlated with the amount of blood lost during surgery. If the anatomy of the spinal cord supply is respected, the risks of embolization are low. Surgery should be performed within the 24 to 72 hours following embolization to allow tumor shrinkage and avoid revascularization.

PEARLS AND PITFALLS

- Preoperative embolization reduces blood loss during radical surgery.
- Nonvisualization of supply to the spinal cord from a segmental artery supplying the lesion may be due to significant tumor blush; therefore, intermediate controls are necessary.

Further Reading

Berkefeld J, Scale D, Kirchner J, Heinrich T, Kollath J. Hypervascular spinal tumors: influence of the embolization technique on perioperative hemorrhage. AJNR Am J Neuroradiol 1999;20(5):757–763

Cloft HJ, Dion JE. Preoperative and palliative embolization of vertebral tumors. Neuroimaging Clin N Am 2000;10(3):569–578

Guzman R, Dubach-Schwizer S, Heini P, et al. Preoperative transarterial embolization of vertebral metastases. Eur Spine J 2005;14(3):263–268

Rehák S, Krajina A, Ungermann L, et al. The role of embolization in radical surgery of renal cell carcinoma spinal metastases. Acta Neurochir (Wien) 2008;150(11):1177–1181, discussion 1181

Shi HB, Suh DC, Lee HK, et al. Preoperative transarterial embolization of spinal tumor: embolization techniques and results. AJNR Am J Neuroradiol 1999;20(10):2009–2015

CASE 42

Case Description

Clinical Presentation

A 29-year-old man presents with progressive chemosis, proptosis, and ophthalmoplegia of the left eye 1 week after sustaining head trauma in a motorcycle accident. He also has pulsatile tinnitus that began the first day after the accident. His neurologic examination is normal. CT and angiography are performed.

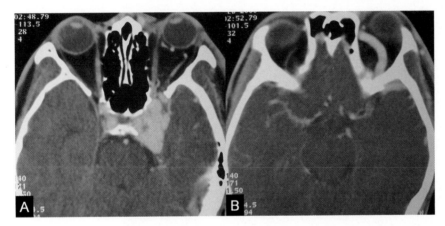

Fig. 42.1 Contrast-enhanced CT scan shows left-sided exophthalmos with bulging of the left cavernous sinus, **(A)** left IOV, and **(B)** left SOV. Prominence of the left sphenoparietal sinus along the anterior aspect of the middle cranial fossa is noted.

Radiologic Studies

CT

Contrast-enhanced CT study showed bulging of the left cavernous sinus with a dilated left superior ophthalmic vein (SOV) and inferior ophthalmic vein (IOV). Exophthalmos of the left orbit was noted with deviation of the left globe medially, likely related to the patient's ophthalmoplegia. There was prominence of the left sphenoparietal sinus along the anterior aspect of the middle cranial fossa, suggestive of cortical venous reflux (**Fig. 42.1**).

DSA

Injection of the left internal carotid artery (ICA) showed a direct high-flow arteriovenous fistula from the cavernous portion of the left ICA to the left cavernous sinus. There was subsequent drainage through the left SOV and left IOV, with cortical venous reflux via the left sphenoparietal sinus to the left superficial sylvian vein and the left deep sylvian vein to the left basal vein of Rosenthal. Collaterals from the left middle meningeal artery to the left ophthalmic artery (left meningo-ophthalmic artery) were seen on lateral view of the left external carotid artery (ECA) injection, with retrograde filling of the left ICA. Enlargement of the left artery of the foramen rotundum from the distal internal maxil-

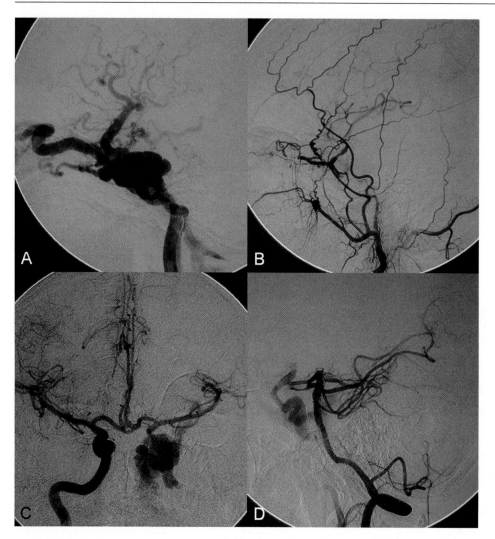

Fig. 42.2 DSA. **(A)** Left ICA angiogram in lateral view. **(B)** Left ECA angiogram in lateral view shows the left meningo-ophthalmic collateral and the artery of the foramen rotundum ICA collateral, with faint opacification of the left ICA. **(C)** Right ICA angiogram in AP view and **(D)** left VA angiogram in lateral view during left CCA compression. Note that the actual site of the fistula is best seen from the left VA injection.

lary artery, serving as a collateral to the left ICA, was also observed. The right ICA injection with compression of the left common carotid artery (CCA) in AP view showed rather good collateral flow through the anterior communicating artery. There was moderate size of the left posterior communicating artery, seen on the left vertebral artery (VA) injection with compression of the left CCA in lateral view. The exact site of the fistula was best demonstrated on this projection (**Fig. 42.2**).

Diagnosis

Left traumatic carotid-cavernous fistula (TCCF) with cortical venous reflux

Treatment

EQUIPMENT

- Standard 8F access (puncture needle, 8F vascular sheath)
- Standard 8F guiding catheter (Cordis, Warren, NJ) with continuous flush and a 0.038-in hydrophilic guidewire (Terumo, Somerset, NJ)
- No. 9 gold valve detachable balloons (Nycomed, Melville, NY) and GOLDBAL5 gold valve detachable balloon (Balt International, Montmorency, France)
- Microcatheter system (Baltacci microcatheters for detachable balloons; Balt)
- Isotonic contrast solution for balloon inflation
- Contrast material
- Heparin 3000 units, protamine 30 mg

DESCRIPTION

After diagnostic angiography, 3000 units of heparin were given intravenously. The 8F guiding catheter was advanced carefully into the proximal left ICA. (A coaxial system may be used to facilitate navigation of the large guiding catheter and to avoid possible dissection of the ICA.) The detachable balloon was prepared and mounted onto the microcatheter system. A roadmap was done, followed by introduction of the balloon and detachable system into the guiding catheter. After the balloon was within the left ICA, it was slightly inflated with 0.1 mL of isotonic contrast solution to facilitate navigation into the fistula. After the balloon entered the cavernous sinus, it was slightly inflated while several injections via the guiding catheter were performed to check its position. When the balloon was correctly placed within the first venous pouch, closest to the left ICA, it was fully inflated and detached. The microcatheter was then removed, and a final control run was performed. The heparin was reversed with 30 mg of protamine at the end of the procedure. Unfortunately, the balloon deflated 2 days after the embolization, with early reopening of the TCCF. The patient underwent a second embolization 1 month later in which two balloons were placed in a similar procedure. The first balloon was navigated more distally within the cavernous sinus and detached while not fully inflated to facilitate placement of the second balloon, which was then detached fully inflated within the first venous pouch. Final control angiograms showed complete closure of the fistula, which was confirmed on follow-up MRA 2 months after the second embolization session (**Fig. 42.3**). The patient

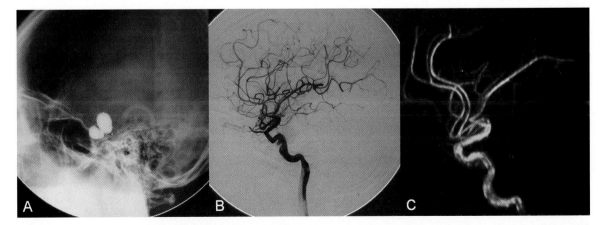

Fig. 42.3 **(A)** Plain radiography after the second embolization demonstrates the position of the two balloons within the cavernous sinus. Note that the first balloon is not fully inflated and is placed more distally within the cavernous sinus. **(B)** Control left ICA angiogram in lateral view shows complete closure of the fistula, which was confirmed on **(C)** the 2-month follow-up MRA.

was prescribed absolute bed rest for 3 days before being discharged home and was advised to limit his activities for at least 1 month to avoid dislocation of the balloons.

Discussion

Background

The most common cause of a direct carotid-cavernous fistula is trauma. A TCCF may also be iatrogenic, usually following skull base surgery, or result from rupture of an underlying cavernous aneurysm or a disease of the vascular wall, such as Ehlers-Danlos syndrome or neurofibromatosis type 1. The pathologic mechanism of a TCCF is tearing and rupture of the ICA, which is fixed at the cavernous level by fibrous trabeculae and by small dural arteries into the cavernous sinus. The clinical symptoms depend on the drainage pathways. Anterior drainage toward the SOV and IOV will lead to exophthalmos and chemosis; posterior drainage into the inferior petrosal vein results in pulsatile tinnitus; and cortical venous reflux through the sphenoparietal sinus into the superficial middle cerebral vein or the superior petrosal vein into the posterior fossa may cause venous congestion with subsequent delayed hemorrhage.

Noninvasive Imaging Workup

PHYSICAL EXAMINATION

- A loud bruit at the orbit or region behind the ear together with a history of significant head trauma makes the diagnosis.
- Exopthalmos and chemosis are classically seen.

CT/MRI

- Because a TCCF can be diagnosed from the clinical history and physical examination, CT and MRI are used mainly to rule out other possible causes of chemosis and proptosis and associated brain injuries.
- Bulging of the cavernous sinus and dilatation of the SOV are best seen on contrast-enhanced CT or T2-weighted images.
- The presence of an enhancing lesion within the sphenoid sinus in the context of a TCCF suggests an associated sphenoid pouch/pseudoaneurysm, a situation in which emergency treatment is indicated.
- Cortical venous reflux is typically seen as prominence of the sphenoparietal sinus located along the anterior aspect of the middle cranial fossa and dilated vessels along the sylvian fissure or cerebellar folia.

CTA/MRA

- CT, MRI, and static CTA and MRA cannot identify the side or exact site of the fistula. Static CTA and MRA may not be helpful because of the high-flow nature of the TCCF and multiple drainage routes.
- Dynamic CTA and dynamic MRA may be able to identify the side of the fistula, which is seen as early filling of the cavernous sinus.

Invasive Imaging Workup

- Angiography is required in the pre-treatment evaluation of TCCFs and may be performed in the same session as the endovascular treatment.

- Both CCAs should be checked first with hand injections before the catheter is advanced into the ICAs to look for associated arterial dissection.
- The ICA angiogram on the suspected side of the TCCF is performed first, in both AP and lateral views, to determine the drainage pathways of the fistula. The ipsilateral ECA is then injected to rule out associated vascular injuries and evaluate the ophthalmic artery collaterals in case the ICA must be sacrificed.
- The contralateral ICA angiogram is performed in AP view during manual compression of the ipsilateral CCA to evaluate the collateralization through the anterior communicating artery. This is followed by injection of the VA in lateral view, also during manual compression of the ipsilateral CCA, to evaluate the size of the posterior communicating artery. The exact site of the fistula is usually best seen on the lateral view of the VA angiogram.

Treatment Options

SURGICAL TREATMENT

- In the past, TCCFs were treated with carotid ligation or muscle embolization through surgical exposure of the carotid artery. Because this was often done blindly, the procedure was associated with a high risk for complications and low cure rates; therefore, it is rarely practiced nowadays.
- Other surgical options include direct packing of the carotid-cavernous fistula and surgical disconnection of the cortical venous reflux.

ENDOVASCULAR TREATMENT

- Balloon embolization is the first choice in the treatment of TCCFs. If balloons are not available or the tear in the ICA is too small, then platinum coils (see Case 45) and/or liquid embolic materials may be considered.
- Heparin is routinely given to all patients; it is reversed with protamine at the end of the procedure.
- The goal of treatment is to close the first venous pouch, which is the one closest to the ICA tear.
- If more than one balloon is required, then the first balloon is navigated further into the cavernous sinus and detached **not** fully inflated.
- In our institution, all patients are prescribed absolute bed rest for at least 72 hours after the procedure to avoid migration of the balloon. Aggressive medication for nausea, vomiting, hiccups, and coughing may be needed.
- If early deflation of the balloon occurs within this period, then the bed rest is cancelled and another embolization is rescheduled after 1 month. This waiting period is often necessary to allow the first balloon to deflate enough that placement of the second or third balloon will not be obstructed.
- If the TCCF recurs after the second embolization, the period of bed rest may be extended to 5 days, or other embolic materials, such as coils and/or liquid agents, are considered.
- After discharge from the hospital, patients are usually advised to limit their activities for at least 1 month following the procedure.

Possible Complications

- Standard angiographic complications (at the puncture site: bleeding, false aneurysms, fistula; in catheterized vessels: emboli, dissections; systemically: contrast reaction, renal failure)
- Migration and/or early deflation of the balloon

- Transient worsening of ophthalmoplegia and exophthalmos occurs after complete closure because of progressive thrombosis of the SOV, which usually regresses after medical management with steroids

Published Literature on Treatment Options

In 1981, Debrun et al published the first large series of patients with TCCFs treated with detachable balloon embolization via both transarterial and transvenous approaches. Since then, embolization has replaced the older surgical methods, with the advantages of a lower risk for complications, higher rate of ICA preservation, and much higher cure rates. In a large series of 100 patients reported by Lewis et al, the cure rate was 86%, and the ICA was preserved in 75% of cases, with a complication rate of only 4%. Many cases in which different techniques were used have been reported, but in our opinion, the easiest route is still a transarterial route with a detachable balloon. If this fails, other embolic materials, such as coils and liquid agents, or a transvenous route may be considered. Reports of successful reconstruction of the ICA with covered stents have recently been published by several groups, and this may be the ideal treatment in the future; currently, however, there are still no dedicated covered stents for intracranial use, and the long-term patency of these stents has yet to be determined.

PEARLS AND PITFALLS _____

- TCCFs are diagnosed clinically by the history and the presence of a bruit. CT, MRI, and static CTA/MRA cannot determine the side and site of the fistula.
- A medial sphenoid pouch, like a sphenoid pseudoaneurysm, is an indication for emergency treatment, given the risk for life-threatening epistaxis.

Further Reading

Debrun G, Lacour P, Vinuela F, Fox A, Drake CG, Caron JP. Treatment of 54 traumatic carotid-cavernous fistulas. J Neurosurg 1981;55(5):678–692

Gupta AK, Purkayastha S, Krishnamoorthy T, et al. Endovascular treatment of direct carotid cavernous fistulae: a pictorial review. Neuroradiology 2006;48(11):831–839

Lewis AI, Tomsick TA, Tew JM Jr. Management of 100 consecutive direct carotid-cavernous fistulas: results of treatment with detachable balloons. Neurosurgery 1995;36(2):239–244, discussion 244–245

Wang C, Xie X, You C, et al. Placement of covered stents for the treatment of direct carotid cavernous fistulas. AJNR Am J Neuroradiol 2009;30(7):1342–1346

CASE 43

Case Description

Clinical Presentation

A 34-year-old man is admitted to the hospital with the history of a severe head injury and loss of consciousness following a motor vehicle accident. Initial CT scan shows crushing skull base fractures and traumatic subarachnoid hemorrhage. His initial neurologic examination reveals no motor or sensory deficits. He has massive facial swelling related to the extensive facial and skull base fractures, so that the clinical development of progressive right proptosis is not noticed. Two weeks after admission, the new onset of left hemiparesis is noted. Another CT scan is performed, followed by angiography.

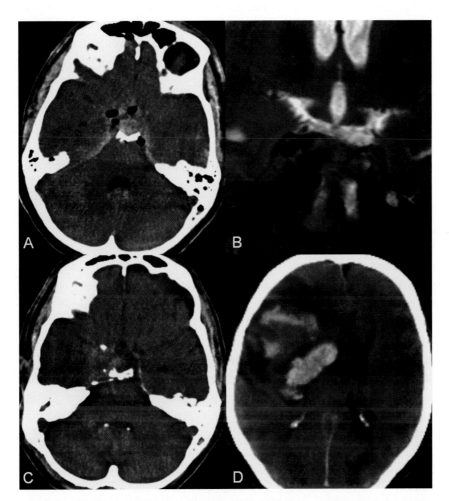

Fig. 43.1 **(A)** Initial unenhanced CT shows hyperdensity along the suprasellar cistern and the hypodensity of air within the subarachnoid space and right cavernous sinus. **(B)** Follow-up coronal T2-weighted MRI 1 week later demonstrates bulging of the right cavernous sinus with multiple internal flow-void structures. **(C)** Follow-up unenhanced CT at 2 weeks reveals bulging of the right cavernous sinus at the level of the skull base. **(D)** Unenhanced CT done one day later after the acute onset of left hemiparesis shows a large hyperdense hematoma involving the right frontotemporal lobe and basal ganglia with marked surrounding hypodensity due to edema.

249

Radiologic Studies

CT/MRI

Initial unenhanced CT showed traumatic subarachnoid hemorrhage and air within the subarachnoid space and right cavernous sinus. Multiple fractures at the right side of the skull base were noted. Follow-up MRI 1 week later showed bulging of the right cavernous sinus with multiple internal flow-void structures on T2-weighted images. The follow-up unenhanced CT study at 2 weeks after admission, when the patient exhibited neurologic deterioration, revealed a new, large intraparenchymal hemorrhage along the right frontotemporal lobe and basal ganglia, with marked surrounding edema and mass effect. Bulging of the right cavernous sinus was noted at the level of the skull base. These findings suggested the diagnosis of a traumatic carotid-cavernous fistula (TCCF) with cortical venous reflux and secondary venous infarction (**Fig. 43.1**).

DSA

Injection of the right internal carotid artery (ICA) showed a direct high-flow arteriovenous fistula from the cavernous portion of the right ICA to the right cavernous sinus. Drainage through the right superior ophthalmic vein (SOV) and right inferior ophthalmic vein (IOV) with cortical venous reflux via the right sphenoparietal sinus to the right frontal cortical veins and the right deep sylvian vein toward the right basal vein of Rosenthal was noted (**Fig. 43.2 A,B**). Poor collateralization through the anterior communicating artery and right posterior communicating artery was observed (not shown).

Diagnosis

Right TCCF with cortical venous reflux

Treatment

EQUIPMENT

- Standard 8F access (puncture needle, 8F vascular sheath)
- Standard 8F guiding catheter (Cordis, Warren, NJ) with continuous flush and a 0.035-in hydrophilic guidewire (Terumo, Somerset, NJ)
- GOLDBAL1 gold valve detachable balloon (Balt International, Montmorency, France)
- Magic BD PE 1.8F catheter for detachable balloon (Balt)
- Isotonic contrast solution for balloon inflation
- A 0.019-in over-the-wire microcatheter (Excelsior 10–18; Boston Scientific, Natick, MA) with a 0.014-in hydrophilic guidewire (Synchro 14; Boston Scientific)
- Bare and fibered detachable platinum coils (GDC 360-degree SR 10 and GDC VortX; Boston Scientific)
- Contrast material
- Heparin 5000 units

DESCRIPTION

After diagnostic angiography, 5000 units of heparin was given intravenously. An 8F guiding catheter was advanced carefully into the proximal right ICA. A roadmap was done. Several attempts to place a small balloon into the fistula failed because of the small size of the tear within the right ICA. Two separate tears were identified with hand injections during gentle inflation of the balloon within the cavernous ICA. The balloon and microcatheter were removed, and an over-the-wire microcatheter was introduced into the first tear along the inferior wall of the right ICA. A 360-degree bare platinum coil was placed and detached in the first venous pouch as a frame, followed by careful placement of multiple fibered platinum coils to introduce further thrombosis until stagnation of the contrast

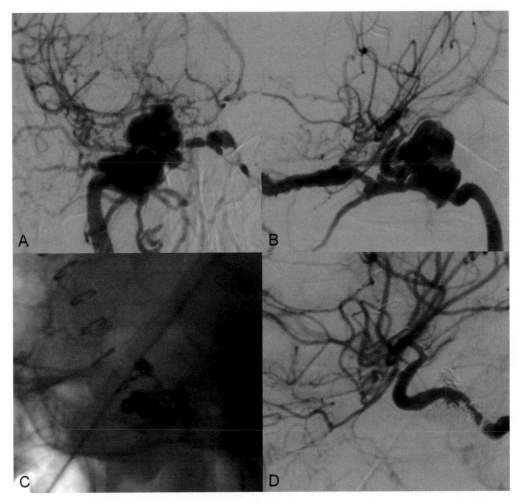

Fig. 43.2 DSA. Right ICA angiogram in **(A)** AP and **(B)** lateral views shows a high-flow arteriovenous fistula from the cavernous portion of the right ICA to the cavernous sinus. **(C)** Plain skull radiography and **(D)** right ICA angiogram after coil embolization demonstrate the position of the two coil meshes and confirm complete closure of the fistula.

within the cavernous sinus was observed on the hand injections. The microcatheter was then gently removed and maneuvered into the second tear within the superior wall of the right ICA. A frame was formed by placement of a 360-degree bare platinum coil within the first venous pouch closest to the ICA tear, followed by packing with fibered platinum coils until no filling of the cavernous sinus was seen on the hand injection. The microcatheter was then removed, and the final control run revealed complete obliteration of the fistula (**Fig. 43.2 C,D**).

Discussion

Background

TCCFs occur secondary to rupture of the ICA or its cavernous branches. Occasionally, rupture of an intra-cavernous branch from the external carotid artery (ECA) may result in similar symptoms. Cavernous dural arteriovenous fistulae, also known as indirect carotid cavernous fistulae, are a separate entity (see Case 30). Significant head trauma is typically required for a TCCF; in some cases with no history of trauma or only minor trauma, an underlying lesion such as a cavernous aneurysm or a vessel wall disease should be suspected. The clinical symptoms are typically related to the drainage pathways. In rare instances, fracture of an adjacent wall of the sphenoid sinus may lead to the development of an associated sphenoid aneurysm and result in massive epistaxis; these situations are life-threatening emergencies. Aneurysmal dilatations of the venous pouches may also project intradurally, and subsequent rupture can produce subarachnoid hemorrhage. Intraparenchymal hemorrhage and venous infarctions are usually caused by cortical venous reflux through either the sphenoparietal sinus to the superficial sylvian vein or the superior petrosal sinus to the posterior fossa veins. Because the cavernous sinuses are anastomosed in the midline, TCCFs can produce symptoms contralaterally or bilaterally.

Noninvasive Imaging Workup

PHYSICAL EXAMINATION

- In patients with crushing skull base fractures, proptosis or chemosis may be difficult to recognize. However, a bruit at the orbit or region behind the ear may help in making the diagnosis.

CT/MRI

- A crushing skull base fracture that crosses the ICA canal as well as air within the ICA canal should raise suspicion of a carotid artery laceration.
- Progressive bulging of the cavernous sinus is a good indicator of the development of a TCCF.
- If a TCCF is suspected from the imaging findings, CTA or MRA is indicated to rule out cortical venous reflux.

CTA/MRA

- CT, MRI, and static CTA and MRA cannot identify the side or exact site of the fistula. Static CTA and MRA may not be helpful at all because of the high-flow nature of the TCCF and multiple drainage routes.
- Dynamic CTA and dynamic MRA may be able to identify the side of the fistula, which is seen as early filling of the cavernous sinus and venous drainage pathways.

Invasive Imaging Workup

- Angiography is required in the pre-treatment evaluation of TCCFs and may be performed in the same session as the endovascular treatment.
- Ipsilateral and contralateral injections of the ICA and ECA as well as an injection in the dominant vertebral artery constitute the protocol for the evaluation of a TCCF, to assess for cross-flow, the exact site of the fistula, and the presence of venous congestion.
- To determine the exact location of a carotid wall tear, 3D rotational angiography may be helpful.

Differential Diagnosis

- Delayed intraparenchymal hemorrhage following trauma can have a variety of causes, including the following: delayed rupture of a traumatic aneurysm, traumatic arteriovenous fistulae of the ECA into cortical veins with venous congestion, hemorrhagic transformation of an ischemic stroke resulting from arterial dissection, and venous injury with delayed venous congestion.

Treatment Options

SURGICAL TREATMENT

- If the ICA cannot be preserved and there are insufficient collaterals, bypass surgery may be required.

ENDOVASCULAR TREATMENT

- Balloon embolization is the first preferred treatment of a TCCF (see Case 44). If balloons are not available or the tear in the ICA is too small, then platinum coils and/or liquid embolic materials may be considered.
- The goal of treatment is to close the first venous pouch, which is the one closest to the ICA tear.
- In our experience, a bare platinum coil is typically placed first as a frame within the first venous pouch, followed by subsequent packing with fibered coils to induce thrombosis.
- If only bare platinum coils are used, a dense coil mesh is required to close the fistula because of its high flow.
- Occasionally, injection of glue is also needed to induce thrombosis within the venous pouch.

Possible Complications

- Coil protrusion into the parent artery with thromboembolic complications
- Transient worsening of ophthalmoplegia and exophthalmos occurs after complete closure because of progressive thrombosis of the SOV, which usually regresses after medical management with steroids.

Published Literature on Treatment Options

The success rate for the balloon embolization of TCCFs in the literature ranges from 85 to 98%. Embolization with coil or liquid agents may be required in ~5 to 10% of cases, when the tear is too small or the flow is too slow for the use of balloons. Dense packing is often needed to close the fistula with bare platinum coils; several authors have reported the use of coils coated with hydrogel to facilitate TCCF closure via coil swelling and therefore a denser occlusion, with good results. In fewer than 3 to 5% of cases, a transarterial route may fail, so that a transvenous route is required. Several small case series have been reported in which covered stents were used to treat TCCFs, with promising results. However, at present, there are still no dedicated cover stents for intracranial use, and long-term follow-up results are pending.

PEARLS AND PITFALLS _____

- CT, MRI, static CTA, and MRA cannot determine the side and site of a fistula because of midline intercavernous anastomoses.
- The goal of treatment for TCCFs is to close the fistula with preservation of the parent ICA.

Further Reading

Higashida RT, Halbach VV, Tsai FY, et al. Interventional neurovascular treatment of traumatic carotid and vertebral artery lesions: results in 234 cases. AJR Am J Roentgenol 1989;153(3):577–582

Tjoumakaris SI, Jabbour PM, Rosenwasser RH. Neuroendovascular management of carotid cavernous fistulae. Neurosurg Clin N Am 2009;20(4):447–452

Wang ZG, Ding X, Zhang JQ, et al. HydroCoil occlusion for treatment of traumatic carotid-cavernous fistula: preliminary experience. Eur J Radiol 2009;71(3):456–460

CASE 44

Case Description

Clinical Presentation

A 72-year-old patient who has a history of squamous cell carcinoma with head and neck invasion, multiple previous surgeries, and neck irradiation has an acute episode of arterial bleeding from an ulcerative lesion in the neck.

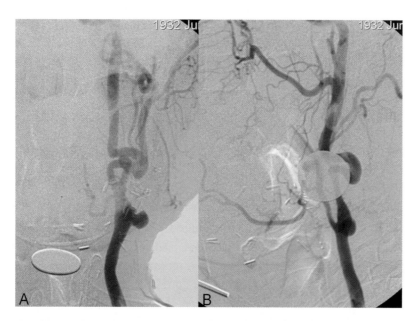

Fig. 44.1 DSA. Left CCA angiogram in **(A)** AP and **(B)** lateral views demonstrates a pseudoaneurysm at the left common carotid bifurcation.

Radiologic Studies

DSA

Injection of the left common carotid artery (CCA) showed a large pseudoaneurysm at the level of the left CCA bifurcation. No other abnormalities were observed after injection of the right internal carotid artery (ICA) and the left cervical vertebral artery (**Fig. 44.1**).

Diagnosis

Carotid blowout with a pseudoaneurysm at the left carotid artery bifurcation

Treatment

EQUIPMENT

- Standard 5F access (puncture needle, 5F vascular sheath)
- 5F Berenstein multipurpose catheter (Boston Scientific, Natick MA) with continuous flush and a 0.035-in hydrophilic guidewire (Terumo, Somerset, NJ)
- 6F Shuttle Sheath (Cook Medical, Bloomington, IN)
- A 260-cm exchange guidewire (Cook)
- Straight microcatheter (Turbo Tracker 18; Boston Scientific) with a 0.014-in guidewire (Synchro 14; Boston Scientific)
- Coil selection: six GDC 18 fibered coils (Boston Scientific)
- Wallstent Symbiot 45/5 mm (Boston Scientific)
- Contrast material
- Heparin
- Abciximab (ReoPro; Eli Lilly, Indianapolis, IN) 5 mg

DESCRIPTION

Following catheterization of the left CCA with a 5F multipurpose catheter, a 6F shuttle sheath was placed in the left CCA over a 260-cm exchange wire. The external carotid artery (ECA) was catheterized with a microcatheter and subsequently occluded with six GDC 18 fibered coils as verified by control runs. Complete occlusion of the left ECA distal to the lingual branch was demonstrated. Via a micro-guidewire placed into the left ICA, a Wallstent was advanced to the bifurcation, with the radiopaque marks distal to the left carotid artery bifurcation and proximal to the pseudoaneurysm, and deployed. The final runs showed correct placement of the stent with complete occlusion of the pseudoaneurysm (**Fig. 44.2**). No abnormalities or clots were observed in the vessel lumen. The shuttle sheath was exchanged for a short 7F sheath; this was left in place, to be removed later. The patient was given 5 mg of abciximab and transferred to the recovery room. He had an uneventful recovery and no further bleeding.

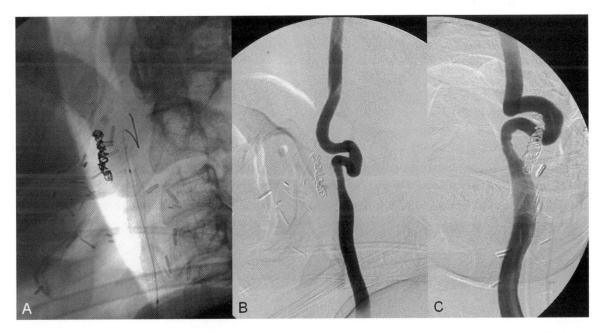

Fig. 44.2 Plain radiography of the neck in **(A)** lateral view demonstrates the coil mesh within the ECA and the stent position. Left CCA angiograms in **(B)** AP and **(C)** lateral views after coiling and stent placement show occlusion of the pseudoaneurysm.

Discussion

Background

Carotid blowout is defined as the rupture of the extracranial carotid arteries or their major branches. It is a feared complication of head and neck cancer and its treatment. Following neck dissection, carotid blowout develops in 3 to 5% of patients. Historically, carotid blowout had morbidity rates of up to 60% and mortality rates of 40%, which have been reduced to less than 8% with recent advances in endovascular techniques. The most common cause of carotid blowout is squamous cell carcinoma or its treatments; other causes include other tumors, blunt or penetrating trauma to the neck, and functional endoscopic surgery for refractory epistaxis. Irradiation of the neck increases the risk for carotid blowout approximately sevenfold because of vessel wall weakening related to obliteration of the vasa vasorum, adventitial fibrosis, or atherosclerosis.

Noninvasive Imaging Workup

CLINICAL AND IMAGING FINDINGS

- Three entities can be distinguished clinically and on imaging: threatened, impending, and acute carotid blowout.
- Threatened carotid blowout is defined as evidence on physical examination and radiologic studies suggestive of inevitable hemorrhage from one of the carotid arteries in the immediate future if no action is taken. However, hemorrhage has not yet occurred. Exposure of the carotid artery or one of its major branches, neoplastic invasion of the carotid system, and nonhemorrhagic pseudoaneurysm are the salient clinical and imaging findings.
- Impending blowout is characterized by an episode of transcervical or transoral hemorrhage, typically from a pseudoaneurysm, that resolves either spontaneously or with packing or pressure.
- During acute blowout, hemorrhage is present that cannot be stopped with packing or pressure.
- The most commonly affected sites are the ICA (43.6%), followed by the ECA (23.4%), CCA (11.7%), buccal artery (3.2%), inferior thyroid artery (3.2%), and superior thyroid artery (2.1%).
- CTA can demonstrate the pseudoaneurysm and define its exact parent vessel in most instances.

Invasive Imaging Workup

- Angiography is considered the gold standard and will demonstrate the pseudoaneurysm with potentially active extravasation or stagnation of contrast.
- The vessel wall may be irregular, especially in patients who have undergone irradiation.
- The study should also include an evaluation of the patency of the circle of Willis. Balloon test occlusions should be performed at a level where the vessel wall is healthy.
- ECA branches that may possibly be used for subsequent EC-IC bypass surgery must be identified.
- Studies should include the venous phase because the site of bleeding may also be at the jugular vein.

Differential Diagnosis

- Bleeding from the tumor itself and hemorrhage from venous structures (most notably the jugular veins) must also be considered as reasons for acute bleeding in patients with head and neck tumors.

Treatment Options

CONSERVATIVE OR MEDICAL MANAGEMENT

- Given the very high rate of rebleeding, conservative management is not an option in acutely symptomatic patients.
- In the acute setting, before endovascular or surgical management, control of the airway, control of the bleeding with pressure, and crossmatch and typing for blood and intravenous fluid management will be required.

SURGICAL TREATMENT

- Exploration of the neck and ligation of the vessel are surgical options that rarely play a role nowadays, given the high rate of complications, discussed below, in the acute setting.
- Surgery with arterial bypass of the affected region and flap coverage (with vascular tissue) of the exposed artery in the subacute phase are important measures to achieve a permanent solution and to avoid infection of any implanted foreign bodies.

ENDOVASCULAR TREATMENT

- Parent vessel occlusion with coils or balloons, endovascular trapping, and stent-assisted treatments (including stent-grafts) must be considered, depending on the individual location of the carotid blowout.

Possible Complications

- Thromboembolic complications during parent vessel occlusion
- High risk for repeated rupture of the pseudoaneurysm if an endosaccular coil deposition is performed
- Risk for infection and delayed recurrence of hemorrhage in implanted materials

Published Literature on Treatment Options

Because of the difficulties encountered in operating on an infected and often tumor-laden wound, with postoperative scars and fibrosis due to irradiation, the complication rates of surgical exploration during the acute phase of carotid blowout are high, with morbidity and mortality ranging from 9 to 100% (median, 60% for morbidity and 40% for mortality). Endovascular treatment is therefore considered the method of choice in the acute setting. Depending on the location of the blowout, different strategies must be adopted. Simple parent vessel occlusion with detachable coils, which may be fibered or expanding (hydrocoils), or liquid embolic agents can be used in the ECA or the jugular vein (if the contralateral jugular vein is patent). If the CCA or ICA is affected, though, evaluation of the patency of the circle of Willis is necessary. If there is sufficient cross-flow via the anterior and posterior communicating arteries, parent vessel occlusion (both distal and proximal to the blowout!) can be performed. In cases in which the ICA or CCA is involved and test balloon occlusion has failed, stenting must be performed. Endovascular stents or stent-grafts are effective in arresting the acute hemorrhage; however, in a contaminated wound with an exposed stent, infection of the stent and occlusion or repeated hemorrhage may occur over time. Therefore, some authors view endovascular techniques more as a temporary solution and advocate surgical bypass to the intracranial vasculature and subsequent proximal parent vesselocclusion as a more permanent solution. Finally, if hemorrhage occurs from the tumor itself, tumor embolization (with particles and subsequent parent vessel occlusion) is advocated.

PEARLS AND PITFALLS

- In most instances, noninvasive imaging can determine the site of a carotid blowout and whether the blowout is threatened, impending, or acute.
- Treatment strategies depend on the location of the blowout and patency of the circle of Willis. They include deconstructive therapies with parent vessel occlusion (both distal and proximal to the blowout) and reconstructive therapies with stents or stent-grafts.

Further Reading

Chang FC, Lirng JF, Luo CB, et al. Patients with head and neck cancers and associated postirradiated carotid blowout syndrome: endovascular therapeutic methods and outcomes. J Vasc Surg 2008;47(5):936–945

Cohen J, Rad I. Contemporary management of carotid blowout. Curr Opin Otolaryngol Head Neck Surg 2004;12(2):110–115

Mazumdar A, Derdeyn CP, Holloway W, Moran CJ, Cross DT III. Update on endovascular management of the carotid blowout syndrome. Neuroimaging Clin N Am 2009;19(2):271–281

Pyun HW, Lee DH, Yoo HM, et al. Placement of covered stents for carotid blowout in patients with head and neck cancer: follow-up results after rescue treatments. AJNR Am J Neuroradiol 2007;28(8):1594–1598

Simental A, Johnson JT, Horowitz M. Delayed complications of endovascular stenting for carotid blowout. Am J Otolaryngol 2003;24(6):417–419

CASE 45

Case Description

Clinical Presentation

A 26-year-old man presents with recurrent, severe, right-sided epistaxis requiring blood transfusion. He has a history of a car accident 6 months before admission with loss of consciousness for 2 days and immediate blindness in his right eye. His neurologic examination is normal. CT and angiography are performed.

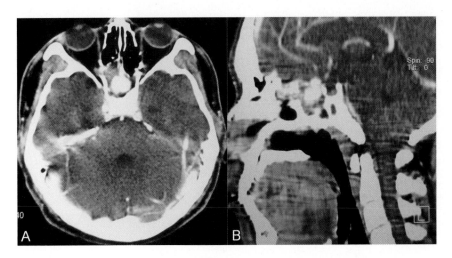

Fig. 45.1 Contrast-enhanced CT scan in **(A)** axial and **(B)** sagittal reconstruction.

Radiologic Studies

CT

Contrast-enhanced CT revealed a rather round enhancing structure within the sphenoid sinus (**Fig. 45.1**). Hyperdensity surrounding this lesion suggested blood clot. Erosion of the right lateral sphenoid wall was also noted. These findings were suggestive of a pseudoaneurysm of the right internal carotid artery (ICA).

DSA

Injection of the right ICA showed an irregular outpouching along the medial wall of the cavernous portion of the right ICA, just proximal to the origin of the ophthalmic artery and pointing medially into the sphenoid sinus. Layering and stagnation of contrast were seen within the sac, with delayed washout of contrast, in keeping with a pseudoaneurysm (**Fig. 45.2**).

Diagnosis

Traumatic pseudoaneurysm of the right ICA with extension into the sphenoid sinus

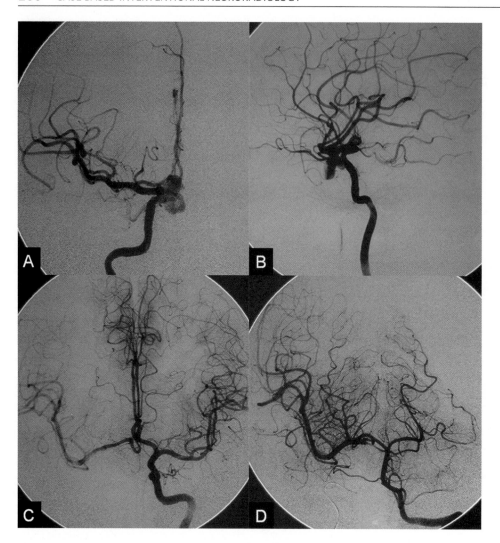

Fig. 45.2 DSA. Right ICA angiogram in **(A)** AP and **(B)** lateral views. **(C)** Left ICA angiogram and **(D)** left vertebral angiogram in AP view during balloon occlusion of the right ICA.

Treatment

EQUIPMENT

- Bilateral 5F and 8F access (puncture needles, 5F and 8F vascular sheaths)
- 5F Berenstein catheter (Boston Scientific, Natick, MA)
- Standard 8F guiding catheter (Cordis, Warren, NJ) with continuous flush and a 0.038-in hydrophilic guidewire (Terumo, Somerset, NJ)
- Nondetachable balloon for balloon occlusion test (BALTACCIB1, 6 × 9 mm; Balt International, Montmorency, France)
- No. 9 gold valve detachable balloons (Nycomed, Melville, NJ) and GOLDBAL5 gold valve detachable balloon (Balt)
- Minitorque detachable system (Baltacci microcatheters for detachable balloons; Balt)
- Isotonic contrast solution for balloon inflation
- Contrast material

DESCRIPTION

Following diagnostic angiography, an 8F guiding catheter was advanced carefully into the proximal right ICA. A nondetachable balloon was then placed at the petrous segment under roadmap and inflated to close the right ICA. Subsequent runs of the left ICA and left vertebral artery (VA) were performed through the diagnostic catheter, which demonstrated good collaterals to the right anterior cerebral artery (ACA) through the anterior communicating artery and to the right middle cerebral artery (MCA) through the right posterior communicating artery without any delayed venous phase.

After the balloon occlusion test, the nondetachable balloon was removed, and the detachable balloons were prepared and mounted onto the detachable microcatheter system. A roadmap was performed before insertion of the detachable balloons. When the first balloon reached the proximal right ICA, it was slightly inflated with 0.1 mL of isotonic contrast solution to facilitate navigation into the proper position. The first balloon was placed distally in the supraclinoid portion of the ICA, distal to the aneurysm and proximal to the origin of the right posterior communicating artery. A second balloon was then placed across the neck of the aneurysm, and a third balloon, which was used as a safety balloon, was placed within the proximal right ICA. Final control angiogram showed occlusion of the right ICA and no filling of the pseudoaneurysm (**Fig. 45.3**). Post-procedural blood pressure monitoring and absolute bed rest for 3 days were prescribed, and the patient was discharged home after 4 days without any complications.

Discussion

Background

Traumatic aneurysms of the head and neck can be extracranial or intracranial in location. Intracranial traumatic aneurysms can be subdivided into three types, according to their location: skull base (ICA); subcortical (ACA-falx, MCA-sphenoid ridge, PCA-tentorium); and distal (associated with a skull fracture). The most frequent location (48% of cases) is the cavernous segment of the ICA. The most dangerous form is a medial tear of the ICA with rupture into the sphenoid sinus through a fracture of the lateral sphenoid wall. Delayed hemorrhage from traumatic aneurysms can occur anywhere from 5 days to 9 weeks after the initial trauma. The mortality rate associated with these hemorrhagic episodes is reported to be as high as 50%. Aneurysms of the sphenoid portion of the ICA that point medially are not constrained by a bony wall; they extend freely into the sphenoid sinus and constitute a life-threatening emergency.

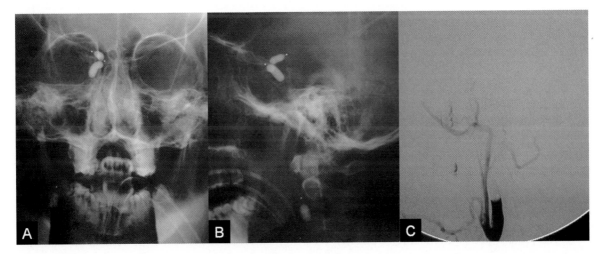

Fig. 45.3 Plain radiography in **(A)** AP and **(B)** lateral views demonstrates the position of the three balloons. The first balloon is placed distally in the supraclinoid portion of the ICA distal to the aneurysm and proximal to the origin of the right posterior communicating artery, the second bal- loon is placed across the neck of the aneurysm, and the third balloon is placed as a safety balloon within the proxi- mal right ICA. Right common carotid artery angiogram in **(C)** lateral view after sacrifice of the ICA with detachable balloons shows closure of the ICA and pseudoaneurysm.

Noninvasive Imaging Workup

CT/MRI

- Traumatic aneurysms are typically associated with a surrounding hematoma within the sphenoid sinus, which can be seen on unenhanced CT as an area of hyperdensity and on MRI as a hyperintense T1 signal and a hypointense T2 signal.
- The aneurysm can be seen as an enhancing lesion on post-contrast CT or as a flow-void structure on T1- or T2-weighted MR sequences. Occasionally, it may have a high signal on T1-weighted images caused by turbulent flow and/or stagnation within the aneurysm sac.
- The aneurysm may not be well seen on cross-sectional imaging in the acute phase of trauma.

CTA/MRA

- Static CTA and MRA can be used to demonstrate the aneurysm; however, dynamic CTA and MRA are more useful in the evaluation of a possible associated arteriovenous fistula.

Invasive Imaging Workup

- Both common carotid arteries should be checked first with hand injections before the catheter is advanced into the ICA to exclude the possibility of an associated dissection.
- An outpouching representing the aneurysm, usually with stagnation or layering of contrast within the false sac, can be seen from the ICA wall on venous phases. If angiography is performed during the acute stage, the aneurysm sac may not be visualized, and only mild irregularity of the ICA, representing dissection, is seen.
- A balloon occlusion test is required to evaluate the option of sacrificing the ICA; this can be carried out under local anesthesia with neurologic monitoring of the patient or under general anesthesia with evaluation of the cross-flow pattern.
- Heparin is not routinely given to patients with traumatic aneurysms undergoing a balloon occlusion test. If a balloon occlusion test is performed for other reasons, then 3000 units of heparin is given intravenously before the balloon is inflated.
- A balloon occlusion test is considered "passed" by angiographic criteria if there is a venous phase delay of less than 2 seconds compared with the normal side, "borderline" if the venous phase delay is between 2 and 4 seconds, and "failed" if the venous phase is delayed for more than 4 seconds.
- The contralateral ICA angiogram is performed in AP view, and the VA angiogram may be performed in either AP or lateral view, or both.

Treatment Options

SURGICAL TREATMENT

- Surgical bypass may be necessary if the patient fails the balloon occlusion test.
- Surgical ligation may also be performed; however, it may be more difficult to close the ICA distal to the aneurysm.

ENDOVASCULAR TREATMENT

- If the patient passes the balloon occlusion test, then sacrifice of the ICA with detachable balloons is the best treatment option.
- Placement of the first balloon beyond the origin of the aneurysm neck is usually attempted; however, if this does not succeed because of difficulty navigating the balloon beyond the ICA curve at the ophthalmic artery, then coils may be used to close the ICA distal to the aneurysm. If this is

done after placement of the balloon proximal to the aneurysm neck, then an approach via either the anterior communicating artery or the posterior communicating artery may be used.

- The next balloon is placed just proximal to the aneurysm neck. Inflation of the balloon within the aneurysm itself **must** be avoided because traumatic aneurysms have no true wall.

- In our experience, we often place a third balloon at the proximal cervical ICA as a safety balloon, to prevent migration of the first or second balloon if deflation occurs.

- After the procedure, the blood pressure has to be monitored closely and intravenous fluids administered to maintain the blood pressure above 90/60 mm Hg. The patient is prescribed absolute bed rest for at least 72 hours to prevent migration of the balloons and is observed in the hospital for at least 4 days.

- A plain skull radiograph is typically obtained at 24 hours to evaluate for early deflation of the balloon.

- If early deflation of the balloons is detected, further investigation with CTA is done to detect recurrence of the aneurysm, which warrants repeated embolization with coils.

Possible Complications

- Arterial dissection during the balloon occlusion test
- Embolic complications
- Migration and/or early deflation of the balloon
- Watershed stroke due to insufficient collaterals and/or low blood pressure

Published Literature on Treatment Options

The treatment of certain intracranial vascular diseases, such as giant aneurysms, direct carotid-cavernous fistulae, and tumors of the skull base, may involve therapeutic sacrifice of the parent artery. A balloon occlusion test is usually performed before the sacrifice to evaluate the patient's ability to tolerate permanent occlusion. The reported risk of this diagnostic procedure is ~3%. The test can be done with the patient under general anesthesia by a simple evaluation of the blood flow pattern, or with the patient conscious by continuous neurologic monitoring over a prolonged period (classically, 15–30 minutes). Several authors have reported the use of additional tests in conjunction with the balloon occlusion test, including transcranial Doppler ultrasound, quantitative cerebral blood flow measurements with xenon, HMPAO SPECT (single-photon emission computed tomography with hexamethylpropylene amine) perfusion imaging, and MRI to evaluate tolerance of the occlusion. Some of these tests require the patient to be moved while the balloon is inflated, which may be considered dangerous. In our experience and in various reports in the literature, evaluation of the venous delay is sufficient to determine whether or not a patient has passed a balloon occlusion test. If the venous delay is less than 2 seconds, occlusion of the ICA is considered safe; on the other hand, ICA sacrifice is contraindicated without prior bypass surgery if the venous delay is more than 4 seconds. For borderline cases, immediate sacrifice may be considered in emergency situations; however, for elective cases, a bypass should be contemplated. Despite the techniques or criteria used for the balloon occlusion test, the risk for ischemic complications, mainly due to stump emboli, following permanent occlusion still ranges between 2 and 22%.

Traumatic pseudoaneurysms of the ICA presenting with epistaxis require emergent treatment because of their associated high mortality rate. A balloon occlusion test can be done within the same session as the endovascular treatment. Both balloons and coils have been used to sacrifice the ICA. Because these false aneurysms do not have a true wall, the visualized "sac" is actually surrounded only by hematoma, so that intrasaccular coiling of these aneurysms is neither appropriate nor sufficient to stop the bleeding. In fact, this maneuver is associated with a high risk for repeated rupture during the procedure. Several case reports have been published of the use of covered stents to treat these lesions; however, the use of anticoagulants in an acutely traumatized patient may be inappropriate. Currently, there are still no dedicated covered stents for intracranial use, and the rate of in-stent thrombosis is reported to range between 15 and 50%.

PEARLS AND PITFALLS

- Traumatic ICA aneurysms with a sphenoid pouch require emergency treatment.
- If the balloon occlusion test is passed according to angiographic criteria, then endovascular sacrifice of the ICA with either balloons or coils is the best treatment option.
- Surgical bypass is required if the patient fails the balloon occlusion test.

Further Reading

Abud DG, Spelle L, Piotin M, Mounayer C, Vanzin JR, Moret J. Venous phase timing during balloon test occlusion as a criterion for permanent internal carotid artery sacrifice. AJNR Am J Neuroradiol 2005;26(10):2602–2609

Bavinzski G, Killer M, Knosp E, Ferraz-Leite H, Gruber A, Richling B. False aneurysms of the intracavernous carotid artery—report of 7 cases. Acta Neurochir (Wien) 1997;139(1):37–43

Chen D, Concus AP, Halbach VV, Cheung SW. Epistaxis originating from traumatic pseudoaneurysm of the internal carotid artery: diagnosis and endovascular therapy. Laryngoscope 1998;108(3):326–331

Krings T, Geibprasert S, Lasjaunias PL. Cerebrovascular trauma. Eur Radiol 2008;18(8):1531–1545

McIvor NP, Willinsky RA, TerBrugge KG, Rutka JA, Freeman JL. Validity of test occlusion studies prior to internal carotid artery sacrifice. Head Neck 1994;16(1):11–16

CASE 46

Case Description

Clinical Presentation

A 57-year-old woman with underlying hereditary hemorrhagic telangiectasia (HHT) has a history of recurrent epistaxis since the age of 16 years. In the past, the epistaxis could be controlled with compression and tamponade, but it has gradually worsened. Over the past 2 weeks, her hemoglobin has dropped from 117 to 74 g/L because of recurrent significant episodes of epistaxis, and she is referred to our institution for embolization.

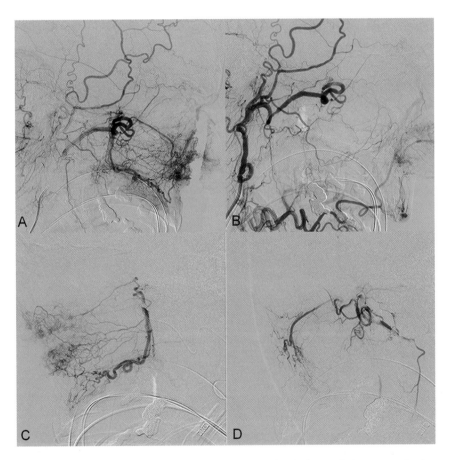

Fig. 46.1 DSA. Right ECA angiograms **(A)** before and **(B)** after embolization and selective microcatheter injections of the distal left IMA **(C)** before and **(D)** after embolization show hyperemia and several areas of telangiectasia of the nasal cavity, supplied predominantly by the sphenopalatine branches of the IMAs. No early venous drainage or extravasation of contrast is identified.

Radiologic Studies

DSA

The study demonstrated hyperemia with a slightly prominent capillary blush of the nasal cavity, including several areas of telangiectasia supplied predominantly by the sphenopalatine branches of the internal maxillary arteries (IMAs) bilaterally **(Fig. 46.1 A,C)**. Minimal supply from branches of the distal facial arteries was also observed bilaterally.

Diagnosis

Epistaxis related to HHT

Treatment

EQUIPMENT

- Standard 5F access (puncture needle, 5F vascular sheath)
- Standard 5F multipurpose catheter (Guider Soft Tip; Boston Scientific, Natick, MA) with continuous flush and a 0.035-in hydrophilic guidewire (Terumo, Somerset, NJ)
- A 0.021-in over-the-wire microcatheter (Prowler Plus; Cordis, Warren, NJ) with a 0.014-in hydrophilic guidewire (Synchro 14; Boston Scientific)
- Polyvinyl alcohol particles, 355 to 500 μm (Contour; Boston Scientific)
- Contrast material

DESCRIPTION

Following diagnostic angiography, a 5F multipurpose catheter was advanced into the proximal right external carotid artery (ECA). An over-the-wire microcatheter was introduced over a micro-guidewire into the distal IMA at the origin of the sphenopalatine artery. A mixture of 300- to 500-μm polyvinyl alcohol particles with contrast media was injected slowly under a blank roadmap until stagnation of the distal branches was observed. The microcatheter was then introduced into the distal right facial artery, which was embolized with the same technique. A control run of the right ECA was done after removal of the microcatheter. The 5F multipurpose catheter was moved into the proximal left ECA, and the procedure was repeated for the distal left IMA and distal left facial artery. Control runs of the ECAs showed obliteration of the previously seen hyperemia within the nasal cavity **(Fig. 46.1 B,D)**.

Discussion

Background

Epistaxis is one of the most common ear, nose, and throat emergencies and occurs in up to 60% of persons within their lifetime. Only 6% of these cases are severe enough to require medical attention. There is a bimodal distribution, with a small peak just before the age of 20 years and another peak after the age of 40 years. Cases of epistaxis can be subdivided etiologically as having a local or systemic cause. Up to 80 to 90% of cases are idiopathic. Some local causes are trauma (including picking the nose), inflammation, tumors, and vascular lesions (e.g., HHT, arteriovenous malformations). Iatrogenic epistaxis, such as that related to surgery or nasogastric tube placement, also has a local cause. Common systemic causes of epistaxis are hypertension, hematologic conditions, the use of anticoagulation or antiplatelet medications, and liver failure. Cases of epistaxis are also usually classified according to the site of origin as anterior or posterior. The majority of cases are located anteriorly, arising from the anterior septal area (also known as Little's area), which receives its vascular supply from the Kiesselbach plexus. The major supply to this region is from the sphenopalatine artery (of the IMA), the descending palatine artery (of the IMA), the superior labial artery (of the facial artery), and the anterior and posterior ethmoidal arteries, arising from the distal ophthalmic artery. Anterior epistaxis can usually be managed with pressure applied to the nose, anterior packing, chemical cautery or electrocautery, and topical vasoconstrictors, in addition to control of any underlying risk factors, such as hypertension and the use of anticoagulation medication. In ~5% of cases, epistaxis arises posteriorly, so that initial management measures fail. These cases may require more aggressive management, such as surgical ligation or embolization.

HHT is an autosomal-dominant disorder characterized by vascular abnormalities of the nose, skin, lungs, gastrointestinal tract, and central nervous system. Epistaxis from telangiectasia of the nasal mucosa is a common presentation in these patients, typically in the second or third decade of life. Various options, including embolization, have been used to treat epistaxis in patients with HHT. However, the recurrence rate in these patients following embolization is generally higher than in those without HHT.

Noninvasive Imaging Workup

PHYSICAL EXAMINATION

- If possible, the source of the bleeding (anterior or posterior, right or left) should be determined before embolization.
- Patients with HHT may have typical telangiectasia involving the tongue and lip regions and a family history of epistaxis.

CT/MRI

- Cross-sectional imaging is usually not indicated for the investigation of epistaxis unless there is any reason to suspect a tumor as an underlying cause.
- CT is indicated in cases of arterial epistaxis after acute trauma.

CTA/MRA

- CTA and MRA may be useful in patients with traumatic epistaxis and patients in whom an underlying vascular cause is suspected (arterial bleeding).

Invasive Imaging Workup

- It is important to obtain a diagnostic angiogram of both the internal carotid arteries (ICAs) and the ECAs before embolization; however, this can be performed within the same session.
- In a minority of cases, the cause (e.g., vascular malformation, traumatic aneurysm) and location (e.g., extravasation of contrast, tumoral blush) of epistaxis may be identified.
- An evaluation of potential anastomoses between the ECA and ICA or ophthalmic artery must be done before embolization to avoid a risk for stroke and blindness.

Treatment Options

CONSERVATIVE AND MEDICAL MANAGEMENT

- Resuscitation and treatment of any underlying systemic cause of epistaxis, such as hypertension or a coagulation disorder, are performed.
- Nasal preparation with a local anesthetic and a vasoconstrictor is followed by a local examination to determine the cause of epistaxis. Chemical cauterization with silver nitrate or electrocautery may be performed.

- If the bleeding continues, then anterior packing is usually performed. Posterior packing is reserved for patients in whom all of the above-mentioned initial measures fail or who are bleeding from a more posterior source.

SURGICAL TREATMENT

- The surgical management of epistaxis includes diathermy, septal surgery, and arterial ligation.
- Anterior/posterior ethmoidal artery ligation is typically performed if the bleeding is mainly from the supply through the ophthalmic artery, which may be the case if epistaxis continues after proper embolization of both IMAs and both facial arteries.
- ECA ligation, including IMA ligation, is no longer recommended because it is associated with a high rate of long-term recurrence and prevents re-treatment via an endovascular route.
- Surgery may be performed after other management options have failed to control the bleeding.

ENDOVASCULAR TREATMENT

- The goal of embolization is to stop active bleeding. Because of the rich vascular network of the facial arteries, mucosal perfusion will return to normal within 2 to 8 days after embolization. Therefore, the procedure does not eliminate the chance of recurrent bleeding, particularly in patients with HHT.
- Embolization is typically performed under general anesthesia to avoid patient discomfort and possible movement during the procedure.
- In cases of unilateral epistaxis, both distal IMAs and the ipsilateral facial artery are embolized. The contralateral facial artery may be spared as a collateral pathway to the nasal mucosa. If the source of the bleeding is bilateral, then both IMAs and both facial arteries must be embolized.
- The most important anatomic variant to be aware of during embolization for epistaxis is an anastomosis between the ECA and ophthalmic artery. The landmark for the central retinal artery is the choroidal blush, which can be identified in the capillary phase on the lateral view. This may arise from the ICA and/or the ECA injection, depending on its origin.
- The most common anastomosis between the ECA and ophthalmic artery is through the middle meningeal artery (MMA), either a meningo-ophthalmic artery or the meningolacrimal variant. If the ophthalmic artery is visualized only through the ECA injection, the MMA must be preserved, the position of the catheter or microcatheter must be beyond the origin of the MMA, and no reflux is allowed during particle injection (**Fig. 46.2**). In a case with a dual supply to the ophthalmic artery from both the ICA and the ECA, the proximal MMA can be closed with large embolic material (coil, large Gelfoam particles) before embolization with smaller particles to prevent emboli from entering the ophthalmic artery (**Fig. 46.3**). When the anastomosis is located more distally from the IMA (i.e., through the anterior deep temporal artery to the lacrimal artery or the sphenopalatine artery to the ethmoidal arteries), a dual supply with the dominant supply from the ICA is typically present. In this instance, the anastomosis can be closed safely with large particles before embolization. However, if the supply from the ICA is occluded, as in cases of severe atherosclerosis (**Fig. 46.4**), then embolization of the IMA on that side must be avoided.
- Apart from the anastomoses to the ophthalmic artery, the IMA branches also form multiple anastomoses at the skull base with the intrapetrous and intracavernous branches of the ICA. These are usually too small to be visualized on a routine angiogram and can be avoided by using particles larger than 80 to 100 μm. In our experience, we prefer particles with a size of 250 to 500 μm.

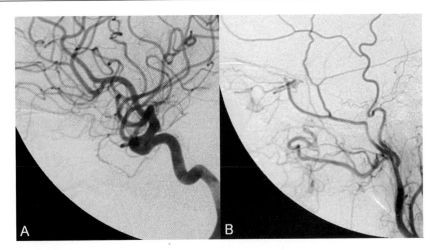

Fig. 46.2 DSA. Angiograms of **(A)** the right ICA and **(B)** the right ECA in lateral view demonstrate a classic meningo-ophthalmic artery variant in which the ophthalmic artery arises only from the MMA. Note the absence of the "normal" ophthalmic artery from the ICA. The MMA must be preserved during embolization by the use of distal catheterization beyond its origin, and no reflux of the embolic material is allowed.

Possible Complications

- Blindness, stroke, and cranial nerve palsies may occur after distal embolization through the ophthalmic and skull base anastomotic channels.
- Skin and mucosal necrosis are often temporary. Ischemic sialadenitis has been reported.
- Minor complications include headaches, facial pain, jaw pain, trismus, facial edema, facial numbness, facial hypersensitivity to cold, paresthesias, mild ulceration of the palate, and fever.

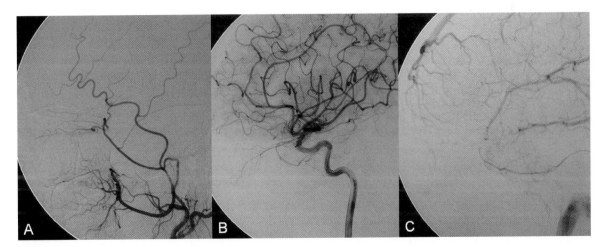

Fig. 46.3 DSA. Angiograms of the left ICA in **(A)** arterial and **(B)** early venous phases and of **(C)** the left ECA in lateral view reveal a dual supply to the ophthalmic artery from both the ICA and the ECA. Note the crescent-shaped choroidal blush on the capillary-early venous phase of the ICA angiogram. When a dual supply is present, either a distal catheterization technique or occlusion of the proximal MMA can be used to prevent the distal migration of emboli into the ophthalmic artery.

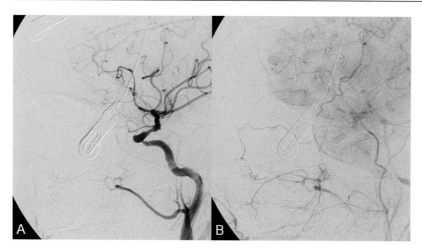

Fig. 46.4 DSA. Right common carotid artery angiograms in **(A)** early arterial and **(B)** capillary phases in lateral view show irregularity of the cavernous segment of the right ICA, likely related to atherosclerosis. The origin of the ophthalmic artery from the ICA is not visualized and is likely to be occluded. There is late retrograde filling of the ophthalmic artery through anastomoses between the sphenopalatine artery and ethmoidal branches. In this case, the IMA cannot be embolized.

Published Literature on Treatment Options

In the literature, embolization stops active bleeding in ~93 to 100% of all cases of acute epistaxis; however, early rebleeding is reported to occur in ~5 to 25% of cases, with a delay of 72 hours to 33 days after embolization. Success rates of bleeding control depend on the embolization protocol. If only the IMAs are embolized, the success rate is 87%; however, this increases to 97% if the facial arteries are also embolized. More than half of long-term failures are in patients with HHT. The larger series report minor transient complications in ~25 to 60% and major complications in 1 to 3%, including skin necrosis, hemiparesis, visual field loss, blindness, facial nerve paralysis, and ischemic sialadenitis requiring surgery.

PEARLS AND PITFALLS_____

- Knowledge of the anastomoses between the ophthalmic artery, ICA, and ECA is necessary to avoid potential major complications of embolization.
- Embolization is useful for stopping active bleeding but not for preventing recurrent bleeding.

Further Reading

Elden L, Montanera W, Terbrugge K, Willinsky R, Lasjaunias P, Charles D. Angiographic embolization for the treatment of epistaxis: a review of 108 cases. Otolaryngol Head Neck Surg 1994;111(1):44–50

Geibprasert S, Pongpech S, Armstrong D, Krings T. Dangerous extracranial-intracranial anastomoses and supply to the cranial nerves: vessels the neurointerventionalist needs to know. AJNR Am J Neuroradiol 2009;30(8):1459–1468

Willems PW, Farb RI, Agid R. Endovascular treatment of epistaxis. AJNR Am J Neuroradiol 2009;30(9):1637–1645

CASE 47

Case Description

Clinical Presentation

A 68-year-old previously healthy woman experiences the acute onset of aphasia and right-sided hemiplegia. She is brought to the emergency department within the first hour after symptom onset, and emergency CT is performed.

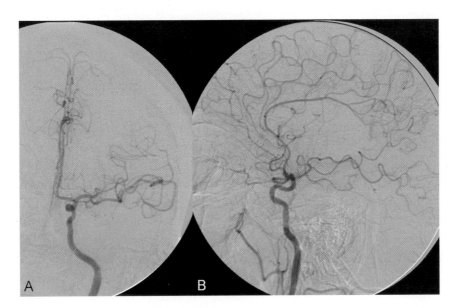

Fig. 47.1 DSA. Left ICA angiogram in **(A)** AP and **(B)** lateral views demonstrates occlusion of the proximal middle branch of the left MCA.

Radiologic Studies

CT

CT was unremarkable and did not demonstrate any signs of acute stroke, especially no hyperdense middle cerebral artery (MCA) sign. CTA demonstrated an M2 occlusion on the left side.

Diagnosis

Acute left-sided MCA branch occlusion

Treatment

EQUIPMENT

- Standard 6F access (puncture needle, 6F vascular sheath)
- 6F multipurpose catheter (Envoy; Cordis, Warren, NJ) with continuous flush and a 0.035-in hydrophilic guidewire (Terumo, Somerset, NJ)

271

- Straight microcatheter (Excel 14; Boston Scientific) with a 0.014-in guidewire (Transend 14; Boston Scientific)
- Recombinant tissue plasminogen activator (Actilyse; Genentech, South San Francisco, CA) 1-mg/mL solution to a total of 22 mg
- Heparin
- Contrast material

DESCRIPTION

After the left common carotid artery had been selected, a roadmap was performed to exclude the possibility of a high-grade stenosis of the internal carotid artery (ICA) origin, and the catheter was advanced via the guidewire into the left ICA. Angiography demonstrated an open M1 but a complete occlusion of the dominant middle trunk of the MCA trifurcation, which left a large perfusion deficit within the left hemisphere (**Fig. 47.1**). A bolus of 2000 units of heparin was given, and the heparin was continued with the injection of 450 units per hour. Following this, a standard Excel 14 microcatheter equipped with a Transend 14 Soft Tip was advanced via the guiding catheter, which was continuously flushed with heparinized saline. The microcatheter was also continuously flushed and advanced with caution under roadmap conditions distal to the thrombus into the distal M2 branch, as verified by a gentle microcatheter injection (**Fig. 47.2**). Subsequently, 1 mg of recombinant tissue plasminogen activator (rtPA) dissolved in 2 mL of saline was injected distal to the clot over 1 minute. The microcatheter was then slowly withdrawn into the proximal part of the thrombus, where another bolus of 1 mg of rtPA was administered. A continuous injection of 10 mg of rtPA per hour was performed at this point (proximal part of the thrombus). Control runs via the guiding catheter were performed every 15 minutes. After 1 hour and the administration of a total of 12 mg of rtPA intra-arterially, there was still no change visible at catheter angiography, with complete occlusion of the proximal M2 branch. After the administration of another 2.5 mg of rtPA, however, the control run demonstrated complete reopening of the distal and proximal M2 branch, with minimal stagnation of contrast in distal M4 branches. The microcatheter was removed, and the final control run demonstrated complete reopening of the M2 branch with reperfusion of more than 90% of its territory (**Fig. 47.3**). The guiding catheter was removed, and the sheath was sutured to the groin. During a neurologic examination on the table, the patient was able to speak again, and the hemiplegia had completely resolved. Follow-up CT 1 day later demonstrated no area of ischemia.

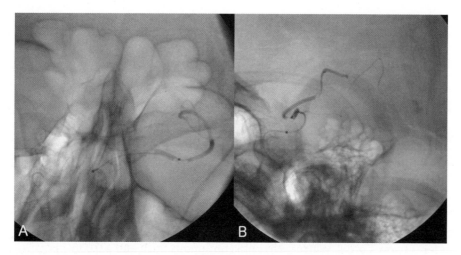

Fig. 47.2 Unsubtracted gentle microcatheter injection in **(A)** AP and **(B)** lateral views reveals a filling defect, representing thrombus in the MCA branch.

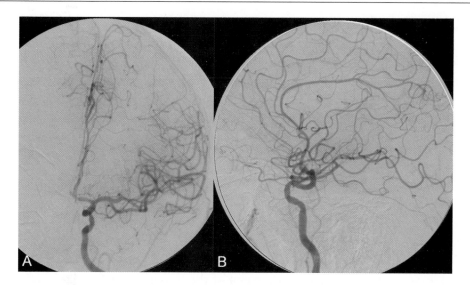

Fig. 47.3 DSA. Left ICA angiogram in **(A)** AP and **(B)** lateral views after successful thrombolysis shows complete reopening of the entire MCA.

Discussion

Background

Stroke is one of the leading causes of death or long-term disability, and demographic changes are likely to result in an increase in both the incidence and prevalence of stroke. Stroke is a common cause of dementia, epilepsy, and depression in the elderly. More than 85% of all strokes are ischemic in nature. Up to 30 to 35% of ischemic strokes are due to extracranial or intracranial large-artery atherosclerosis. Cardioembolic strokes account for 25 to 30% of all cerebral ischemic events. Small-vessel disease accounts for 15 to 20% of all ischemic strokes. The remaining ischemic strokes have either another, uncommon cause or an undetermined origin. Nearly 10% of patients with acute stroke die, and of those who survive, about 50% are disabled. Older age, a poor neurologic score on admission, high blood levels of glucose, and a large clot burden increase the chance of a poor outcome.

Ischemic stroke is caused by a critical reduction in the blood supply to the brain for a prolonged period. Following the occlusion of a brain-supplying artery, a core of infarcted tissue will develop, surrounded by tissue that is initially only functionally impaired because of a reduced blood supply. The amount of functionally impaired tissue depends on the location of the occluded vessel and the collateral blood supply. Reperfusion can salvage those cells at risk for critical hypoperfusion.

In a recent Cochrane Database Review of more than 7000 patients, Wardlaw et al stated that thrombolytic therapy, mostly administered up to 6 hours after ischemic stroke, significantly reduced the proportion of patients who died or became dependent (modified Rankin Scale score of 3–6) at 3 to 6 months after stroke (odds ratio [OR], 0.81; 95% confidence interval [CI], 0.73–0.90). However, the route of administration remains controversial (i.e., intravenous, intra-arterial, or bridging therapy, which is started with the intravenous administration and continued with the intra-arterial administration of a drug).

Noninvasive Imaging Workup

PHYSICAL EXAMINATION

- The clinical syndrome in a patient with stroke will indicate the location and size of affected brain tissue and therefore the affected vessel

- Infarction of the anterior circulation may lead to hemiparesis, hemisensory loss, homonymous hemianopia, aphasia, or neglect, whereas stroke affecting the posterior circulation causes ipsilateral cranial nerve palsies with contralateral motor or sensory deficits, conjugate eye movement disorders, cerebellar dysfunction, cortical blindness, or a decreased level of consciousness.
- Lacunar strokes must be differentiated from large-vessel occlusions. They are often clinically silent; however, when they affect the internal capsule, they may lead to a purely motor or a purely sensory stroke without associated symptoms such as neglect or aphasia.

CT/MRI

- Unenhanced CT is often the first-choice modality, given its wide availability. It can detect intracranial hemorrhage and may demonstrate early signs of ischemia, including hyperdense vessel signs (at the site of the vessel occlusion), and early markers of cytotoxic edema, including loss of the cortical ribbon, loss of gray/white differentiation at the level of the basal ganglia, and brain swelling.
- CTA can demonstrate the site of the occluded vessel, extent of the thrombus, and, if the carotid arteries are also imaged, potential sources of the acute thrombus.
- Perfusion CT can differentiate functionally impaired brain tissue from already infarcted brain tissue by differences in the cerebral blood volume (< 2 mL/100 g in the infarcted core). Compared with areas of the brain that are not impaired, both irreversibly and reversibly impaired brain tissue will show increases in mean transit time and decreases in blood flow.
- MRI is more sensitive than CT; however, it is not as widely available, and longer delays before imaging is completed may be encountered, depending on the clinical setting. A comprehensive MR stroke protocol comprises FLAIR-weighted scans to demonstrate old infarctions, diffusion-weighted scans to demonstrate the amount of acutely and irreversibly damaged brain tissue, perfusion-weighted MRI to evaluate the tissue at risk, and MRA to demonstrate the site of vessel occlusion.
- For many authors, a diffusion-perfusion mismatch serves as a rational criterion for the selection of therapeutic strategies. This concept is based on the assumption that diffusion-weighted imaging demonstrates irreversibly damaged brain tissue, whereas perfusion defects indicate the area that may progress to infarction if recanalization does not occur.
- Alternatives to diffusion-perfusion mismatch are diffusion-clinical findings mismatch (based on differences between the extent of diffusion-weighted imaging changes and the clinical severity of the stroke symptoms) and diffusion-MRA mismatch (in which MRA methods are used to estimate the tissue at risk).
- Infarctions are often first seen in subcortical areas (i.e., striatocapsular infarctions) because of the persistence of cortical collateral blood flow.

Invasive Imaging Workup

- DSA can demonstrate the site of occlusion and potential leptomeningeal collaterals, as well as collaterals from the anterior and posterior communicating arteries.
- If not already done during prior CTA or MRA, injections of the common carotid arteries and the subclavian arteries to evaluate the origins of the ICA and the vertebral artery are essential because high-grade stenoses in these regions may be the cause of the stroke.
- In most instances, invasive imaging is performed immediately before intra-arterial therapies are administered.

Differential Diagnosis

- Depending on the clinical findings, onset of symptoms, and imaging findings, the differential diagnosis of stroke (based on both clinical and imaging findings) can be extensive and includes neoplastic, inflammatory, and metabolic disorders.
- Rare causes of stroke must also be considered, especially in younger patients.

Treatment Options

CONSERVATIVE OR MEDICAL MANAGEMENT

- Intravenous thrombolysis with rtPA within a 4.5-hour therapeutic window has proved to be beneficial for patients with acute ischemic stroke.
- Antiplatelet therapies have proved beneficial for patients with acute stroke, and most authors recommend starting acetylsalicylic acid within the first 48 hours after acute ischemic stroke.
- Anticoagulation is not associated with clinical benefits in most patients with acute ischemic stroke.
- Neuroprotective agents have not proved beneficial thus far.

ENDOVASCULAR TREATMENT

- Intra-arterial thrombolysis with either rtPA or urokinase may be administered.
- Different strategies of drug delivery may be chosen. The microcatheter can be positioned at the proximal aspect of the clot, into the clot, or beyond the clot. The protocol employed in our institution is described in greater detail in the earlier section, "Description of Treatment."
- Mechanical treatments may be administered. (These are discussed in greater detail in later cases.)

Possible Complications

- Reperfusion hemorrhage
- Distal embolism during recanalization
- Nonresponsiveness of the clot to the thrombolytic drug

Published Literature on Treatment Options

It is beyond doubt that longer periods of time between the onset of symptoms of ischemic stroke and the initiation of treatment are associated with a progressively lower likelihood of clinical benefit. Likewise, the probability of a good clinical outcome decreases as the time to angiographic reperfusion increases. However, the way to reach the goal of rapid recanalization remains controversial.

Physicians who favor the use of intravenous therapy alone base their arguments mostly on the fact that it is the only FDA-approved therapy for improving the outcome of acute stroke. Data to support this came from the National Institute of Neurological Disorders and Stroke trial of intravenous thrombolysis conducted in 1995. Intravenous rtPA was given in a dose of 0.9 mg/kg of body weight, with a maximum dose of 90 mg, within the first 3 hours after symptom onset. Compared with patients in the placebo arm of the study, patients in the treatment arm were 30% more likely to have minimal or no disability at 90 days. The rate of symptomatic intracranial hemorrhage was higher in those receiving treatment (6.4%) than in the controls (0.6%). However, the mortality rates at 90 days were similar. The recent European Cooperative Acute Stroke Study (ECASS III), a randomized, double-blind, multicenter, placebo-controlled trial of rtPA in acute ischemic stroke in which thrombolysis was initiated between 3 and 4.5 hours after stroke onset, extended even further the time window in which the intravenous administration of rtPA was proven beneficial. The arguments against intra-arterial therapies that are often put forward are the greater complexity of the procedure, lack of availability, potential delays in initiating treatment, added risks of an invasive procedure, and higher expenses.

In intra-arterial thrombolysis, the drug is given only to those patients who have an occluded artery; the dosage to be given is usually smaller and may therefore be safer. Further data in favor of endovascular therapies are derived from the Prolyse in Acute Cerebral Thromboembolism (PROACT) trials, which demonstrated good outcomes for patients with large-vessel occlusion given intra-arterial therapy. A significant 15% increase in the chance of a good outcome was noted when patients with M1 occlusion were treated with intra-arterial thrombolysis within a 6-hour time window without an increase in mortality in comparison with those who did not receive this intervention. In a recent observational study that compared data from two stroke units where the management of stroke was similar, except that one unit performed intra-arterial thrombolysis with urokinase and the other intravenous thrombolysis with plasminogen activator, intra-arterial thrombolysis was more beneficial than intravenous thrombolysis, even though intra-arterial thrombolysis was started later.

A bridging strategy between intravenous and intra-arterial thrombolysis has the advantage of not delaying lytic therapy while identifying nonresponders with persistent large-artery occlusion. Initial positive results for this treatment strategy have been reported by the RECANALISE study, which compared recanalization rates, neurologic improvement, and functional outcome in patients treated within the first 3 hours after stroke onset either with intravenous thrombolysis alone or with a combined intravenous-endovascular approach. The authors found that an intravenous-endovascular approach was associated with higher recanalization rates than intravenous alteplase in patients with stroke and confirmed arterial occlusion. The clinical outcome was more often favorable in the intravenous-endovascular group, whereas mortality rates and rates of hemorrhagic stroke were similar in the two groups. The bridging approach is currently being tested in the Interventional Management of Stroke (IMS III) trial, in which initial intravenous tPA is followed by artery reopening with thrombolytic agents or clot retrieval if vessel occlusion is demonstrated.

According to the presently available data, intravenous thrombolysis within the first 3 hours after stroke onset will result in less than a 30% chance of reopening large arteries with a large clot burden, versus a 60% to 70% chance of recanalization with intra-arterial thrombolysis. Given these data, one may be inclined to reassess current management strategies for patients with acute stroke in the 3-hour time period. If a patient has a major large-vessel occlusion and considerable mismatch, intra-arterial treatment may be considered. If significant delays in starting intra-arterial treatment are anticipated, intravenous thrombolysis can be initiated, followed by intra-arterial treatment if recanalization does not occur. For other cases in the early time window, intravenous thrombolysis may still be considered. After the 3- (or 4.5-) hour time window, treatment should be guided by the results of the PROACT II trial, which indicated a better outcome for patients treated with intra-arterial thrombolysis within up to 6 hours after stroke onset.

PEARLS AND PITFALLS
- Early recanalization can improve the prognosis in acute ischemic stroke.
- Although intra-arterial thrombolysis has been shown to be effective, the time delay required for cerebral angiography and microcatheter positioning is a handicap that can be overcome with "bridging" therapies.

Further Reading

Furlan A, Higashida R, Wechsler L, et al. Intra-arterial prourokinase for acute ischemic stroke. The PROACT II study: a randomized controlled trial. Prolyse in Acute Cerebral Thromboembolism. JAMA 1999;282(21):2003–2011

Jahan R, Vinuela F. Treatment of acute ischemic stroke: intravenous and endovascular therapies. Expert Rev Cardiovasc Ther 2009;7(4):375–387

Mattle HP, Arnold M, Georgiadis D, et al. Comparison of intraarterial and intravenous thrombolysis for ischemic stroke with hyperdense middle cerebral artery sign. Stroke 2008;39(2):379–383

Mazighi M, Serfaty JM, Labreuche J, et al; RECANALISE investigators. Comparison of intravenous alteplase with a combined intravenous-endovascular approach in patients with stroke and confirmed arterial occlusion (RECANALISE study): a prospective cohort study. Lancet Neurol 2009;8(9):802–809

Schonewille WJ, Wijman CA, Michel P, et al; BASICS study group. Treatment and outcomes of acute basilar artery occlusion in the Basilar Artery International Cooperation Study (BASICS): a prospective registry study. Lancet Neurol 2009;8(8):724–730

Tissue plasminogen activator for acute ischemic stroke. The National Institute of Neurological Disorders and Stroke rt-PA Stroke Study Group. N Engl J Med 1995;333(24):1581–1587

Wardlaw JM, Murray V, Berge E, Del Zoppo GJ. Thrombolysis for acute ischaemic stroke. Cochrane Database Syst Rev 2009; (4):CD000213

CASE 48

Case Description

Clinical Presentation

A 68-year-old woman presents to the emergency department 5 hours after the sudden onset of left hemiparesis. Her baseline National Institutes of Health Stroke Scale (NIHSS) score is 19. Risk factors include chronic hypertension and heavy smoking. Emergency CT, including CTA and CT perfusion, is performed.

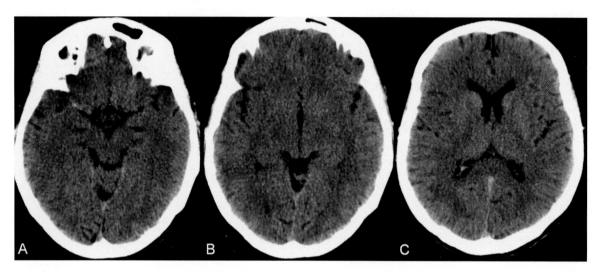

Fig. 48.1 **(A)** Unenhanced axial CT scan demonstrates a hyperdense right MCA sign and **(B,C)** slight hypodensity within the right insular and fronto-opercular regions.

Radiologic Studies

CT

Plain CT of the brain demonstrated a hyperdense right middle cerebral artery (MCA) sign and mild right insular and fronto-opercular hypodensity in less than one-third of the MCA territory. CTA confirmed occlusion of the distal M1 and corresponding hypoperfusion (**Fig. 48.1**).

DSA

The common carotid artery (CCA) and the internal carotid artery (ICA) origins were unremarkable. Intracranially, there was a right MCA occlusion. During late arterial phases, mild pial collateral filling of the distal MCA via the anterior cerebral artery (ACA) was seen (**Fig. 48.2**).

Diagnosis

MCA occlusion at the M1 (Thrombolysis in Cerebral Infarction [TICI] grade, 0).

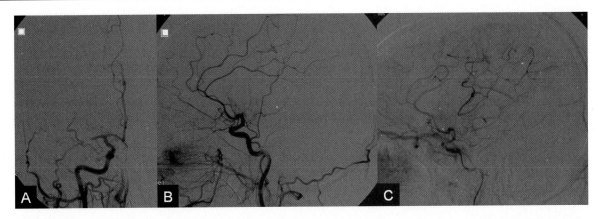

Fig. 48.2 DSA. Right CCA angiogram in **(A)** AP and **(B,C)** lateral views in **(B)** early arterial and **(C)** late arterial phases reveals occlusion of the right MCA. There is minimal filling of the distal MCA through leptomeningeal collaterals from the ACA branches.

Treatment

EQUIPMENT

- Standard 8F access (puncture needle, 8F vascular sheath)
- Standard 8F multipurpose catheter (Cordis, Warren, NJ) with continuous flush and a 0.035-in hydrophilic guide wire (Terumo, Somerset, NJ)
- Preparation for the aspiration procedure
    - Penumbra Aspiration Catheter 041, curved at vapor (30 degrees) with continuous flush (Penumbra Inc, Alameda, CA)
    - A 0.016-in hydrophilic micro-guidewire
    - Connector to the pump (pretested at –20 mm Hg)
    - Penumbra Separator 041
- Contrast material
- Recombinant tissue plasminogen activator (Actilyse; Genentech, South San Francisco, CA) 1-mg/mL solution

DESCRIPTION

Following diagnostic angiography, an 8F multipurpose catheter was advanced into the right ICA. A Penumbra Aspiration Microcatheter 041 with a 30-degree angled curve was introduced with a 0.016-in guidewire and advanced gently to the MCA proximal to the clot under roadmap guidance. The guidewire was removed, and the Penumbra Separator 041 was advanced. The connection to the pump was opened at a pressure of –20 mm Hg. When refluxed blood started to appear in the connecting tubes to the pump, the separator was advanced and used to disperse the thrombus while the microcatheter was slowly advanced. An intermediate control demonstrated a persistent M2 branch occlusion and some distal emboli in frontal branches. A solution of recombinant tissue plasminogen activator (rtPA) was then infused through the microcatheter, which was positioned at the M1. Progressive reperfusion was observed during infusion of a total of 12 mg until a TICI grade of 2b was achieved (**Fig. 48.3**). After the procedure, the patient was taken to the intensive care unit and extubated. A small residual motor deficit of the left arm was noted. At 24 hours, the NIHSS score was 2. The patient recovered completely and was discharged at day 7 (**Fig. 48.4**).

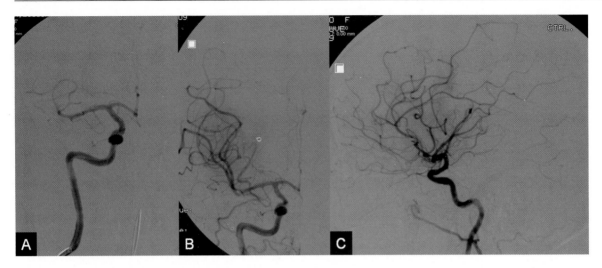

Fig. 48.3 DSA. **(A)** Right ICA angiogram in AP view during the revascularization procedure shows the position of the Penumbra aspiration system (aspiration catheter 041 plus separator 041) in the distal M1 segment. Right CCA angiogram in **(B)** AP and **(C)** lateral views after the procedure reveals complete recanalization of the M1 segment (TICI grade, 2b).

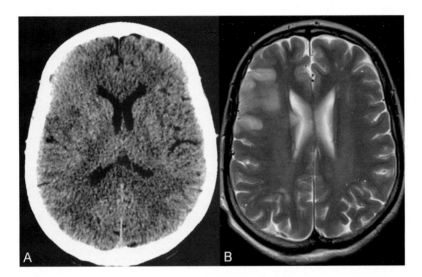

Fig. 48.4 (A) Unenhanced axial CT scan at 24 hours after treatment reveals no evidence of intracranial hemorrhage. There is mild effacement of the cortical sulci in the right fronto-opercular region. **(B)** Axial T2-weighted MR image 3 days after treatment shows a small right frontal infarction.

Discussion

Background

As stated in the previous case, ischemic stroke is one of the leading causes of disability and mortality in the world. Intravenous thrombolysis is at present the only approved treatment of this devastating disease, with the therapeutic window extended to 4.5 hours after symptom onset. With intravenous thrombolysis, however, recanalization rates in patients with proximal large-vessel occlusions are low; reported rates are 10% for the ICA and 30% for the proximal MCA. In addition, more than 80% of patients with an NIHSS score of 10 or higher have persistent arterial occlusion on subsequent angiography, even after initial treatment with intravenous tPA. Therefore, there is keen interest in intra-arterial therapies for acute stroke that may extend the therapeutic window and make it possible to treat patients who have contraindications to or who have failed intravenous thrombolysis. Advantages of intra-arterial thrombolysis are higher rates of recanalization, smaller doses of rtPA, and immediate confirmation of recanalization; disadvantages are the limited availability of this technique in the community and the slightly higher rate of hemorrhagic complications. Given the risk for hemorrhage and the time constraints associated with thrombolytic agents, alternate means for removing a clot have been proposed that are discussed here and in the next case.

Noninvasive Imaging Workup

PHYSICAL EXAMINATION

- The NIHSS score is commonly used to indicate the clinical impact of an occlusion and is strongly correlated with the prognosis (**Table 48.1**).

CT

- In the European Cooperative Acute Stroke Study (ECASS), CT hypodensity in more than one-third of the MCA territory was considered a contraindication to acute treatment. However, the one-third of the MCA territory rule is a poorly defined volumetric estimate of the size of a cerebral infarction of the MCA territory.
- Therefore, a 10-point quantitative topographic CT score, the Alberta Stroke Program Early CT Score (ASPECTS), has been developed, in which 10 regions are identified on two nonadjacent CT slices. One slice is at the level of the basal ganglia, in which seven regions are identified: the caudate head, the lentiform nucleus, the internal capsule, the insular ribbon, and the cortical MCA territories M1, M2, and M3 (anterior MCA cortex, cortex lateral to the insular ribbon, and posterior MCA cortex). A second slice 2 cm superior to M1 through M3 and rostral to the basal ganglia comprises M4, M5, and M6 as the anterior, lateral, and posterior MCA territories, respectively. A score of 10 is a normal scan, and one point is deducted for each area of hypoattenuation in the above-mentioned 10 areas. A sharp increase in dependence and death occurs with an ASPECTS of 7 or less. This CT evaluation method is now being used in many centers.

Invasive Imaging Workup

- Classically, a four-vessel workup was recommended (including both vertebral arteries and both carotid arteries to evaluate the collateral circulation and brain perfusion). More recently, prior noninvasive vascular and perfusion imaging allows immediate catheterization of the affected axis to start recanalization.
- Revascularization is measured with the primary arterial occlusive lesion (AOL) recanalization grade, and reperfusion is measured with a modified TICI grade, as described below (**Table 48.2**).

Treatment Options

MEDICAL OR SURGICAL TREATMENT

- The role of medical treatment was discussed in the previous case. There is no place for surgery in acute stroke except in extremely rare circumstances (e.g., removal of iatrogenic materials, coils).

ENDOVASCULAR TREATMENT

- Mechanical thrombectomy or intra-arterial medical thombolysis can be performed.
- For mechanical thrombectomy, many different devices are available. These can be placed proximal to the clot for aspiration or distally for retrieval.

Table 48.1 National Institutes of Health Stroke Scale

Category	Results	Score
1a. LOC (Patients with a score of 2 or 3 for this item should be assessed with the Glasgow Coma Scale.)	Alert, keenly responsive	0
	Not alert (arousable–minor stimulation)	1
	Not alert (arousable–painful stimulation)	2
	Unresponsive	3
1b. LOC questions (month, age)	Answers both correctly	0
	Answers one correctly	1
	Answers neither correctly	2
1c. LOC commands (open and close eyes, make and release fist)	Performs both tasks correctly	0
	Performs one correctly	1
	Performs neither correctly	2
2. Best gaze	Normal	0
	Partial gaze palsy	1
	Forced deviation	2
3. Visual	No visual loss	0
	Partial hemianopia	1
	Complete hemianopia	2
	Bilateral hemianopia	3
4. Facial palsy	Normal	0
	Minor paralysis	1
	Partial paralysis	2
	Complete paralysis	3
5. Motor function (arm) a. Left b. Right	No drift	0
	Drift before 5 seconds	1
	Drift before 10 seconds	2
	No effort against gravity	3
	No movement	4
6. Motor function (leg) a. Left b. Right	No drift	0
	Drift before 5 seconds	1
	Drift before 10 seconds	2
	No effort against gravity	3
	No movement	4
7. Limb ataxia	No ataxia	0
	Ataxia–one limb	1
	Ataxia–two limbs	2
8. Sensory function	No sensory loss	0
	Mild sensory loss	1
	Severe sensory loss	2
9. Language	Normal	0
	Mild aphasia	1
	Severe aphasia	2
	Mute or global aphasia	3
10. Articulation	Normal	0
	Mild-to-moderate dysarthria	1
	Severe dysarthria	2
11. Extinction and inattention	Absent	0
	Mild	1
	Severe	2

Abbreviation: LOC, level of consciousness

Table 48.2 TICI Reperfusion and AOL Recanalization Grades

Post-treatment TICI Reperfusion Grade

0	No perfusion
1	Perfusion past the initial obstruction but limited distal branch filling with little or slow distal perfusion
2a	Perfusion of less than half of the vascular distribution of the occluded artery (e.g., filling and perfusion through one M2 division)
2b	Perfusion of half or more of the vascular distribution of the occluded artery (e.g., filling and perfusion through two or more M2 divisions)
3	Full perfusion with filling of all distal branches

Post-treatment AOL Recanalization Grade

0	No recanalization of the occlusion
1	Incomplete or partial recanalization of the occlusion, with no distal flow
2	Incomplete or partial recanalization of the occlusion, with any distal flow
3	Complete recanalization of the occlusion with any distal flow

Abbreviations: AOL, arterial occlusive lesion; TICI, Thrombolysis in Cerebral Infarction

- Thrombolytic therapy can be used primarily to dissolve the clot or at the end of a mechanical procedure to treat distal emboli. Although there is no consensus in the literature about what constitutes a safe dose, most authors quote a maximum of 22 mg of intra-arterial rtPA within the first 6 hours after stroke onset.

Possible Complications

- Distal emboli (which can be treated with further intra-arterial injection of rtPA)
- Intracranial vascular dissection, subarachnoid hemorrhage, and vessel rupture
- Reperfusion syndrome and hemorrhagic transformation of acute stroke

Published Literature on Treatment Options

The goal of recanalization therapy in acute ischemic stroke is to improve the clinical outcome by restoring antegrade perfusion and salvaging brain tissue at risk. Early vessel recanalization is linked to a good clinical outcome. Mechanical clot removal is an alternative to intravenous or intra-arterial medical thrombolysis, especially in patients with failed medical treatment, those with contraindications to rtPA (e.g., recent surgery), and those with a large clot burden. In this case, we focus on the two devices that are currently approved by the FDA; in the next case, we discuss additional new and promising devices for the mechanical treatment of stroke.

The MERCI device consists of a flexible, tapered nitinol wire with five helical loops that can be embedded within the thrombus for retrieval. Two major trials, Mechanical Embolus Removal in Cerebral Ischemia (MERCI) and Multi MERCI, have demonstrated its usefulness, especially in large-vessel occlusions. In these two trials, 48 to 68% of occluded vessels were recanalized, with a 5 to 7% rate of clinically significant procedural complications, an 8 to 10% rate of symptomatic hemorrhage, and a 34 to 44% mortality rate.

The Penumbra System is specifically designed to remove thrombus in large intracranial vessels. Revascularization with thrombus debulking and aspiration is followed by direct extraction of thrombus if clot remains. Once the catheter is positioned just proximal to the clot, the aspiration pump is connected to the catheter, and a vacuum of −20 mm Hg is produced that will facilitate aspiration of the clot. The separator is then advanced through the catheter into the proximal part of the clot, aiding the aspirating and debulking process, until the distal aspect of the clot is reached. In a preliminary clinical trial, recanalization was achieved in 82% of occluded vessels, with a 3% rate of clinically significant complications, an 11% rate of symptomatic hemorrhage, and a mortality rate of 33%.

The present trials do not have a nontreatment arm and so cannot directly demonstrate the superiority of mechanical treatment versus no treatment or medical treatment. However, the rate of artery recanalization far exceeds the expected rate of spontaneous or drug-induced early recanalization. Therefore, mechanical thrombectomy for acute stroke is likely to be beneficial in appropriate patients.

PEARLS AND PITFALLS

- An intra-arterial procedure after intravenous thrombolysis requires careful attention to the puncture site. A one-wall technique or a micro-puncture set can be used. Heparin is not indicated when a previous dose of rtPA has been given because it increases the risk for hemorrhage.
- For aspiration procedures, the following should be noted:
  - Larger catheters work better and faster (Penumbra 041 and 054).
  - Do not allow the aspiration system to be blocked for a long time. Continuous reflux should be maintained to avoid the formation of clot inside the catheter system, which decreases the efficacy of aspiration or permanently blocks the catheter.
  - *Always* start aspirating at the proximal aspect of the clot, precisely at the zone between the clot and the vessel to be opened.
  - The separator is used to break up the clot, so that it enters the microcatheter more easily. It should *never* be used as a guidewire.
  - If the tip of the microcatheter is inside the thrombus and aspiration suddenly stops, the separator should be kept in position while the microcatheter is pulled back until reflux starts again.
  - For distal emboli, intra-arterial rtPA can be administered through the microcatheter or guiding catheter.

Further Reading

Gandhi CD, Christiano LD, Prestigiacomo CJ. Endovascular management of acute ischemic stroke. Neurosurg Focus 2009;26(3):E2

Nogueira RG, Liebeskind DS, Sung G, Duckwiler G, Smith WS; MERCI; Multi MERCI Writing Committee. Predictors of good clinical outcomes, mortality, and successful revascularization in patients with acute ischemic stroke undergoing thrombectomy: pooled analysis of the Mechanical Embolus Removal in Cerebral Ischemia (MERCI) and Multi MERCI Trials. Stroke 2009;40(12):3777–3783

Nogueira RG, Schwamm LH, Hirsch JA. Endovascular approaches to acute stroke, part 1: Drugs, devices, and data. AJNR Am J Neuroradiol 2009;30(4):649–661

Penumbra Pivotal Stroke Trial Investigators. The penumbra pivotal stroke trial: safety and effectiveness of a new generation of mechanical devices for clot removal in intracranial large vessel occlusive disease. Stroke 2009;40(8):2761–2768

Pexman JH, Barber PA, Hill MD, et al. Use of the Alberta Stroke Program Early CT Score (ASPECTS) for assessing CT scans in patients with acute stroke. AJNR Am J Neuroradiol 2001;22(8):1534–1542

Rha JH, Saver JL. The impact of recanalization on ischemic stroke outcome: a meta-analysis. Stroke 2007;38(3):967–973

Tomsick T, Broderick J, Carrozella J, et al; Interventional Management of Stroke II Investigators. Revascularization results in the Interventional Management of Stroke II trial. AJNR Am J Neuroradiol 2008;29(3):582–587

CASE 49

Case Description

Clinical Presentation

A 48-year-old man with a known patent foramen ovale presents to the emergency department with left hemiparesis 2 hours after symptom onset. His baseline National Institutes of Health Stroke Scale (NIHSS) score is 12. Emergency CT is performed.

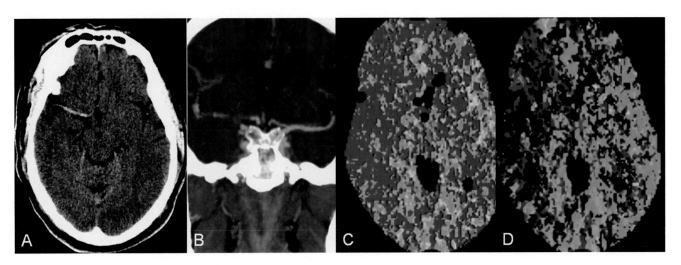

Fig. 49.1 **(A)** Unenhanced axial CT scan demonstrates a hyperdense right MCA sign and no evidence of hypodensity or intracranial hemorrhage. **(B)** CTA in coronal view shows occlusion of the right ICA bifurcation and the right MCA. **(C,D)** CT perfusion reveals hypoperfusion of the right MCA territory (blue).

Radiologic Studies

CT

Plain CT of the brain demonstrated no evidence of hypodensity (Alberta Stroke Program Early CT Score [ASPECTS] of 10), but a dense right middle cerebral artery (MCA) was noted. CTA and CT perfusion demonstrated an occlusion of the right internal carotid artery (ICA) bifurcation, occlusion of the MCA, and hypoperfusion of the right MCA territory (**Fig. 49.1**).

DSA

The patient received 0.6 mg of recombinant tissue plasminogen activator (rtPA) per kilogram of body weight intravenously over 30 minutes and was re-evaluated clinically and with transcranial Doppler ultrasound. His clinical status was unchanged, and the transcranial Doppler study showed complete occlusion of the right MCA (Thrombolysis in Cerebral Infarction [TICI] grade, 0). Intra-arterial treatment was initiated.

Injection of the right ICA showed a carotid T occlusion with the clot burden starting beyond the posterior communicating artery. Reflux via the posterior communicating artery into the basilar artery was noted (**Fig. 49.2**).

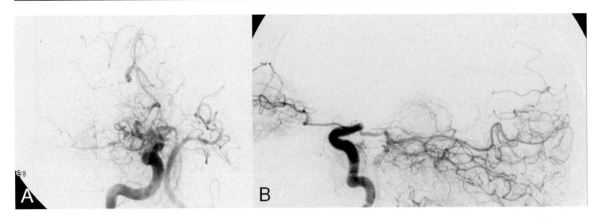

Fig. 49.2 DSA. Right ICA angiogram in **(A)** AP and **(B)** lateral views demonstrates a carotid T occlusion starting beyond the origin of the right posterior communicating artery. There is retrograde flow of contrast into the basilar artery.

Diagnosis

Acute occlusion of the carotid termination

Treatment

EQUIPMENT

- Standard 8F access (puncture needle, 8F vascular sheath)
- Standard 8F balloon guide catheter (Concentric Medical, Mountain View, CA) with continuous flush and a 0.035-in hydrophilic guidewire (Terumo, Somerset, NJ)
- Preparation for acute stenting procedure
  - Rebar 18 Micro Catheter (ev3, Plymouth, MN), curved at vapor (30 degrees) with continuous flush
  - A 0.014-in hydrophilic micro-guidewire (Synchro2 14; Boston Scientific, Natick, MA)
  - Solitaire FR Revascularization Device 4 × 20 mm (ev3)
- Contrast material
- Recombinant tissue plasminogen activator (Actilyse; Genentech, South San Francisco, CA) 1-mg/mL solution

DESCRIPTION

The patient was taken to the angiography suite and put under general anesthesia. Based on the vascular information obtained from the angiographic CT, complete diagnostic angiography was not performed. The 8F, 90-cm balloon guide catheter was placed directly into the right ICA. Under fluoroscopic control, an 18-in microcatheter was manipulated over a 14-in micro-guidewire across the occlusion site until it was distal to the thrombus. A 4 × 20-mm Solitaire FR Revascularization Device was deployed across the thrombus, and an angiographic control run was performed. Immediate reperfusion (TICI grade, 1) was achieved on deployment of the Solitaire FR Device, which was followed by the intra-arterial infusion of 5.0 mg of rtPA for 5 minutes through the balloon guide catheter (**Fig. 49.3**). Because the clot was not dissolving with the proximal injection of rtPA, the next step was to use the Solitaire FR Device as a retriever. The device was recovered during carotid occlusion with the balloon guide catheter and continuous aspiration from the Y connector of the

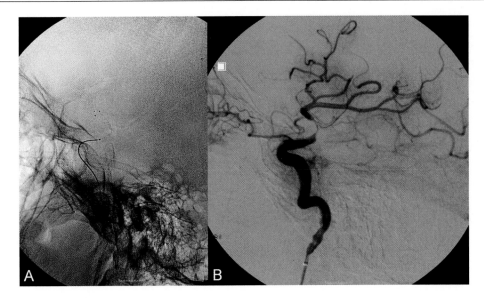

Fig. 49.3 (A) Plain radiography in lateral view reveals the position of the Solitaire FR Revascularization Device. **(B)** Right ICA angiogram in lateral view after deployment of the Solitaire Device shows immediate restoration of flow to the MCA branches.

guiding catheter to remove the parts of the clot that could be detached from the device. The procedure was repeated twice, resulting in complete removal of the residual clot (**Fig. 49.4**). The final control angiogram showed complete recanalization of the MCA, and follow-up MRI 3 days after the procedure demonstrated a small residual infarction at the right basal ganglion (**Fig. 49.5**). The patient was discharged from the hospital and was able to return to his normal activities with rehabilitation.

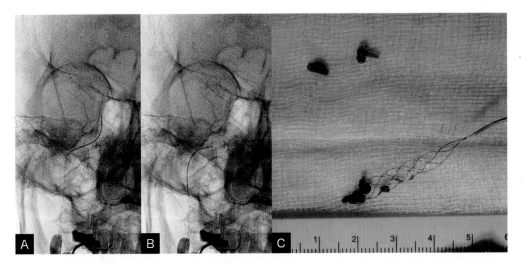

Fig. 49.4 (A,B) Plain radiography in AP view during recovery of the device. Note inflation of the balloon guide catheter to stop flow in the ICA during recovery of the device. **(C)** The recovered device and retrieved clot.

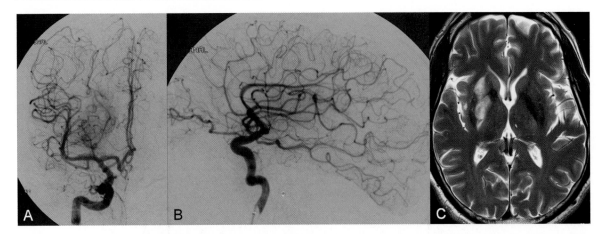

Fig. 49.5 DSA. Right ICA angiogram in **(A)** AP and **(B)** lateral views after the procedure shows complete recanalization (TICI grade of 3). **(C)** Axial T2-weighted MR image 3 days after the procedure demonstrates a small residual infarction at the right basal ganglion.

Discussion

Background

In the treatment of acute stroke, the major concerns at present are the limited treatment window, the risk for hemorrhage associated with intravenous and intra-arterial thrombolytic agents, and the disappointing rates of recanalization reported with mechanical embolectomy. These shortcomings, together with the successful application of angioplasty and stenting in acute cardiac ischemia, have prompted the application of intracranial angioplasty and stenting in the acute phase of cerebral ischemia. However, caution must be exercised because the vasculature and circulation of the cardiac system differ significantly from those of the cerebrovascular system. In the present case, a relatively new device is described that has demonstrated good recanalization rates without being overly aggressive.

Noninvasive Imaging Workup

TRANSCRANIAL DOPPLER ULTRASOUND

- Together with the clinical evaluation, transcranial Doppler ultrasound is a helpful tool to determine noninvasively at the bedside whether a vessel has reopened following the intravenous administration of rtPA.

CT/MRI

- Unenhanced CT is at present the most widely used screening tool for patients with acute stroke. However, modern MRI and CT techniques (i.e., diffusion- and perfusion-weighted imaging and perfusion CT) have been introduced that allow a comprehensive, noninvasive survey of patients with acute stroke. They accurately demonstrate the site of arterial occlusion and its hemodynamic and pathophysiologic effects on the brain parenchyma. After the onset of ischemic stroke, potentially viable tissue may be salvageable for as long as 48 hours. A combination of diffusion-weighted and perfusion-weighted MRI or perfusion CT may improve the selection of patients with potentially salvageable tissue and should therefore be used as soon as patients arrive in the emergency department.

Treatment Options

ENDOVASCULAR TREATMENT

- Current reperfusion strategies are many, and some are still in the investigational phase. The following strategies are available.
  - Endovascular thrombectomy with distal devices: MERCI (Concentric), CATCH (Balt), Phenox clot retriever (Phenox), Neuronet (Guidant Endovascular), Attractor 18 (Target Therapeutics); endovascular thrombectomy with proximal devices: Alligator (ev3), InTime Retriever (Boston Scientific), snares
  - Endovascular mechanical aspiration with large catheters (Penumbra stroke system, Possis AngioJet) that have been shown to be effective in patients with a large clot burden (carotid T and M1 portion of the MCA)
  - Mechanical disruption of thrombus with micro-guidewires, snares, or balloon angioplasty
  - Transcranial augmented fibrinolysis (transcranial Doppler ultrasound) or endovascular augmented fibrinolysis (EKOS)
  - Endovascular entrapment of thrombus with balloon-expandable stents
  - Temporary endovascular bypass with resheathable stents

Possible Complications

- Distal embolic events, intracranial vascular dissection, rupture with subarachnoid hemorrhage
- Reperfusion syndrome and hemorrhagic transformation of acute stroke

Published Literature on Treatment Options

In addition to the previously mentioned techniques, the present case illustrates the possibility of treating acute stroke with a retractable stent that can also serve as a retrieval device. Intracranial stents are currently used for aneurysms and intracranial atherosclerotic disease. Their use for acute stroke was initially reported after failure of thrombolysis or other mechanical devices. Because high rates of recanalization (78–92%) of acute intracranial occlusions treated with intracranial stents have been reported, their use as a first-line treatment must be considered. A major shortcoming of acute stent deployment is the need to start immediate and aggressive anti-aggregation therapy to prevent secondary occlusion, with a concomitant risk for symptomatic intracranial hemorrhage as high as 38% and an associated mortality of 11%. Present data therefore confirm the efficacy of the stent technique for acute stroke but also demonstrate the major disadvantages—high rates of morbidity and mortality related to antiplatelet therapy after procedures in which a stent is permanently deployed. The present system has the major advantage of being completely retrievable; at the same time, it offers rapid reopening of the vessel and a high recanalization rate because of its ability to function as a clot retriever. It permits rapid recanalization of the occluded vessel, and because it increases the surface of the clot, tPA is better able to dissolve the clot. As demonstrated here, clot retrieval is also possible, which makes this device a promising alternative to current endovascular treatments for stroke.

PEARLS AND PITFALLS

- Heparin is not indicated for intra-arterial procedures after intravenous thrombolysis because it increases the risk for hemorrhage.
- Resheath the Solitaire FR Device ~25 to 30% before starting recovery.
- Lock the "Y" valve (the Solitaire FR Device with the Rebar Micro Catheter) and remove slack from the system.

- Inflate the balloon on the guide catheter to provide proximal occlusion and stop the flushes.
- Recover the Solitaire FR Device and Rebar Micro Catheter during aspiration through the balloon guide catheter.
- This sequence can be repeated.
- Some practical considerations:
  - Evaluate the balloon guide catheter after each pass.
  - Continue aspiration after removing the Solitaire FR Device.
  - Confirm backflow and make sure the guide catheter is clear before doing the control. If not, then aspirate more (actively).
  - Confirm that the Y connector is clean and clear.

Further Reading

Brekenfeld C, Schroth G, Mattle HP, et al. Stent placement in acute cerebral artery occlusion: use of a self-expandable intracranial stent for acute stroke treatment. Stroke 2009;40(3):847–852

Donnan GA, Baron JC, Ma H, Davis SM. Penumbral selection of patients for trials of acute stroke therapy. Lancet Neurol 2009;8(3):261–269

Ledezma CJ, Fiebach JB, Wintermark M. Modern imaging of the infarct core and the ischemic penumbra in acute stroke patients: CT versus MRI. Expert Rev Cardiovasc Ther 2009;7(4):395–403

Levy EI, Mehta R, Gupta R, et al. Self-expanding stents for recanalization of acute cerebrovascular occlusions. AJNR Am J Neuroradiol 2007;28(5):816–822

Nogueira RG, Schwamm LH, Hirsch JA. Endovascular approaches to acute stroke, part 1: Drugs, devices, and data. AJNR Am J Neuroradiol 2009;30(4):649–661

Williams M, Patil S, Toledo EG, Vannemreddy P. Management of acute ischemic stroke: current status of pharmacological and mechanical endovascular methods. Neurol Res 2009;31(8):807–815

Zaidat OO, Wolfe T, Hussain SI, et al. Interventional acute ischemic stroke therapy with intracranial self-expanding stent. Stroke 2008;39(8):2392–2395

CASE 50

Case Description

Clinical Presentation

A 73-year-old patient presents with left-sided amaurosis fugax. Ultrasound of the neck vessels demonstrates a high-grade, left-sided stenosis of the internal carotid artery (ICA) at its origin.

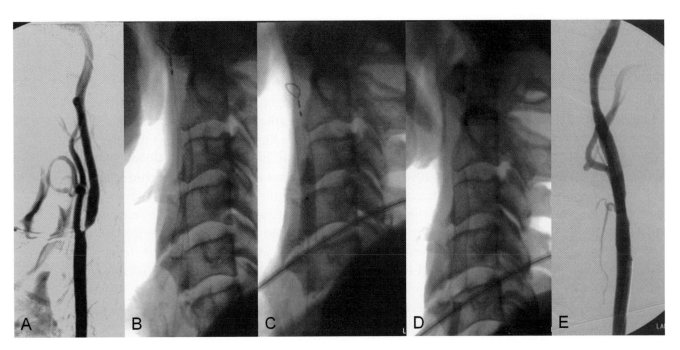

Fig. 50.1 Stent-assisted percutaneous transluminal angioplasty with distal protection of a symptomatic ICA stenosis. Left CCA angiogram in **(A)** lateral view before the procedure demonstrates a proximal ICA stenosis. **(B)** Plain radiography following deployment of the stent **(C)** during and **(D)** after the balloon angioplasty shows complete reopening of the residual stenosis. **(E)** Left CCA angiogram in lateral view following the procedure reveals restoration of flow within the left ICA.

Radiologic Studies

CT AND CTA

CT demonstrated no acute infarctions of the brain; CTA confirmed the diagnosis of a left-sided ICA stenosis and also demonstrated an elongated aortic arch. The patient was scheduled to undergo carotid artery stenting and was premedicated for 3 days with acetylsalicylic acid and clopidogrel.

Diagnosis

Symptomatic stenosis of the origin of the left ICA

Treatment

EQUIPMENT

- Standard 5F access (puncture needle, 5F vascular sheath)
- 7F Shuttle Sheath (Cook Medical, Bloomington, IN)
- Extra-long (125-cm) SIM2 5F catheter (Cook Medical) with a 0.035-in stiff hydrophilic guidewire (Terumo, Somerset, NJ)
- FilterWire EZ Embolic Protection System 3.5–5.5 mm (Boston Scientific, Natick, MA)
- Carotid Wallstent Monorail Endoprosthesis 7 × 30 mm (Boston Scientific)
- RX Aviator Plus PTA Balloon Dilation Catheter 6.0 × 20 mm (Cordis, Warren, NJ)
- Balloon inflation device (manometer)
- Heparin
- Contrast material

DESCRIPTION

With the patient under conscious sedation, a 5F sheath was inserted following single-hole puncture of the femoral artery. Heparin was initiated with an activated clotting time of 275 seconds. A stiff guidewire was advanced via the sheath into the aorta. The short sheath was exchanged via the guidewire with the 7F shuttle sheath, which was advanced to the aortic arch. With the extra-long SIM2 catheter, the left common carotid artery (CCA) was catheterized, and a roadmap was obtained. The stiff guidewire was introduced into the external carotid artery, and the shuttle sheath was advanced over the guidewire into the CCA. Control runs demonstrated the stenosis. Under roadmap guidance, the FilterWire EZ System was advanced via the delivery sheath into the distal ICA and deployed. The Wallstent was back-loaded and advanced without prior dilation and deployed over the stenosis. Fluoroscopic control demonstrated residual stenosis, and a dilation balloon was inserted and slowly inflated with a 50:50 mixture of saline and contrast to a maximum inflation pressure of 6 atm, which resulted in complete reopening of the vessel (**Fig. 50.1**). After removal of the balloon, the protection device was recaptured with the retrieval sheath.

Discussion

Background

Stroke is the second most common cause of death in developed countries. It results in 4.5 million deaths every year and is a major source of morbidity and long-term disability. Extracranial ICA stenosis accounts for 15 to 25% of ischemic strokes, with an incidence as high as 10% in people older than 80 years of age. The risk for stroke in patients with extracranial ICA stenosis is associated with the degree of narrowing; for asymptomatic patients with less than 75% stenosis, the yearly risk for stroke is less than 1%, but the risk increases to 2 to 5% for patients with more than 75% stenosis. In symptomatic patients (previous transient ischemic attack or stroke), the risk is considerably higher: nearly 10% in the first year and 30 to 35% over the next 5 years for patients with stenoses larger than 70%. Currently, the three major treatment modalities for extracranial ICA stenosis are medical management, carotid endarterectomy (CEA), and carotid angioplasty with stenting (CAS).

Noninvasive Imaging Workup

PHYSICAL EXAMINATION

- Carotid artery stenoses, particularly those involving the origin of the ICA, are a frequent clinical problem. These stenoses are almost invariably atherosclerotic in origin. They can present with bruits discovered on physical examination, with one or more transient ischemic attacks or ischemic strokes related to thromboembolism from stenotic lesions, or with hypoperfusion, especially if the circle of Willis is incomplete.

IMAGING FINDINGS

- Doppler ultrasound is well established as an accurate, noninvasive, and inexpensive method to assess carotid stenosis. It provides reliable information about the location and extent of stenosis, flow dynamics, plaque structure, and vessel wall characteristics. Shortcomings are interoperator variability, artifacts from calcified plaques, and difficulties distinguishing pseudo-occlusions from total occlusions. The surrounding anatomy and the brain are not imaged. The low false-negative rate makes it an ideal screening test before a confirmatory test such as MRA or CTA.
- CT and CTA are widely available and can visualize the vessels reliably. Calcifications are better demonstrated than with MRI, and the circle of Willis can be evaluated as well as the origin of the brain-supplying arteries. A volumetric acquisition during continuous rotation of the radiographic source and simultaneous table movement is required. Limitations of this technique are the radiation dose and artifacts caused by extensive, circumferential calcifications of plaque.
- MRI has the major advantages of being able to provide high-quality imaging of the vessels as well as the brain parenchyma and to detect small or clinically silent areas of recent or remote ischemia. Contrast-enhanced MRA is less dependent on flow-related artifacts and can image the brain-supplying vessels from the arch to the circle of Willis. It is the most accurate of the available MRA techniques. In addition to MRI and MRA of the brain and its supplying vessels, advances in imaging techniques have made it possible to visualize the vessel wall and carotid plaque, which may in the future help to risk-stratify patients depending on the characteristics of their plaque.

Invasive Imaging Workup

- With the advent of the previously mentioned accurate, noninvasive imaging techniques, DSA is no longer the diagnostic gold standard for the presurgical assessment of carotid artery stenosis.
- DSA may still be used to visualize collateral flow patterns and to differentiate pseudo-occlusions from true occlusions; however, in most instances noninvasive imaging techniques will suffice for a determination of whether and what type of treatment is required.

Treatment Options

CONSERVATIVE OR MEDICAL MANAGEMENT

- Medical management is by far the most commonly used treatment of extracranial ICA stenosis, traditionally with low-dose aspirin (81–325 mg) taken orally on a daily basis. It is the only modality considered an essential aspect of management for any patient with extracranial ICA stenosis and is used either alone or in conjunction with more invasive treatment modalities.

SURGICAL TREATMENT

- CEA with exposure of the bifurcation, occlusion of flow, arteriotomy, and plaque dissection can be performed.
- Shunting of the CCA to the distal ICA during flow occlusion can be performed.
- Patching of the ICA may reduce perioperative and later stroke.
- An eversion technique does not significantly alter the incidence of stroke but does lower the risk for re-stenosis or occlusion.

ENDOVASCULAR TREATMENT

- Stent-assisted carotid angioplasty is performed with or without distal protection devices.

- Dilation may be necessary before stent insertion.
- Following stent insertion, angioplasty is performed to reopen the vessel.
- Before endovascular treatment, the patient is loaded with acetylsalicylic acid and clopidogrel. The procedure itself is performed under full heparinization.
- Before balloon inflation, atropine is administered intravenously to prevent reflex bradycardia or asystole.

Possible Complications

- The most significant risk associated with carotid artery stenosis is periprocedural stroke, which results from the embolization of debris released during treatment of the carotid artery stenosis. This has fueled the interest in the use of protection devices, which are discussed in greater detail in the next case, as are the technical considerations regarding the treatment of carotid artery stenosis and the influence of stent geometry and design.
- Periprocedural bradycardia or reflex asystole is classically controlled with intravenous atropine.
- Bleeding from the groin is a feared complication, given the large diameter of the inserted sheaths, the dual antiplatelet medication, and the additional heparinization.
- Delayed hyperperfusion hemorrhage may be controlled by lowering the blood pressure following the intervention.

Published Literature on Treatment Options

The first question to answer in the treatment of extracranial ICA stenosis is, Who should be treated? For patients with symptomatic stenoses, the pooled analysis of three major trials—the North American Symptomatic Carotid Endarterectomy Trial (NASCET),the European Carotid Surgery Trial (ECST), and the Veterans Affairs Cooperative Studies Program Trial—clearly demonstrated the benefits of surgery versus medical treatment in the group with stenosis larger than 70%; an absolute risk reduction of 16% was noted after 5 years of follow-up. Patients with moderate stenosis (50–69%) still benefited from surgery, although the overall gains were more modest, with an absolute risk reduction of 4.6% after 5 years. In patients with mild stenosis (≤ 50%), the risks incurred during CEA outweighed the benefits of surgery. For asymptomatic patients with stenoses, there was always considerably more debate about whom to treat until three major trials evaluated CEA versus best medical treatment—the Veterans Affairs Cooperative Studies Program Trial, the Asymptomatic Carotid Atherosclerosis Study (ACAS), and the Asymptomatic Carotid Surgery Trial (ACST). These studies demonstrated that CEA is beneficial for patients younger than 75 years of age with asymptomatic stenoses larger than 70% because it approximately halves the net 5-year risk for stroke from ~12% to ~6%.

The second question to be answered is, When should a (symptomatic) patient be treated in relation to the qualifying event? Increasing evidence from observational and epidemiologic studies shows that the risk for subsequent stroke in patients with carotid stenosis is highest in the first few weeks after the qualifying event, and this risk declines rapidly thereafter. In a recent post hoc analysis of the NASCET and ECST data, the 30-day perioperative risk for stroke and death was unrelated to time since the last symptomatic event and was not increased in patients operated on 2 weeks after a nondisabling stroke. In contrast, the risk for ipsilateral ischemic stroke in the medical group fell rapidly with time since the event, as did the absolute benefit of surgery. This decline in benefit is more pronounced in women than in men. It is therefore suggested that revascularization should occur within 2 weeks following a qualifying event.

The previous studies have established CEA as the gold standard for the invasive management of symptomatic carotid stenosis and have established its role in asymptomatic patients. Therefore, if CAS is to become competitive with CEA, prospective randomized controlled trials are required to demonstrate the noninferiority of CAS to CEA. In a recent systematic Cochrane Database Review of 10 trials involving 3178 patients, a primary outcome comparison of any stroke or death within 30 days after treatment favored surgery; however, the difference was not statistically significant when the random effects model was used. Endovascular treatment was significantly better than surgery in avoiding cranial neuropathy and myocardial infarction, and there was no significant difference between endovascular treatment and surgery in the following comparisons: 30-day stroke, myocardial infarction, or death; 30-day disabling stroke or death; 30-day death, 24-month death, or stroke; and 30-day death or stroke in patients given endovascular treatment with or without protection devices. However, these studies did not include the data of the recently completed International Carotid Stenting Study (ICSS), which demonstrated a rather striking advantage of CEA versus CAS, with a risk for stroke or death following CAS of 8.5% versus 5.1% after CEA. In most centers, therefore, CEA is currently performed as the method of choice unless contraindications to surgery are present, which are addressed in the next case. However, this practice may change when data from the Carotid Revascularization Endarterectomy versus Stenting Trial (CREST) become available, especially because the lead-in phase of this trial suggests that CAS can be competitive with CEA, with a 30-day rate of stroke or death of only 4.4%.

The significant differences between rates of stroke or death following CAS in different studies (4.4% for CREST, 6.9% for SPACE [Stent-Supported Percutaneous Angioplasty of the Carotid Artery versus Endarterectomy], 8.5% for ICSS, and 9.6% for EVA3S [Endarterectomy Versus Angioplasty in Patients with Severe Symptomatic Carotid Stenosis]), compared with the rather constant rates of stroke or death for CEA (between 4 and 6%), have raised concern that the experience of the interventionalists may have affected the results of these trials. In fact, a subgroup analysis of SPACE demonstrated that centers with low recruitment rates have profoundly (and negatively) affected the results for CAS. A second subgroup analysis of both the SPACE data and the data from the lead-in phase of CREST, regarding the dependence of primary outcome events (stroke or death) on the patient's age, seems noteworthy. In patients younger than 68 years of age, CAS had only a 2.7% rate of stroke or death, whereas in patients older than 68 years, this rate increased to 10.8%; the results for CEA were not affected by age (7.0% vs. 5.9% in SPACE). In the CREST lead-in phase, patients younger than 70 years had risks for stroke or death of less than 2%; in those 70 to 79 years old, the risk increased to 5.3%; and in those older than 80 years, the risk for CAS was 12.1%. This indicates that stenting becomes more dangerous with increasing age, and one may argue that CAS should be reserved for younger patients. However, long-term results will be necessary to prove the durability of stenting compared with CEA. Preliminary data suggest that the rate of in-stent re-stenosis is slightly higher; however, most of these cases are asymptomatic.

At present, the question of what is the best invasive treatment cannot be answered, and as with many of the other treatments described in this book, the respective experiences of the local treating team of interventionalists and surgeons as well as the anatomy and pathology of the individual patient will likely influence what kind of treatment is offered.

PEARLS AND PITFALLS _____

- Extracranial ICA stenosis accounts for 15 to 25% of ischemic strokes and has a high incidence, especially in the elderly population.
- Patients with symptomatic stenoses and high-grade asymptomatic stenoses do benefit from revascularization.
- Although CEA is the established therapeutic strategy, CAS and balloon angioplasty are promising alternatives, especially when performed in experienced hands

Further Reading

Eckstein HH, Ringleb P, Allenberg JR, et al. Results of the Stent-Protected Angioplasty versus Carotid Endarterectomy (SPACE) study to treat symptomatic stenoses at 2 years: a multinational, prospective, randomised trial. Lancet Neurol 2008;7(10):893–902

Ederle J, Featherstone RL, Brown MM. Randomized controlled trials comparing endarterectomy and endovascular treatment for carotid artery stenosis: a Cochrane systematic review. Stroke 2009;40(4):1373–1380

Lal BK, Brott TG. The Carotid Revascularization Endarterectomy vs. Stenting Trial completes randomization: lessons learned and anticipated results. J Vasc Surg 2009;50(5):1224–1231

Lanzino G, Rabinstein AA, Brown RD Jr. Treatment of carotid artery stenosis: medical therapy, surgery, or stenting? Mayo Clin Proc 2009;84(4):362–387, quiz 367–368

McClelland S III. Multimodality management of carotid artery stenosis: reviewing the class-I evidence. J Natl Med Assoc 2007;99(11):1235–1242

Rothwell PM, Eliasziw M, Gutnikov SA, Warlow CP, Barnett HJ. Sex difference in the effect of time from symptoms to surgery on benefit from carotid endarterectomy for transient ischemic attack and nondisabling stroke. Stroke 2004;35(12):2855–2861

Touzé E, Calvet D, Chatellier G, Mas JL. Carotid stenting. Curr Opin Neurol 2008;21(1):56–63

U-King-Im JM, Young V, Gillard JH. Carotid-artery imaging in the diagnosis and management of patients at risk of stroke. Lancet Neurol 2009;8(6):569–580

van der Vaart MG, Meerwaldt R, Reijnen MM, Tio RA, Zeebregts CJ. Endarterectomy or carotid artery stenting: the quest continues. Am J Surg 2008;195(2):259–269

Wardlaw JM, Chappell FM, Best JJ, Wartolowska K, Berry E; NHS Research and Development Health Technology Assessment Carotid Stenosis Imaging Group. Non-invasive imaging compared with intra-arterial angiography in the diagnosis of symptomatic carotid stenosis: a meta-analysis. Lancet 2006;367(9521):1503–1512

Wholey MH, Wu WC. Current status in cervical carotid artery stent placement. J Cardiovasc Surg (Torino) 2009;50(1):29–37

CASE 51

Case Description

Clinical Presentation

A 60-year-old woman with a previous history of carcinoma of the tonsil was treated with radiation and tonsillectomy 10 years ago. Subsequent follow-up visits demonstrated no recurrence; however, a progressive but asymptomatic stenosis of the right internal carotid artery (ICA) developed that led to asymptomatic occlusion of the artery 3 years ago. At the present visit, a new mass lesion in the left posterolateral oropharynx is discovered, and she undergoes surgery for recurrent oropharyngeal carcinoma. Because of the postoperative development of neurologic deficits and reduced consciousness, CT and CTA imaging of the head and neck area are performed.

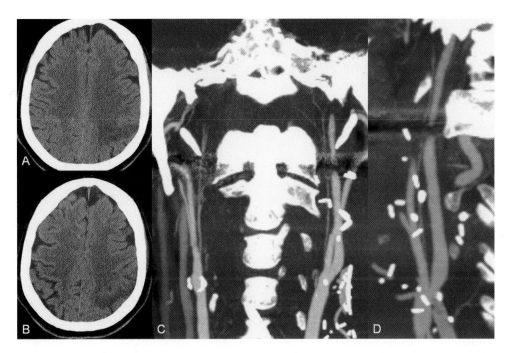

Fig. 51.1 (A,B) Unenhanced axial CT scan demonstrates a well-defined hypodensity within the left parietal region, representing an acute infarct. CTA in **(C)** coronal and **(D)** sagittal views reveals changes after radical neck dissection, with multiple clips within the soft tissues. There is complete occlusion of the right ICA. A filling defect is noted at the left cervical ICA ~3 cm below the skull base, resulting in a severe stenosis.

297

Radiologic Studies

CT AND CTA

CT demonstrated a well-defined hypodensity within the left parietal lobe region compatible with acute infarction. There was complete occlusion of the right ICA at its origin, and a filling defect within the cervical portion of the left ICA ~3 cm from the skull base was causing a severe stenosis at this site. The cervical ICA measured 4 mm in diameter below the stenosis and 2 mm above the stenosis, indicating a marked decrease in flow distal to the stenosis. The stenosis measured 4 to 5 mm in length and was believed to be related to a focal dissection following surgery (**Fig. 51.1**). Posterior communicating arteries were not present. Postoperative changes were seen within the neck on the left side, with numerous surgical clips.

Diagnosis

Post-surgical symptomatic high-grade ICA stenosis

Treatment

EQUIPMENT

- Standard 5F access (puncture needle, 5F vascular sheath)
- 5F Berenstein catheter (Boston Scientific, Natick, MA) and a 0.035-in hydrophilic guidewire for diagnostic angiography (Terumo, Somerset, NJ)
- A 300-cm Amplatz exchange guidewire (Boston Scientific)
- 6F Shuttle Sheath multipurpose catheter (Shuttle Select; Cook Medical, Bloomington, IN) with continuous flush
- Synchro2 microwire (Boston Scientific)
- Precise Stent 6 × 40 mm (Cordis, Warren, NJ)
- Heparin, acetylsalicylic acid, clopidogrel
- Contrast material
- Short 7F sheath

DESCRIPTION

A 5F Berenstein catheter was introduced into the left common carotid artery (CCA). AP and lateral images were obtained of both the cervical and cranial areas. The left ICA demonstrated a midcervical focal stenosis with post-stenotic narrowing. The intracranial ICA was reconstituted at the level of the inferolateral trunk by multiple branches from the external carotid artery (ECA). A combination of slow antegrade and retrograde flow subsequently filled the entire ICA trajectory, which showed no further irregularity or narrowing (**Fig. 51.2**). The cranial run showed the ECA to be slowly opacifying the ICA, as previously described. Filling of the distal intracranial territories was sluggish. Cross-flow to the opposite side was not demonstrated. The ICA stenosis appeared to be most consistent with an intimal flap resulting from a dissection.

Heparinization was initiated. An Amplatz exchange wire was introduced into the ECA through a Berenstein catheter, which was subsequently exchanged for a 6F shuttle sheath with its tip just proximal to the CCA bifurcation. After removal of the exchange wire, a Synchro2 microwire was introduced into the shuttle sheath and used to traverse the stenosis, with its tip lying in the petrous ICA. A 6 × 40-mm Precise Stent was then introduced over the Synchro2 wire and deployed across the stenosis. The stent instantly restored the original diameter of the ICA, and no secondary percutaneous transluminal angioplasty (PTA) was necessary.

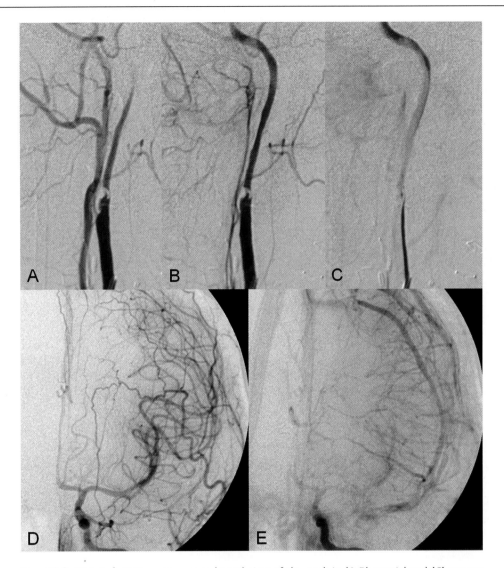

Fig. 51.2 DSA. Left CCA angiogram in lateral view of the neck in **(A,B)** arterial and **(C)** venous phases demonstrates a focal midcervical stenosis with post-stenotic narrowing of the ICA. Left CCA angiogram in AP view of the brain in **(D)** arterial and **(E)** venous phases shows slow antegrade filling of the remaining left ICA without any other irregularity or narrowing.

Control runs were performed through the shuttle sheath, centered on both the neck and head area. The cervical runs now showed the ICA to be fully patent, with restored normal flow into the distal territories (**Fig. 51.3**). The cranial runs demonstrated normal rapid flow into all intracranial territories supplied by the anterior circulation, including flow across the anterior communicating artery into the contralateral anterior cerebral artery and middle cerebral artery territories (**Fig. 51.4**). Heparin was not reversed; the 6F shuttle sheath was exchanged for a short 7F sheath and removed after heparin was discontinued (after 24 hours). The patient was given aspirin and clopidogrel via a gastric tube while on the angiography table, and this medication was continued afterward. The patient had a dramatic recovery, with return to a normal level of consciousness immediately after the procedure.

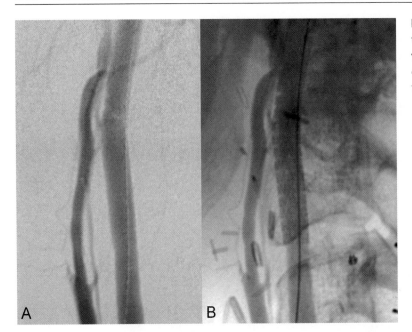

Fig. 51.3 (A) DSA and **(B)** unsubtracted left CCA angiogram in lateral view following stent insertion demonstrate immediate reconstitution of the normal luminal diameter.

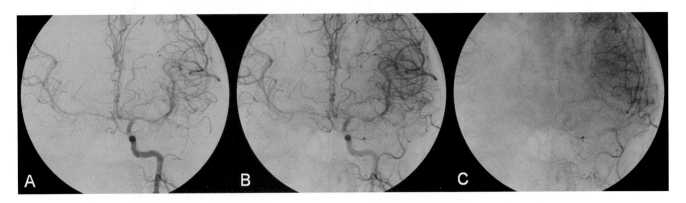

Fig. 51.4 DSA. Left CCA angiogram, AP view in **(A)** early arterial, **(B)** late arterial, and **(C)** capillary phases reveals good cross-flow through the anterior communicating artery and normal flow within both cerebral hemispheres.

Discussion

Background

Despite controversy about what is the best treatment for symptomatic high-grade carotid artery stenosis, current well-accepted indications for carotid artery stenting are situations in which endarterectomy is contraindicated: previous anterior neck surgery (previous carotid endarterectomy [CEA] or other neck dissection), previous neck irradiation (**Fig. 51.5**), a prohibitive medical risk, carotid artery stenosis in hyperacute stroke, a high bifurcation, a long segment of stenosis, or a tandem stenosis. In the present case, the previous surgery, the high location of the stenosis, the presumed pathologic mechanism, the previous neck irradiation, and the contralateral occlusion were all factors strongly favoring endovascular management. In this case, we focus on the indications for carotid artery stenting and discuss technical issues, including stent design and the use of protection devices.

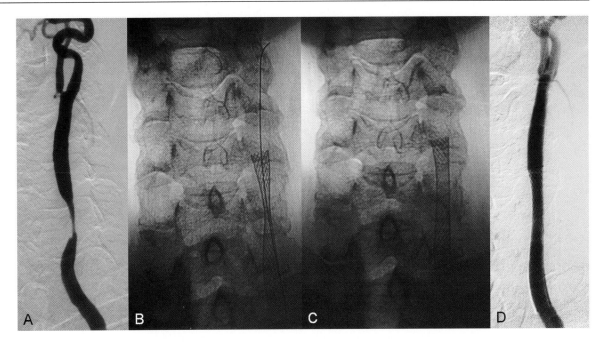

Fig. 51.5 Symptomatic high-grade stenosis in a patient with previous neck radiation. Left CCA angiogram in **(A)** lateral view demonstrates a focal high-grade stenosis at the midleft CCA. Plain radiography in AP view after stent deployment **(B)** during and **(C)** after balloon angioplasty shows reopening of the residual stenosis. No residual stenosis is seen on the final control run of the left CCA angiogram in **(D)** lateral view.

Noninvasive Imaging Workup

PHYSICAL EXAMINATION

- An acute hypoperfusion syndrome is characterized by a decreased level of consciousness and may be present in patients with insufficient collateral supply through the circle of Willis.

IMAGING FINDINGS

- Angiographic evaluation should demonstrate the brain-supplying arteries from the arch to the M2 and A2 level. Maximum-intensity projections and multiplanar reconstructions are helpful to evaluate the morphology and extent of the stenosis.
- The hemodynamic relevance and the age of the stenosis can sometimes be deduced from the diameter of the artery distal to the stenosis; a collapsed vessel suggests a significant stenosis.
- In addition to an evaluation of the stenosis, the report should include a description of potential collateral pathways, such as the patency and diameter of the anterior and posterior communicating arteries.
- Distal stenoses should raise suspicion that pathology other than atherosclerosis is the cause.

Invasive Imaging Workup

- DSA can demonstrate the morphology of the stenosis and the flow dynamics. Normally, the ICA should fill before the ECA territories when CCA injections are performed.
- A complete evaluation of the circle of Willis is not necessary if previous noninvasive images are of high quality and have ruled out potential collateral pathways.

Treatment Options

SURGICAL TREATMENT

- CEA following previous surgery or irradiation, as in this case, is generally not recommended.

ENDOVASCULAR TREATMENT

- Self-expandable stents with or without subsequent balloon angioplasty can be used.
- PTA by itself and balloon-mounted stents no longer play a role in extracranial carotid artery disease.
- The use of protection devices is still controversial.
- Dual antiplatelet therapy before and after the procedure is recommended.

Possible Complications

- Acute thromboembolic complications
- Dissections
- Bradycardia
- Delayed re-stenosis

Published Literature on Treatment Options

Carotid angioplasty and stenting (CAS) is indicated for patients in whom CEA is considered high-risk because of medical comorbidities or anatomic considerations (previous CEA, radical neck dissection, radiation). Prior neck irradiation can induce atherosclerosis in the carotid artery. Although CAS is safe and efficacious for the treatment of these patients, previous irradiation may predispose them to the de novo development of stenoses at other locations, and the incidence of thrombosis and re-stenosis is somewhat higher. In patients with re-stenosis following surgery, CAS has demonstrated better outcomes than repeated surgery. Therefore, CAS is the treatment of choice in these circumstances.

Once the decision for endovascular treatment of a stenosis has been made, different techniques and stents can be used. Concerning stent geometry, tapered stents are considered more suitable if the proximal and distal diameters of the vessel differ significantly because they reduce the radial outward force distally while still maintaining sufficient wall apposition proximally. Untapered stents, on the other hand, are more suitable for stenoses in which the proximal and distal diameters of the vessel are similar (as in this case). In addition, the stent design must be taken into account. Recently, there has been significant debate regarding the indications, advantages, and limitations of open-cell stents (e.g., Precise [Cordis] and Acculink [Abbott Vascular]) versus closed-cell stents (e.g., Wallstent [Boston Scientific], Xact [Abbott Vascular], and NexStent [Boston Scientific]), as well as the effects of the size of the open-cell area in symptomatic versus asymptomatic patients. In a retrospective analysis of more than 3000 patients, Bosiers et al found more adverse events associated with open-cell devices and with stents that had a larger open-cell area in symptomatic patients. They explained their findings as a higher rate of embolic events due to a lesser degree of "scaffolding" of the ruptured embologenic plaque by stent struts. However, other groups failed to identify any differences between outcomes with the different types of stents. This controversy highlights the fact that each stent design has specific advantages, and choosing the right stent is an art, similar to choosing the right coil for aneurysm embolization. The desired features of a carotid artery stent include scaffolding strength adequate to control plaque prolapsed, but with acceptable flexibility, conformability, and radial strength to track the lesion, appose the vessel wall, and control recoil. The design of the stent edges must also be carefully considered because the ends tend to induce elevated mechanical stresses and may damage the arterial wall after expansion.

Like the questions about stent design, the questions about whether and when to use a protection device, and what kind, are a matter of controversy. In a secondary analysis of the SPACE (Stent-Supported Percutaneous Angioplasty of the Carotid Artery versus Endarterectomy) trial, Jansen et al found that protection devices did not lead to a significant reduction of ipsilateral strokes. On the other hand, a recent meta-analysis by Garg et al (including more than 10,000 patients undergoing CAS with or without protection) demonstrated a relative risk of 0.59 (95% confidence interval [CI]: 0.47–0.73) for stroke, favoring protected over unprotected CAS (p < 0.001). This analysis concluded that the use of protection devices appears to reduce the risk for stroke during CAS by 38% for both symptomatic and asymptomatic patients. In specific subsets of patients, protection devices do not seem to be indicated, as in our patient, who had no intraluminal atherosclerotic plaque but rather an extraluminal narrowing due to previous surgery. Protection devices in these situations are therefore not necessary. One may argue that advances in neuroimaging, especially the advent of plaque imaging, discussed in the previous case, may help to identify those patients who will benefit most from a protection device.

Finally, some other questions concerning the technique of CAS may arise. Dilation before stenting should in our opinion be avoided, and if it is necessary, we recommend a more liberal use of protection devices. Dilation afterward may not always be necessary, depending on the type of stenosis, and control runs should be performed after stenting to decide whether additional angioplasty is necessary. If balloon angioplasty is performed, we recommend an angioplasty technique similar to that used for intracranial stenosis—very gentle and slow inflation over a prolonged period rather than rapid or vigorous inflation.

PEARLS AND PITFALLS

- Indications for CAS are previous anterior neck surgery (neck dissection or previous CEA), neck irradiation, prohibitive medical risks, a high bifurcation, long stenoses or tandem stenoses, and hyperacute stroke.
- Selection of the stent, protection device, and balloon must be tailored to the specific anatomy and pathologic mechanism of the stenosis.
- Two methods can be used to access the CCA with the shuttle sheath, as described in the previous case and in this case as well: either an exchange guidewire maneuver or an extra-long diagnostic catheter.

Further Reading

Attigah N, Külkens S, Deyle C, et al. Redo surgery or carotid stenting for restenosis after carotid endarterectomy: results of two different treatment strategies. Ann Vasc Surg 2010;24(2):190–195

Bosiers M, de Donato G, Deloose K, et al. Does free cell area influence the outcome in carotid artery stenting? Eur J Vasc Endovasc Surg 2007;33(2):135–141, discussion 142–143

Garg N, Karagiorgos N, Pisimisis GT, et al. Cerebral protection devices reduce periprocedural strokes during carotid angioplasty and stenting: a systematic review of the current literature. J Endovasc Ther 2009;16(4):412–427

Jansen O, Fiehler J, Hartmann M, Brückmann H. Protection or nonprotection in carotid stent angioplasty: the influence of interventional techniques on outcome data from the SPACE Trial. Stroke 2009;40(3):841–846

Sadek M, Cayne NS, Shin HJ, Turnbull IC, Marin ML, Faries PL. Safety and efficacy of carotid angioplasty and stenting for radiation-associated carotid artery stenosis. J Vasc Surg 2009;50(6):1308–1313

Schillinger M, Gschwendtner M, Reimers B, et al. Does carotid stent cell design matter? Stroke 2008;39(3):905–909

Shin SH, Stout CL, Richardson AI, DeMasi RJ, Shah RM, Panneton JM. Carotid angioplasty and stenting in anatomically high-risk patients: Safe and durable except for radiation-induced stenosis. J Vasc Surg 2009;50(4):762–767, discussion 767–768

Siewiorek GM, Finol EA, Wholey MH. Clinical significance and technical assessment of stent cell geometry in carotid artery stenting. J Endovasc Ther 2009;16(2):178–188

CASE 52

Case Description

Clinical Presentation

A 68-year-old previously healthy man presents to the emergency department because of transient episodes of slurred speech, dysarthria, and gait imbalance, as well as fluctuating diplopia. He reports that he has had similar episodes for about 2 months and has been taking aspirin, as recommended by his family physician, for 1 month.

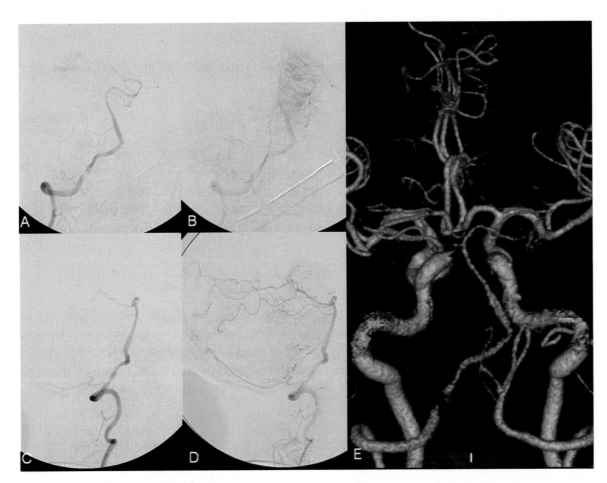

Fig. 52.1 DSA. Right VA angiogram in **(A,B)** AP and **(C,D)** lateral views in **(A,C)** early and **(B,D)** late arterial phases demonstrates a short-segment high-grade stenosis at the intradural portion of the right VA with sluggish flow to the posterior fossa. **(E)** CTA demonstrates the luminal narrowing of the distal right VA.

Radiologic Studies

CT AND CTA

CT demonstrated a remote infarction of the right distal cerebellar hemisphere. CTA demonstrated a high-grade, right-sided intradural stenosis of the dominant vertebral artery (VA). The left VA terminated in a left posterior inferior cerebellar artery that also supplied the left anterior inferior cerebel-

305

lar artery territory. The left V4 segment was aplastic and did not contribute to filling of the basilar circulation. On the right side, a fetal type of posterior cerebral artery (PCA) was noted with an aplastic P1 segment, whereas on the left side, a hypoplastic posterior communicating ramus was noted. Given these findings, the supply to the basilar artery was solely from a severely stenosed right V4 segment, which demonstrated an irregular lumen within the stenosis. The length of the stenosis itself was ~0.8 cm. The vessel lumen proximal to the stenosis measured 4 mm. The vessel lumen distal to the stenosis measured 3 mm. The residual lumen within the stenosis was less than 1 mm. At the origin of the right VA, a small calcified plaque was noted.

Diagnosis

Symptomatic, right-sided intradural VA stenosis without collateral circulation to the basilar artery

Treatment

EQUIPMENT

- Standard 6F access (puncture needle, 6F vascular sheath)
- 4F Berenstein catheter (Boston Scientific, Natick, MA) for diagnostic runs with a 0.035-in hydrophilic guidewire (Terumo, Somerset, NJ)
- 6F multipurpose guide catheter (Envoy MPC; Cordis, Warren, NJ) with continuous flush
- A 2.5 × 30-mm Gateway balloon (Boston Scientific)
- Floppy-tipped, 300-cm, 0.014-in Transend exchange micro-guidewire (Boston Scientific)
- Balloon inflation device (manometer)
- A 4 × 15-mm Wingspan stent (Boston Scientific)
- Heparin
- Contrast material

DESCRIPTION

The patient was premedicated with acetylsalicylic acid and clopidogrel for 3 days. Under sterile technique, a 6F sheath was percutaneously inserted into the right femoral artery with a single-wall puncture technique. A 4F Berenstein catheter was used to evaluate the right VA stenosis. Angiography showed a short-segment, irregular, high-grade luminal narrowing (with a residual luminal diameter of < 0.4 mm) of the intradural portion of the right VA with minimal and sluggish intracranial flow (**Fig. 52.1**).

Heparin was initiated with an activated clotting time (ACT) of 275 seconds. Intracranial stenting of the right VA was performed with a self-expanding stent system and an over-the-wire technique. We started by placing a 6F Envoy MPC guide catheter into the proximal part of the right VA and checked distal flow. Then, with a roadmap technique, we used the 300-cm, floppy-tipped Transend exchange micro-guidewire to cross the stenosis and navigate a 2.5 × 30-mm Gateway balloon over the stenosis, with the tip of the guidewire in the distal PCA. A very gentle dilation with a manometer-controlled balloon was performed over a prolonged period. Control angiography demonstrated significant luminal gain (**Fig. 52.2**). After removal of the balloon, a 4 × 15-mm Wingspan stent was deployed over the narrowed segment of the right VA. Control angiography showed satisfactory dilation of the stenotic segment of the right VA and significantly increased intracranial perfusion (**Fig. 52.3**). There was no evidence of thromboembolic complications.

After the procedure, the right femoral sheath was not removed because systemic heparin was continued for the next 24 hours. The patient woke up without any neurologic deficits.

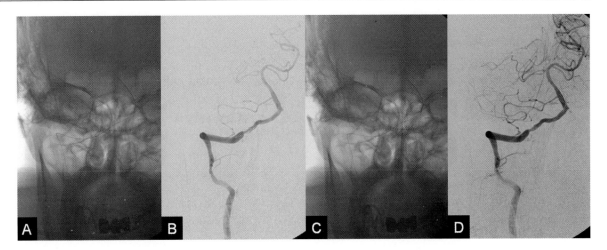

Fig. 52.2 **(A)** Plain radiography in AP view shows the position of the balloon before the dilation procedure. **(B)** Right VA angiogram in AP view after percutaneous transluminal angioplasty shows improved flow to the posterior fossa with residual stenosis. **(C)** Plain radiography in AP view during stent deployment and **(D)** right VA angiogram in AP view after the procedure reveal the stent across the stenosis with significant increased flow to the posterior fossa.

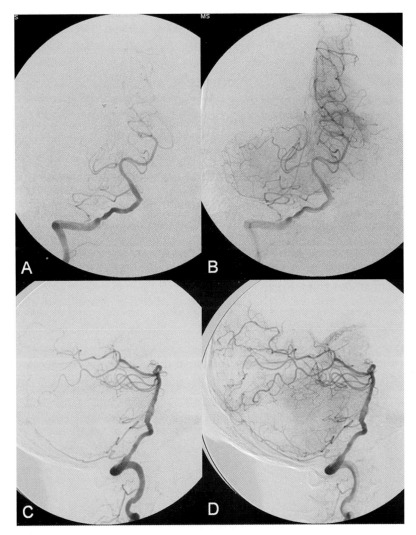

Fig. 52.3 DSA. Right VA angiogram in **(A,B)** AP and **(C,D)** lateral views in **(A,C)** early and **(B,D)** late arterial phases after the procedure has demonstrated satisfactory dilation of the stenotic right VA segment with increased posterior fossa perfusion.

Discussion

Background

Intracranial atherosclerotic disease causes ~8 to 10% of ischemic strokes in Europe and North America and up to 50% of strokes in Asian countries. The risk for stroke in patients with intracranial atherosclerotic disease ranges from 7% to 24% per year. There are some subgroups of patients who are at a high risk for recurrence of stroke despite antithrombotic therapy. In large prospective studies, the degree of stenosis was the most powerful predictor of stroke. Patients with a history of previous transient ischemic attack (TIA) or stroke in the territory of a 70 to 99% stenosis had a stroke rate of 18% at 1 year while on antithrombotic therapy. Therefore, endovascular therapies have been developed to treat these lesions.

Noninvasive Imaging Workup

CLINICAL FINDINGS

- Clinical symptoms of TIA or stroke depend on the affected vascular territory.
- Severe hypoperfusion may be associated with lethargy or a decreased level of consciousness.

IMAGING FINDINGS

- CT and MRI may show the sequelae of recent or remote infarctions. In particular, diffusion-weighted imaging sequences are helpful to determine recent areas of silent ischemia. Embolic events must be differentiated from perforator occlusions.
- CTA and MRA can demonstrate the extent and severity of stenosis. MRA sequences often overestimate the degree of stenosis, and CTA measurements are more accurate.

Invasive Imaging Workup

- DSA is unsurpassed in evaluating potential collateral flow. Therefore, the invasive imaging workup should assess potential collateral routes of supply. Depending on the location of the stenosis, injection into both internal and external carotid arteries, both VAs, and, for mid-VA stenosis, even the ascending and deep cervical arteries may be required.
- To determine the exact diameter of a vessel proximal and distal to a stenosis, the length of the stenosis, and the degree of stenosis, 3D rotational angiography is the gold standard and should be performed to determine the stent and balloon size.

Differential Diagnosis

- In addition to atherosclerosis, inflammatory diseases and intracranial dissections may cause narrowing of intracranial vessels; however, the patient's risk profile and clinical presentation are usually helpful in making the correct diagnosis.
- Other causes of ischemic stroke must be considered, including cardiogenic embolic stroke and proximal large-vessel atherosclerosis.

Treatment Options

CONSERVATIVE OR MEDICAL MANAGEMENT

- Current pharmacologic therapies for secondary prevention include antiplatelet, anticoagulant, and cholesterol-lowering agents, in addition to drugs that reduce elevated blood pressure.

- Patients who fail drug therapy are at even higher risk for subsequent strokes.

SURGICAL TREATMENT

- Extracranial-to-intracranial (EC-IC) bypass surgery has been used for symptomatic intracranial stenosis; however, since the publication of the results of the EC-IC bypass study (described below), most centers have abandoned the use of this technique for this specific indication.

ENDOVASCULAR TREATMENT

- Three treatment options are available: balloon angioplasty alone, balloon-mounted stents, and self-expandable stents following gentle dilation.
- Before endovascular treatment, CTA, MRA or even 3D DSA is necessary to determine what size and type of stent and balloon to use and to determine the best vascular access.
- Pre-procedural dual antiplatelet loading for 3 days is mandatory (300–325 mg of acetylsalicylic acid orally and 75 mg of clopidogrel orally).
- Heparin is given after sheath insertion with an ACT above 250 seconds; following the procedure, heparin should not be reversed until before sheath removal the next day.
- The blood pressure should be kept low after stent insertion to avoid reperfusion hemorrhage.
- Dual antiplatelet therapy is given for at least 3 months (in the authors' practice for 6 months), followed by control angiography (DSA or CTA). If no in-stent stenosis is present, antiplatelet treatment with one agent may be considered.

Possible Complications

- Dissection with acute vessel occlusion
- Perforator occlusion with subsequent stroke or distal embolic events
- Vessel disruption with fatal hemorrhage
- Acute in-stent thrombosis
- Reperfusion hemorrhage
- Delayed in-stent stenosis
- Delayed stroke despite stent treatment

Published Literature on Treatment Options

Concerning antithrombotic therapy, the recent Warfarin-Aspirin Symptomatic Intracranial Disease (WASID) trial showed that aspirin was safer and as effective as warfarin for stroke prevention in patients with symptomatic intracranial stenosis, although the risk for stroke recurrence was still more than 20%. Similar rates of stroke recurrence have been shown for other antiplatelet agents (e.g., clopidogrel and a combination of dipyridamole plus aspirin) in patients with various underlying causes of stroke. Other than aspirin, cilostazol is the only antiplatelet agent that has been studied in a multicenter, double-blind, controlled trial of secondary prevention in patients with symptomatic intracranial stenosis. In the 6-month follow-up period of that study, no strokes occurred in either the cilostazol-plus-aspirin arm or the placebo-plus-aspirin arm. However, progression of intracranial stenosis was less frequent in the cilostazol group (6.7% vs. 28.8%). This finding has led to an ongoing multicenter study comparing cilostazol plus aspirin versus clopidogrel plus aspirin in patients with symptomatic intracranial stenosis. The treatment of risk factors such as elevated low-density lipoprotein (LDL) cholesterol levels and elevated blood pressure also reduces the risk for recurrent stroke. The results of recent studies of risk factor control in stroke patients overall and the results of post hoc analyses of the WASID trial suggest that attempting to lower blood pressure and LDL cholesterol may reduce major vascular events in patients with intracranial stenosis. Some authors even went as far as to say that aggressive risk factor management in patients with stroke and intracranial stenoses might obviate the need for endovascular treatment.

The reluctance to use endovascular treatment may be in part due to the initially reported high risks of complications; however, the results of the WASID trial as well as advances in microcatheter, stent, and balloon technology have made intracranial angioplasty and stenting an alternative to the previously mentioned forms of medical management. In Case 53, we discuss in greater detail the different endovascular techniques that can be employed. Here, we briefly discuss the success and complication rates of endovascular procedures, and the factors related to them. With modern stent systems, technical success rates are higher than 95% and the rates of significant periprocedural or postprocedural complications are lower than 15%, which is considerably better than what is achieved with antithrombotic management alone. Patients who have posterior circulation stenosis, are treated at low-volume sites, undergo stenting soon (< 10 days) after a qualifying event, or have a stroke rather than a TIA as the qualifying event are all at a higher risk for periprocedural or postprocedural complications after endovascular treatments. Patients who have resolved, improving, or stationary symptoms before a stent placement procedure have a significantly better outcome than do patients who have progressive or fluctuating neurologic symptoms. On the other hand, the risk for recurrent stroke is highest within the first 21 days following a qualifying event, which means that the timing of an intervention is a difficult balancing act.

The surgical treatment of intracranial stenoses consists of EC-IC bypass and has been applied for cerebrovascular ischemic disease of both the anterior and posterior circulation. The EC-IC bypass trial is the largest and best data set describing the efficacy of this procedure for anterior circulation disease. In this study, the subset of patients with severe middle cerebral artery stenosis did worse than any other patient subset within the trial after bypass, with a risk for stroke nearly two times higher after surgical bypass than after medical therapy. Smaller series of posterior circulation bypass procedures also described significant complications in more than half of patients despite excellent technical results and high patency rates for the bypasses. On the basis of these data, most authorities agree that surgical bypass therapy is not a reasonable therapeutic option for the vast majority of patients with symptomatic intracranial stenosis.

For the time being, the question of how to treat patients with symptomatic high-grade intracranial stenoses remains unanswered, and one has to await the results of prospective randomized trials of best medical treatment versus best medical treatment with endovascular therapies. In most centers, though, patients who are symptomatic despite best medical treatment and have a stenosis of more than 70% and those patients whose stenosis progresses despite best medical treatment are currently being treated with balloon angioplasty and stenting.

PEARLS AND PITFALLS _____

- Symptomatic intracranial stenosis is a major risk factor for recurrent stroke.
- Patients whose stenoses are larger than 70% have a significantly higher risk for recurrent stroke than do patients with lower-grade stenosis.
- The risk for stroke recurrence is highest immediately after the first stroke.
- Aggressive medical treatment must include not only antithrombotic therapy but also medications that lower LDL cholesterol levels and lower elevated blood pressure.
- Endovascular treatments should be recommended for patients with symptomatic high-grade stenoses in whom best medical therapy fails.

Further Reading

Albuquerque FC, Levy EI, Turk AS, et al. Angiographic patterns of Wingspan in-stent restenosis. Neurosurgery 2008;63(1):23–27, discussion 27–28

Fiorella DJ, Levy EI, Turk AS, et al. Target lesion revascularization after wingspan: assessment of safety and durability. Stroke 2009;40(1):106–110

Kelly ME, Turner RD, Moskowitz SI, et al. Revascularization of symptomatic subacute cerebrovascular occlusions with a self-expanding intracranial stent system. Neurosurgery 2009;64(1):72–78, discussion 78

Nahab F, Lynn MJ, Kasner SE, et al; NIH Multicenter Wingspan Intracranial Stent Registry Study Group. Risk factors associated with major cerebrovascular complications after intracranial stenting. Neurology 2009;72(23):2014–2019

Turan TN, Derdeyn CP, Fiorella D, Chimowitz MI. Treatment of atherosclerotic intracranial arterial stenosis. Stroke 2009;40(6):2257–2261

Turk AS, Levy EI, Albuquerque FC, et al. Influence of patient age and stenosis location on wingspan in-stent restenosis. AJNR Am J Neuroradiol 2008;29(1):23–27

CASE 53

Case Description

Clinical Presentation

A 65-year-old man presents with a 3-month history of nonspecific neurologic events consisting of dizziness and malaise. During the past couple of weeks, he has had episodes of left-sided shaking and ataxia. In the hospital, these events have had a postural component and also have been associated with dysarthria.

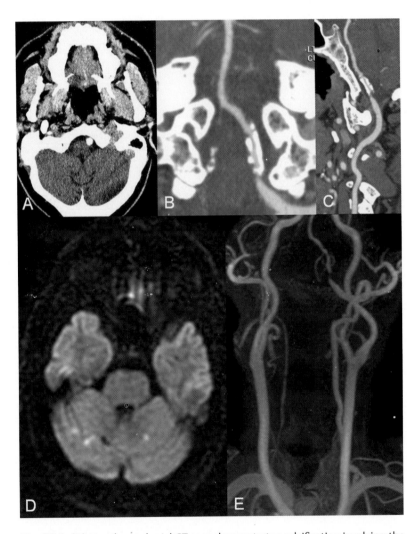

Fig. 53.1 **(A)** Unenhanced axial CT scan demonstrates calcification involving the left VA. CTA in **(B)** coronal and **(C)** sagittal views reveals a high-grade intradural left VA stenosis. **(D)** Axial diffusion-weighted MRI shows multiple foci of diffusion restriction involving both cerebellar hemispheres. **(E)** Contrast-enhanced MRA also reveals the short-segment, high-grade stenosis of the dominant left VA with associated irregularity. The right VA is markedly hypoplastic.

Radiologic Studies

CT demonstrated significant calcifications involving the left vertebral artery (VA) and a high-grade intradural stenosis of the dominant left VA. MRI showed multiple cortical foci of diffusion restriction involving the right and left cerebellar hemispheres. No supratentorial diffusion defects were present. MRA revealed a left-sided dominance of the VA and no significant filling to the basilar system from the right side. A short-segment, high-grade stenosis of the left VA with an irregular lumen was seen just above the dural entry point (**Fig. 53.1**). There was a fetal disposition of the left posterior cerebral artery with an absent or hypoplastic left P1. The right P1 was patent, but there was no evidence of a posterior communicating artery at this site.

Diagnosis

Symptomatic, high-grade calcified stenosis of the left VA, which is the sole supply to the basilar artery

Treatment

EQUIPMENT

- Standard 5F access (puncture needle, 5F vascular sheath)
- 5F Berenstein catheter (Boston Scientific, Natick, MA) and a 0.035-in hydrophilic guidewire (Terumo, Somerset, NJ)
- A 300-cm Amplatz exchange guidewire (Boston Scientific)
- 6F Shuttle Sheath (Shuttle Select; Cook Medical, Bloomington, IN) with continuous flush
- 6F Neuron Delivery Catheter (Penumbra Inc, Alameda, CA) with continuous flush
- Straight microcatheter (Prowler Plus; Cordis, Warren, NJ) with a 0.014-in guidewire (Synchro 14; Boston Scientific)
- Voyager RX 2.5 × 15-mm balloon (Abbott Vascular, Redwood City, CA)
- Driver 3.5 × 9-mm coronary balloon-mounted stent (Medtronic, Minneapolis, MN)
- Balloon inflation device (manometer)
- Heparin
- Contrast material

DESCRIPTION

The patient was premedicated with acetylsalicylic acid and clopidogrel, and heparin was initiated once the 5F sheath had been inserted. Baseline AP and lateral views of the intracranial vertebrobasilar system were obtained with a 5F Berenstein catheter. These confirmed the tight stenosis of the intracranial VA with a short segment of stenosis proximal to the origin of the posterior inferior cerebellar artery (PICA; **Fig. 53.2**). The proximal portion of the vessel was slightly dilated at 4.2 mm, whereas the diameter of the portion of the vessel distal to the stenosis was ~3 mm. An exchange maneuver was performed with an Amplatz wire to bring a 6F shuttle sheath into position in the subclavian artery proximal to the vertebral origin. We then used a 105-cm 6F neuron delivery catheter to access the VA. This was advanced over a glidewire up to the atlantoaxial level. We then used a Prowler Plus microcatheter, which was navigated over a Synchro 14 guidewire, to proceed triaxially and advance the neuron delivery catheter up to the intracranial segment of the VA. The stenosis was crossed with the Synchro 14 guidewire, and this was used to deliver a Voyager 2.5 × 15-mm balloon. We performed angioplasty at the stenotic segment. The balloon was withdrawn, and a Driver 3.5 ×

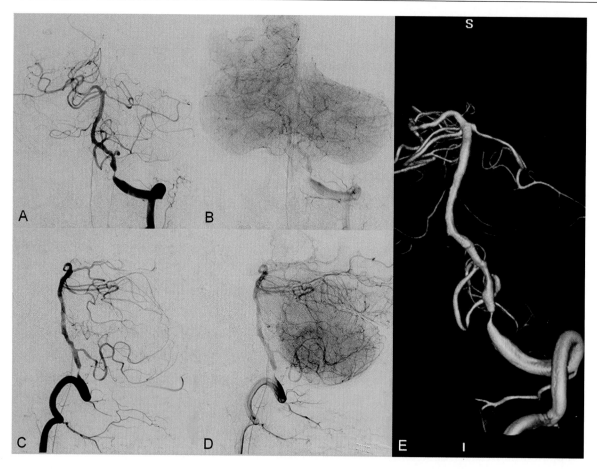

Fig. 53.2 DSA. Left VA angiogram in **(A,B)** AP and **(C,D)** lateral views in **(A,C)** arterial and **(B,D)** venous phases reveals a tight stenosis of the intracranial VA proximal to the origin of the left PICA, which is also seen on **(E)** 3D reconstruction.

9-mm coronary balloon-mounted stent was advanced and centered over the region of stenosis and deployed (**Fig. 53.3**). Control angiography showed good flow through this segment, with appropriate apposition of the stent (**Fig. 53.4**). The delivery catheter was withdrawn, and final PA and lateral views of the intracranial vertebrobasilar system did not reveal any evidence of thromboembolic complications, with good reopening of the VA. The shuttle sheath was exchanged for a 7F sheath, which was sutured in place.

Discussion

Background

As described in the previous case, intracranial atherosclerosis is a major cause of ischemic stroke, with rates of stroke ipsilateral to the intracranial stenosis of 11% at 1 year and 14% at 2 years despite the use of either warfarin or aspirin and possible modifications of vascular risk factors. The risk for subsequent stroke in the territory of the stenotic artery is 23% at 1 year and 25% at 2 years in patients with severe (≥ 70%) stenosis. Because surgery is not considered a viable alternative and data on aggressive medical therapies are lacking, endovascular options, including angioplasty, self-expandable stents, and balloon-mounted stents, have been proposed for the management of these patients. This

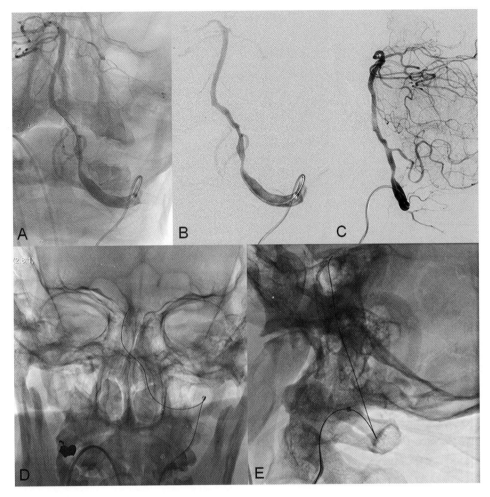

Fig. 53.3 (A) Unsubtracted and **(B,C)** DSA images of the neuron delivery catheter injection within the left VA in **(A,B)** AP and **(C)** lateral views following balloon angioplasty demonstrate the catheter in the distal atlantal loop and partial reopening of the stenosis. Plain radiography in **(D)** AP and **(E)** lateral views reveals the position of the coronal stent within the VA.

case report describes the use of a balloon-mounted stent and discusses the advantages and disadvantages of this treatment modality versus those of self-expandable stents and angioplasty alone.

Noninvasive Imaging Workup

PHYSICAL EXAMINATION

- The indication to treat is determined by the clinical findings, as discussed previously (i.e., symptomatic high-grade stenosis with recurrent symptoms despite best medical treatment).

CTA/MRI

- To decide what treatment option to use, high-quality CTA is necessary to determine whether or not the stenosis is densely calcified and whether a soft plaque is present. In addition, the vascular access, including the origin of the artery to be treated, the tortuosity of the vessel, and the degree of stenosis, are important features to consider in the selection of a treatment modality.
- MRI, including imaging of the vessel wall, may be helpful in the future to determine whether or not a plaque is active; for the time being, though, its findings will not alter treatment strategies as much as those of CTA do.

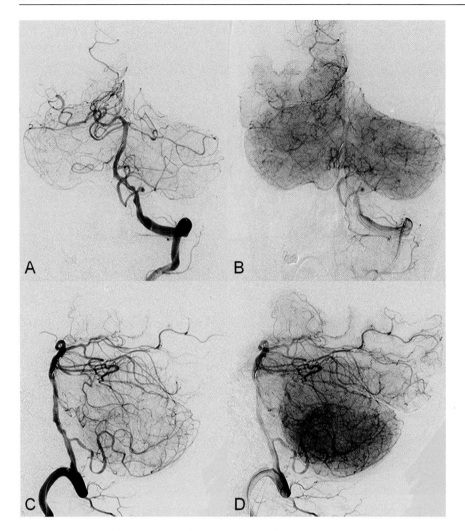

Fig. 53.4 DSA. Left VA angiogram following stent-assisted balloon angioplasty in **(A,B)** AP and **(C,D)** lateral views in **(A,C)** arterial and **(B,D)** venous phases reveals good flow through the previous stenotic segment and appropriate apposition of the stent.

Invasive Imaging Workup

- With high-quality CTA, invasive workup is rarely necessary and plays a role only in the evaluation of the collateral circulation, as stated in the previous case.

Treatment Options

SURGICAL TREATMENT

- As stated in the previous case, surgical treatments only rarely play a role in intracranial arteriosclerotic disease, and medical treatment may still be regarded as the first line of management. Endovascular treatment, however, is recommended once a previously symptomatic stenosis fails best medical management.

ENDOVASCULAR TREATMENT

- The stiffer the stent, the more stable the guiding catheter must be, and the more distal its placement. This can be achieved by using a triaxial system with a shuttle sheath and a flexible guiding catheter, or a transbrachial approach.
- If an exchange wire is used (with a self-expanding stent, as in the present case), a wire tip with a distal J-shape may cause less trauma to the vessel than a wire with a straight tip.
- With self-expanding stents, predilation should be performed with an undersized angioplasty balloon, whereas the stent may be slightly oversized.
- With balloon-mounted stents, the size of the stent should match exactly the size of the unstenosed anchoring segment. Therefore, 3D angiography may be necessary to determine the exact size of the vessel.
- A difference in the diameters of the vessel distal and proximal to the stenosis may be an indication for a self-expandable stent. Alternatively, staged angioplasty can be performed in the proximal and distal parts of the stent.
- Whenever a balloon is inflated in the intracranial circulation, make sure that the inflation is performed very slowly and gently (over minutes).

Possible Complications

In addition to the general complications described in the previous case, more specific procedure-related complications may occur.

- PTA: acute vessel recoil and dissection
- Self-expandable stents: distal guidewire perforations during the exchange maneuver, delayed re-stenosis
- Balloon-mounted stents: mechanical vasospasm, poor apposition to the vessel wall, balloon overhang with dissections

Published Literature on Treatment Options

Three different endovascular techniques can be used: percutaneous transluminal angioplasty (PTA) alone, balloon-mounted stents, and PTA with secondary deployment of a self-expandable stent. There is a general lack of prospective studies of these techniques, results vary (especially given the considerable advances that have been made in endovascular materials over the years), and many studies have a rather limited number of investigated subjects. Still, some general comments about these three techniques are possible.

When the data of 13 different studies involving 418 patients treated with PTA alone were evaluated, a technical success rate of 82% was reported. Periprocedural complications occurred in 15% (ischemia in 9% and hemorrhage in 6%) and postprocedural complications in 22% (delayed stroke in 4%, significant re-stenosis in 18%). However, these results may have been related to the high risk associated with early attempts and nondedicated hardware; in a recent study that took a more conservative approach, with undersizing of the balloon, slow inflation, and better periprocedural management (with dual antiplatelet therapy before and after PTA), the periprocedural morbidity and mortality rate was reduced to 6%, with postprocedural complications occurring in 3%. The available data on intracranial angioplasty suggest that it can be performed relatively safely in stable patients, but the technical drawbacks are numerous, including immediate elastic recoil of the artery, dissection, acute vessel closure, residual stenosis after the procedure, and high rates of re-stenosis.

Self-expanding stents with dilation before stent deployment have the highest technical success rates, given the relative flexibility of the guiding catheter system (nearly 98% in all larger series). The access to the lesion is rather atraumatic. However, at present, the exchange wire operation is not without risk, and distal guidewire perforations have been reported. In addition, predilation without stent protection may result in distal embolization. The chronic radial outward force of self-expanding stents has been related to smooth-muscle cell proliferation and vessel wall thickening, with higher rates of delayed re-stenosis. Stenosis recurs in approximately one-third of all patients treated with self-expanding stents. Of these, more than 80% require re-treatment, in most instances with repeated angioplasty; however, the results are durable in only 50% of patients, and multiple revascularization procedures may be necessary. Re-stenosis is especially common in the anterior circulation in young patients. The supraclinoid carotid artery in younger female patients appears to be the most common site for re-stenosis, which may indicate that lesion pathology at this site is different from "classic" atherosclerotic disease.

Balloon-mounted stents are limited by their rigidity, which makes delivery to intracranial lesions technically more difficult. Oversizing may result in vessel dissection, whereas undersizing can lead to poor apposition to the vessel wall. Vessel wall injury due to balloon overhang with edge dissection may occur (especially with stents that are not specifically designed for navigation in the intracranial vasculature). The higher profile of the stiff balloon-stent delivery system may cause complications when the lesion is crossed, and tortuosity of the vessel wall may hinder distal access. A new generation of low-profile and more flexible stent systems has been developed, though, and with the advent of very flexible guiding catheters, distal access has become possible. These stents are therefore gaining importance, especially in that they do not require an exchange guidewire maneuver, are easy to handle, and do not require predilation. Their major advantage, as demonstrated in this case, is for use in highly calcified lesions, where re-stenosis may occur in self-expanding stents because their radial outward force may not be sufficient to keep the vessel open. The rate of re-stenosis following balloon-mounted stent placement is very low.

Although there are no guidelines concerning what kinds of stents to use in what circumstances, we generally use self-expandable stents for the M1, for very tortuous vessels (given the ease of access compared with the stiffer balloon-mounted stents), and for stenoses in which the diameters of the proximal and distal vessel segments differ significantly. On the other hand, balloon-mounted stents are best used, in our experience, in densely calcified lesions. In our practice, PTA alone is not used.

PEARLS AND PITFALLS

- In most centers, PTA alone is no longer performed for the treatment of symptomatic intracranial stenosis.
- Whether to use a self-expandable stent or a balloon-mounted stent depends on the individual features of the vessel anatomy, including proximal access, vessel diameter and tortuosity, and morphology of the stenosis (calcification, vessel diameter distal and proximal to the stenosis).

Further Reading

Blasel S, Yükzek Z, Kurre W, et al. Recanalization results after intracranial stenting of atherosclerotic stenoses. Cardiovasc Intervent Radiol 2009 Nov 12. [Epub ahead of print]

Fiorella D, Chow MM, Anderson M, Woo H, Rasmussen PA, Masaryk TJ. A 7-year experience with balloon-mounted coronary stents for the treatment of symptomatic vertebrobasilar intracranial atheromatous disease. Neurosurgery 2007;61(2):236–242, discussion 242–243

Fiorella D, Woo HH. Emerging endovascular therapies for symptomatic intracranial atherosclerotic disease. Stroke 2007;38(8):2391–2396

Hartmann M, Jansen O. Angioplasty and stenting of intracranial stenosis. Curr Opin Neurol 2005;18 (1):39–45

Lutsep HL. Symptomatic intracranial stenosis: best medical treatment vs. intracranial stenting. Curr Opin Neurol 2009;22(1):69–74

SSYLVIA Study Investigators. Stenting of Symptomatic Atherosclerotic Lesions in the Vertebral or Intracranial Arteries (SSYLVIA): study results. Stroke 2004;35(6):1388–1392

Suh DC, Kim JK, Choi JW, et al. Intracranial stenting of severe symptomatic intracranial stenosis: results of 100 consecutive patients. AJNR Am J Neuroradiol 2008;29(4):781–785

CASE 54

Case Description

Clinical Presentation

A 73-year-old man has had multiple episodes of double vision, difficulty walking, and dysarthria. He experiences strange sensations involving his left arm. On examination, a difference between blood pressure measurements in the right and left arms is noted. CTA and MRA are performed.

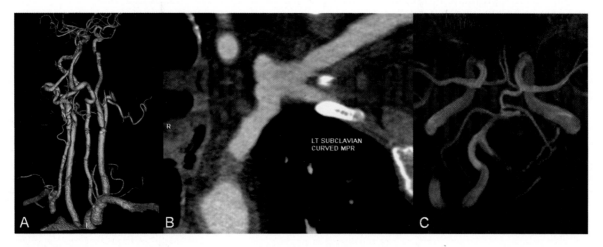

Fig. 54.1 CTA. **(A)** 3D reconstruction and **(B)** coronal view demonstrate occlusion of the proximal left subclavian artery with a "fading phenomenon," indicative of retrograde flow, in **(C)** the left VA on TOF MRA.

Radiologic Studies

CT/MRI

CTA revealed occlusion of his proximal left subclavian artery before the takeoff of the left vertebral artery (VA). Subsequent MR examination, including phase contrast MRA, demonstrated reversed flow within the left VA, which supplied the left upper extremity (**Fig. 54.1**). An additional stenosis with a 60 to 70% diameter was present at the origin of the right internal carotid artery.

Diagnosis

Subclavian steal syndrome

Treatment

EQUIPMENT

- Standard femoral 5F access and sheath and brachial 4F access (micropuncture set)
- 6F Shuttle Sheath (Shuttle Select; Cook Medical, Bloomington, IN) with continuous flush
- Different (shapeable, stiff) guidewires (Terumo, Somerset, NJ; Boston Scientific, Natick, MA)
- 4F and 5F Berenstein catheters (Boston Scientific)
- Contrast material

320

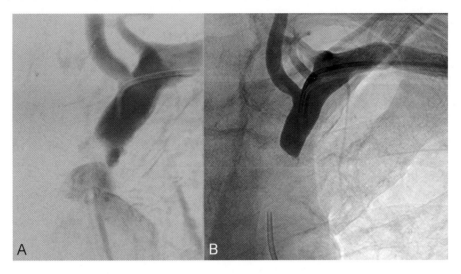

Fig. 54.2 Simultaneous injections into the aortic arch and **(A)** the left subclavian artery and **(B)** unsubtracted angiography of the left subclavian artery in AP view demonstrate complete occlusion of the proximal left subclavian artery.

DESCRIPTION

The left brachial and right femoral arteries were prepared and draped in the usual fashion. A 5F sheath was inserted into the right femoral artery, and a 4F sheath was used for the left brachial artery with a micropuncture technique and ultrasound guidance. A straight 4F catheter was advanced in retrograde fashion through the brachial artery to the stenotic subclavian portion (**Fig. 54.2**). With the guidewire, an unsuccessful attempt was made to pass through the occluded portion, followed by an attempt to pass from below, initially with a 5F Berenstein catheter and a glidewire. The guidewire again came up to the occlusion but would not cross. A shapeable guidewire was used, as well as a stiff guidewire; however, both were unable to cross. In an attempt to create a more stable catheter system, the sheath was exchanged for a 6F shuttle sheath. Next, a Berenstein catheter was passed through the shuttle sheath, and this coaxial system was advanced into the origin of the subclavian artery. Again, multiple attempts to penetrate with the wire were unsuccessful. At this point, the procedure was stopped, the catheters and wires were removed, the patient's heparin was reversed, and manual compression was used to control the puncture sites. The patient was referred to surgery.

Discussion

Background

Arterial steal in general is considered a pathologic process in which an increase in blood flow through a low-resistance vascular bed is sufficient to divert flow away from a region of the central nervous system. In subclavian steal syndrome, a proximal subclavian artery stenosis can lead to the diversion of blood flow from one VA to the other in retrograde fashion, with subsequent posterior fossa hypoperfusion. Subclavian steal is most commonly a marker of generalized atherosclerotic vascular disease, and although it may be associated with claudication of the arm, it is rarely the causative factor in symptoms of cerebral ischemia.

Noninvasive Imaging Workup

PHYSICAL EXAMINATION

- A missing or decreased arterial pulse in the affected arm and a difference in blood pressures between the two arms are noted.
- Isolated symptoms can be present in the extremity: claudication, easy fatigability, paresthesias, and a feeling of coolness.
- Diverse neurologic symptoms may be present that point toward vertebrobasilar insufficiency, including vertigo, ataxia, and visual disturbances.
- Neurologic symptoms can be brought on by arm exercise.

IMAGING FINDINGS

- The radiographic hallmark of subclavian steal is retrograde flow in the affected VA due to stenosis of the subclavian artery proximal to the VA origin. This can be directly visualized with duplex ultrasound or DSA and indirectly imaged by MRI or CT.
- Duplex ultrasound can visualize the effects of subclavian steal on the contralateral VA flow and its possible effect on carotid flow. In cases of subclavian occlusion or stenosis, ultrasound can demonstrate a complete or partial systolic-diastolic steal, with flow reversal in the affected VA. In addition, a significant increase in flow in the contralateral VA and common carotid artery (CCA), in comparison with normal values, can be seen in cases of retrograde vertebral flow. The retrograde flow values, ipsilateral vertebral luminal diameter, and flow values in the CCAs are higher in cases of complete steal in patients with subclavian occlusions than in cases of partial steal in patients with subclavian stenoses.
- CTA can demonstrate the location and degree of subclavian stenosis; however, it cannot provide details of flow direction.
- MRI and MRA with phase contrast can demonstrate flow direction. In routinely used TOF angiography, a "fading phenomenon" may be visualized; this is due to retrograde inflow of unsaturated spins that become progressively saturated during retrograde flow. Contrast-enhanced MRA will present the same problem that CTA does; it can, however, demonstrate the proximal subclavian artery stenosis.

Invasive Imaging Workup

- DSA is considered the gold standard for visualizing arterial steal and will demonstrate retrograde flow in one VA on delayed images. DSA can also demonstrate the location and extent of a proximal subclavian artery stenosis or occlusion.

Differential Diagnosis

- Because stenosis of the subclavian artery is a general marker of atherosclerosis, the patient's symptoms may be related to other vascular stenoses rather than to the visualized steal, which may be asymptomatic.

Treatment Options

CONSERVATIVE OR MEDICAL MANAGEMENT

- Anatomic steal may be present in a large number of asymptomatic patients. Even in patients with neurologic symptoms in whom subclavian steal syndrome is diagnosed, other vascular lesions that are more likely to account for their symptoms may be present, and it is believed that only 10% of patients with anatomically proven steal are truly symptomatic. Therefore, for endovascular or surgical therapies to be indicated, the clinical symptoms must be compelling.

SURGICAL TREATMENT

- Extrathoracic, extra-anatomic bypasses have lower morbidity and mortality rates than those of transthoracic procedures. Therefore, current surgical procedures include subclavian-to-carotid transposition, carotid-to-subclavian bypass, and contralateral subclavian-to-ipsilateral subclavian bypass.
- The choice of procedure is determined by the presence of carotid artery disease.

ENDOVASCULAR TREATMENT

- Endovascular therapies consist of percutaneous transluminal angioplasty (PTA) alone and stenting with balloon-expandable or self-expanding stents.
- Either a retrograde ipsilateral transbrachial approach or an antegrade femoral approach can be attempted.

Possible Complications

- Because flow in the VA ipsilateral to the stenosis is retrograde, thromboembolic complications due to distal embolization into the posterior circulation are rare.
- The most common complications of this procedure are dissection and failure of the attempt to revascularize the subclavian artery.

Published Literature on Treatment Options

The management of occlusive disease of the subclavian artery remains somewhat controversial. Surgical options are challenging procedures with excellent long-term results. Endovascular techniques, on the other hand, are technically easier but, as demonstrated in our case, not always feasible, and their long-term durability is considered to be lower. The primary success rates of endovascular therapies may vary between 70 and 100%, with better results for stenoses than for occlusions. The long-term patency rate is slightly better in patients treated with stenting than in those treated with PTA alone. In larger, long-term series, the primary patency rates at 1, 3, and 5 years are 100%, 98%, and 96%, respectively, for surgical patients versus 93%, 78%, and 70%, respectively, for patients treated with endovascular techniques. Freedom from symptom recurrence is also statistically better in the bypass group than in the stent group. In most centers, endovascular techniques are the procedure of choice for high-risk patients, especially those with a stenosis but no complete occlusion. Surgical management should be offered to patients for whom surgery poses a low risk and who may be seeking a more durable outcome.

PEARLS AND PITFALLS

- Deciding whether treatment is indicated may be the most challenging part of the management of patients with subclavian stenosis and presumed steal because the condition may be an incidental finding in a patient with generalized atherosclerosis and other (truly symptomatic) lesions.
- If endovascular management is chosen, stents should be favored over PTA alone.

Further Reading

AbuRahma AF, Bates MC, Stone PA, et al. Angioplasty and stenting versus carotid-subclavian bypass for the treatment of isolated subclavian artery disease. J Endovasc Ther 2007;14(5):698–704

Brountzos EN, Malagari K, Kelekis DA. Endovascular treatment of occlusive lesions of the subclavian and innominate arteries. Cardiovasc Intervent Radiol 2006;29(4):503–510

Delaney CP, Couse NF, Mehigan D, Keaveny TV. Investigation and management of subclavian steal syndrome. Br J Surg 1994;81(8):1093–1095

Linni K, Ugurluoglu A, Mader N, Hitzl W, Magometschnigg H, Hölzenbein TJ. Endovascular management versus surgery for proximal subclavian artery lesions. Ann Vasc Surg 2008;22(6):769–775

Päivänsalo M, Heikkilä O, Tikkakoski T, Leinonen S, Merikanto J, Suramo I. Duplex ultrasound in the subclavian steal syndrome. Acta Radiol 1998;39(2):183–188

Peeters P, Verbist J, Deloose K, Bosiers M. Endovascular treatment strategies for supra-aortic arterial occlusive disease. J Cardiovasc Surg (Torino) 2005;46(3):193–200

Sixt S, Rastan A, Schwarzwälder U, et al. Results after balloon angioplasty or stenting of atherosclerotic subclavian artery obstruction. Catheter Cardiovasc Interv 2009;73(3):395–403

Taylor CL, Selman WR, Ratcheson RA. Steal affecting the central nervous system. Neurosurgery 2002;50(4):679–688, discussion 688–689

CASE 55

Case Description

Clinical Presentation

A 41-year-old man presents with the new onset of severe headaches. He has no neurologic deficits on physical examination at admission. Initial CT and MRI are performed, and cerebral venous sinus thrombosis of the anterior third of the superior sagittal sinus (SSS) is diagnosed. Further investigation also shows protein C deficiency. He is treated with anticoagulants; however, 48 hours later, progressive right-sided weakness develops and his level of consciousness decreases. CT is again performed, followed by angiography.

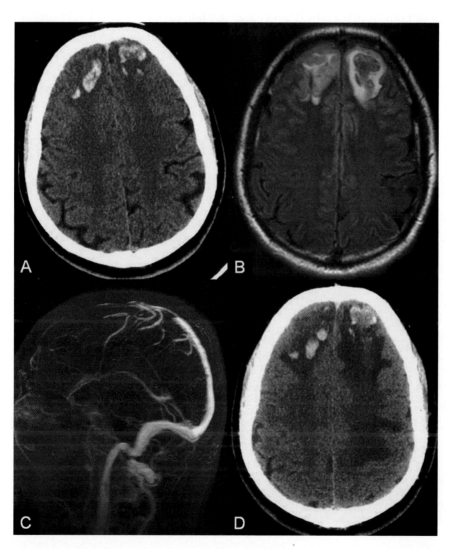

Fig. 55.1 **(A)** Initial unenhanced CT and **(B)** FLAIR MRI reveal small areas of hemorrhage with surrounding edema in both frontal lobes. **(C)** The anterior aspect of the SSS is not visualized on contrast-enhanced MRV. **(D)** Follow-up unenhanced CT 48 hours after anti-coagulation therapy shows progression of the edema, which now extends into the left parietal white matter.

325

Radiologic Studies

CT

Initial CT revealed small areas of hemorrhage with minimal surrounding edema in both frontal lobes (**Fig. 55.1A**). Follow-up CT 48 hours later showed progression of the edema, now extending into the left parietal white matter (**Fig. 55.1D**).

MRI/MRV

FLAIR imaging demonstrated hypersignal within the areas of hemorrhage and edema in both frontal lobes. Sagittal T1-weighted images (not shown) revealed T1 hypersignal of clot within the anterior aspect of the SSS, which corresponded to the findings on contrast-enhanced MRV, in which the anterior SSS was not visualized (**Fig. 55.1 B,C**). These findings are consistent with the diagnosis of cerebral dural sinus thrombosis.

DSA

The arterial phase of the internal carotid artery (ICA) angiograms was normal. The venous phase revealed poor opacification of both frontal cortical veins and the left parietal cortical vein and no opacification of the anterior third of the SSS (**Fig. 55.2A**). The posterior circulation and remainder of the dural sinuses appeared normal.

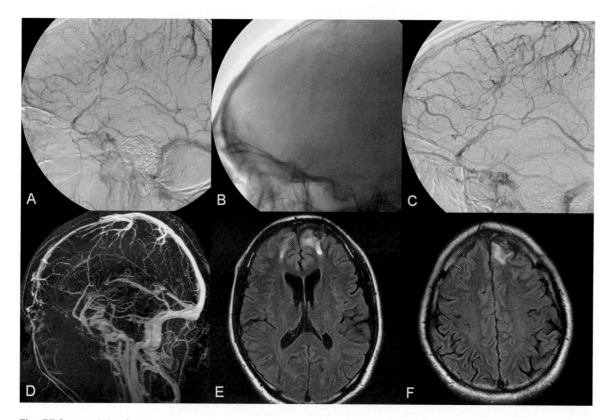

Fig. 55.2 DSA. **(A)** Left ICA angiogram, late venous phase in lateral view. **(B)** Plain radiography shows the position of the microcatheter within the SSS during the thrombolysis procedure. **(C)** Final control run of the left ICA in late venous phase, lateral view after the thrombolysis demonstrates improved opacification of the frontoparietal cortical veins and anterior SSS. **(D)** Follow-up contrast-enhanced MRV and **(E,F)** FLAIR images 2 weeks following the procedure confirm recanalization of the anterior SSS with reduction of the edema.

Diagnosis

Acute thrombosis of the anterior aspect of the SSS, associated with progressive symptoms and signs despite best medical treatment

Treatment

EQUIPMENT

- Standard 5F (arterial) and 6F (venous) access (puncture needle, 5F and 6F vascular sheaths)
- Standard 5F and 6F multipurpose catheters (Guider Soft Tip; Boston Scientific, Natick, MA) with continuous flush and a 0.035-in hydrophilic guidewire (Terumo, Somerset, NJ)
- A 0.021-in over-the-wire microcatheter (Prowler Select Plus; Cordis, Warren, NJ) with a 0.014-in hydrophilic guidewire (Synchro 14; Boston Scientific)
- Contrast material
- Recombinant tissue plasminogen activator 20 mg

DESCRIPTION

The procedure was done under general anesthesia. Following diagnostic angiography, a venous puncture was performed, and a 6F multipurpose catheter was advanced transvenously into the left internal jugular vein and placed at the left jugular bulb. The microcatheter was then advanced through the left transverse-sigmoid sinus into the SSS under a venous phase roadmap. The tip of the microcatheter was placed at the anterior SSS within the most distal aspect of the thrombus. A gentle hand injection through the microcatheter was done to confirm the position, followed by a slow hand infusion of tissue plasminogen activator (tPA); 1 mg was injected every 2 minutes to a total of 20 mg in 40 minutes (**Fig. 55.2 B,C**). During this period, the micro-guidewire was intermittently manipulated to enhance clot fragmentation, and the microcatheter was gradually withdrawn (in a distal-to-proximal direction) through the occluded segment. A control angiogram of the left ICA showed partial recanalization of the anterior SSS, with improved opacification of the frontal cortical veins. The microcatheter was then removed, and the anticoagulation therapy was continued. Follow-up MRI and MRV 2 weeks following the procedure confirmed recanalization of the anterior SSS and a decrease in the edema (**Fig. 55.2 D–F**). The patient made a complete clinical recovery.

Discussion

Background

Cerebral venous sinus thrombosis (CVST) accounts for ~0.5% of all cases of stroke. A bimodal age distribution is observed: a first peak in the pediatric population, particularly in neonates and infants younger than 6 months of age, and a second peak in adults between 20 and 40 years of age. A female predominance is observed in the adult group and is likely to be related to pregnancy, the puerperium, and the use of oral contraceptives. The SSS is the most common location, followed by the transverse sinuses, straight sinus, and cavernous sinus. The cause of and risk factors for CVST are quite extensive. Apart from hormonal disturbances in the female population, prothrombotic states, either genetic or acquired (e.g., antithrombin III, protein C, and protein S deficiencies) also play a major role in the development of CVST. The clinical presentation is highly variable, and symptoms range from a nonspecific minor headache to intracranial hypertension and subsequent brain herniation. Thus, the diagnosis is extremely challenging for the clinician and so may occasionally be delayed.

Noninvasive Imaging Workup

CT/CTV

- Hyperdense intracranial hemorrhage, which may be intraparenchymal, subdural, or subarachnoidal, and/or hypodense brain edema may be seen on unenhanced CT scans. Occasionally, a hyperdense triangle sign may be seen in the region of the dural sinuses or a hyperdense cord sign in the region of the cortical veins; however, several conditions, including dehydration and a high hematocrit, may mimic these findings. These conditions may necessitate further evaluation with post-contrast studies.
- Classic signs of CVST on post-contrast CT and CTV are the empty delta sign, which is seen as an absence of contrast filling within the posterior SSS or torcular and filling defects within the dural sinuses or cortical veins.

MRI/MRV

- The MRI signal of the thrombus varies according to the stage of the clot. During the first 3 to 5 days, the thrombus is typically isointense on T1-weighted images and hypointense on T2-weighted images. After 5 days, high signal on both T1- and T2-weighted images can be expected. The signal of the thrombus changes to isointense on T1-weighted images after 1 month yet remains hyperintense on T2-weighted images and FLAIR images.
- In the acute stage, the thrombus is typically seen as a filling defect on post-gadolinium T1-weighted images; however, in the chronic stage, the thrombus may show a variable degree of enhancement, making the diagnosis more difficult.
- Contrast-enhanced MRV, with a short 21-second delay, may be useful in doubtful cases because the thrombus in both the acute and chronic stages will be seen as a filling defect.
- Venous congestion and infarction are seen as hyperintensity on T2-weighted images and FLAIR images. Areas of hemorrhage and cases with cortical vein thrombosis may be better visualized on gradient-echo T2*-weighted images.

Invasive Imaging Workup

- Angiography is usually not required for the diagnosis of CVST and is performed only if more aggressive treatment (i.e., direct thrombolysis) is indicated.

Treatment Options

CONSERVATIVE OR MEDICAL MANAGEMENT

- Initial management consists of identifying and managing the predisposing factors (antibiotics for infectious causes) and evaluating the prothrombotic state of the patient; other measures include hydration, normalization of elevated intracranial pressure, and the symptomatic treatment of seizures and headaches.
- The role of anticoagulants in the treatment of CVST has been well established, and the presence of intracranial hemorrhage does not contraindicate anticoagulation. Either low-molecular-weight heparin or dose-adjusted intravenous heparin (to twice the normal activated partial thromboplastin time values) can be given in the acute stage. A switch to oral anticoagulants (for an international normalized ratio of 2–3) for 3 to 12 months is then recommended, depending on the prothrombotic state of the patient.

SURGICAL TREATMENT

- Surgery is usually reserved for cases of elevated intracranial pressure that cannot be controlled with medical measures. Surgical management includes external ventricular drainage, insertion of a cerebrospinal fluid shunt, or decompressive craniectomy in patients with large intracerebral hemorrhages whose condition is deteriorating.

ENDOVASCULAR TREATMENT

- No randomized controlled trials have addressed the efficacy and safety of endovascular treatment for CVST. However, it has been suggested that endovascular treatment should be considered for patients presenting with severe neurologic deficits (Glasgow Coma Scale score ≤ 8) and those whose condition deteriorates despite anticoagulation therapy for at least 18 hours.
- Urokinase and tPA are the most commonly used thrombolytic agents in the literature. The dosages for both drugs vary considerably in different studies (urokinase: between 120,000 and 1,600,000 units as a bolus; tPA: between 3 and 70 mg as a bolus or as a continuous infusion for up to 72 hours). In our practice, we generally do a slow hand infusion of 1 mg/min up to 20 mg as a single dose.
- Systemic heparin must be continued during and after the procedure.
- Mechanical thrombolysis/thrombectomy has been described with balloon angioplasty, rheolytic catheters, and stent placement. It is usually combined with thrombolytic agents and in our practice is used in cases in which thrombolytic agents have failed to achieve sufficient recanalization.

Possible Complications

- Venous perforation
- Systemic hemorrhage
- Worsening of intracranial hemorrhage

Published Literature on Treatment Options

Despite the use of anticoagulants, the overall rate of death and dependency related to CVST still ranges from 8.8 to 44.4%. Many case reports and smaller case series support the use of endovascular treatment of CVST in selected patients. Although there is no doubt that medical treatment with intravenous heparin is the first choice, patients with a poor clinical status or clinical deterioration despite heparin treatment for at least 18 hours are classic candidates for more aggressive treatments. Urokinase is the most commonly used thrombolytic agent in the literature, followed by tPA. Streptokinase is no longer used because the rates of systemic hemorrhage are higher than with the other two available drugs. The doses of urokinase and tPA vary in the literature; however, most studies have used a bolus dose, followed by a continuous infusion. Many of these studies combined thrombolytic agents with mechanical thrombectomy devices (balloon angioplasty, stents, rheolytic catheters, microsnares, and Merci clot retrieval devices). These authors agree that the addition of mechanical thrombectomy helps to reduce the dose of the thrombolytic agent required for thrombolysis. In our experience, we prefer a single bolus dose of 20 mg of tPA without any continuous infusion to avoid possible sheath complications. Mechanical thrombectomy is typically considered if the initial attempt with tPA fails. In the few larger series that comprised 10 or more patients, the outcome was good and excellent in ~70%. Hemorrhagic complications were seen in ~10 to 30% of cases. These results of the use of direct thrombolysis seem promising; however, no randomized controlled studies have assessed its efficacy and safety, and therefore in our opinion, the endovascular management of CVST should still be reserved for patients with a poor clinical status or neurologic deterioration.

- The presentation of CVST can be variable, making the diagnosis more challenging. Imaging plays an important role in the diagnosis of CVST, and a delayed diagnosis may lead to major consequences and a poor outcome for the patient.
- Anticoagulants are crucial for the treatment of CVST, and the presence of intracranial hemorrhage does not contraindicate their use.
- Endovascular treatment for CVST is still controversial, although promising, and should be reserved for patients with a poor clinical status or neurologic deterioration despite receiving full medical treatment.

Further Reading

Agid R, Shelef I, Scott JN, Farb RI. Imaging of the intracranial venous system. Neurologist 2008;14(1):12–22

Jonas Kimchi T, Lee SK, Agid R, Shroff M, Ter Brugge KG. Cerebral sinovenous thrombosis in children. Neuroimaging Clin N Am 2007;17(2):239–244

Lee SK, terBrugge K. Clinical presentation, imaging and treatment of cerebral venous thrombosis (CVT). Interv Neuroradiol 2002;8:5–14

Rahman M, Velat GJ, Hoh BL, Mocco J. Direct thrombolysis for cerebral venous sinus thrombosis. Neurosurg Focus 2009;27(5):E7

Stam J, Majoie CB, van Delden OM, van Lienden KP, Reekers JA. Endovascular thrombectomy and thrombolysis for severe cerebral sinus thrombosis: a prospective study. Stroke 2008;39(5):1487–1490

CASE 56

Case Description

Clinical Presentation

A 5-month-old boy has a history of cardiac failure since birth, which has been controlled sufficiently with diuretics, and he is feeding well orally. MRI is performed. His psychomotor development is normal on follow-up visits, and he is now scheduled for angiography and embolization. His physical and neurologic examination findings at admission are normal.

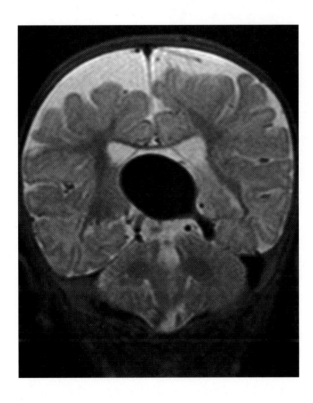

Fig. 56.1 Coronal T2-weighted MRI reveals a midline dilated vascular structure at the vein of Galen region.

Radiologic Studies

MRI

The MRI study showed a midline dilated flow void at the vein of Galen region, representing a vascular structure. The brain parenchymal signal appeared normal. A slightly low-lying position of the cerebellar tonsils was observed (**Fig. 56.1**). Normal myelination was perceived, no abnormal diffusion-weighted changes were seen, and there were no signs of calcifications or brain atrophy.

DSA

Because there is no role for diagnostic angiography without embolization, DSA was performed immediately before embolization. DSA revealed a high-flow arteriovenous shunt fed from a left posterior choroidal artery branch and draining into the dilated median vein of the prosencephalon (the forerunner of the vein of Galen; **Fig. 56.2 A,B**). There were additional collaterals from smaller medial

331

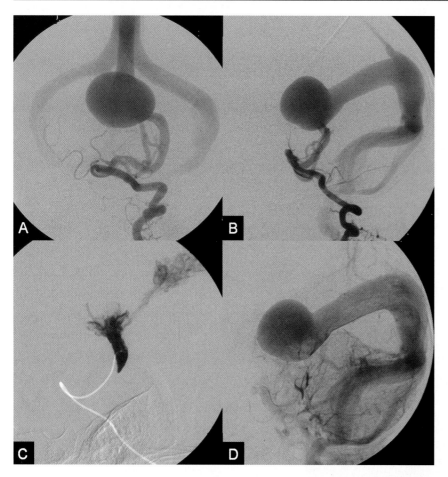

Fig. 56.2 DSA. Left VA angiogram in **(A)** AP and **(B)** lateral views. **(C)** DSA after embolization demonstrates a "mushroom" configuration of the glue cast with minimal penetration into the proximal venous pouch. **(D)** On left VA angiogram in lateral view after embolization, improved visualization of the posterior fossa veins suggests regression of venous congestion.

posterior choroidal branches. A falcine sinus was present, with absence of the straight sinus. Medial occipital and marginal sinuses were also observed. The posterior fossa veins were poorly visualized, suggestive of venous congestion at the level of the posterior fossa structures (which also explained the slightly low-lying tonsils). Internal carotid artery (ICA) injections showed drainage of the cerebral hemispheres through the cavernous sinuses bilaterally (cavernous capture).

Diagnosis

Mural type of vein of Galen aneurysmal malformation

Treatment

EQUIPMENT

- Standard 4F access (puncture needle, 4F vascular sheath)
- Standard 4F multipurpose catheter (Cook Medical, Bloomington, IN) with continuous slow drip and a 0.035-in hydrophilic guidewire (Terumo, Somerset, NJ)
- A 0.018-in flow-directed microcatheter (BALTACCI; Balt International, Montmorency, France) with a steam-shaped 90-degree curve

- A 10% glucose solution
- Histoacryl/Lipiodol/tantalum powder (2 mL/0.1 mL/1 vial)
- Contrast material (maximum number of milliliters, 4 × body weight in kilograms)

DESCRIPTION

Following diagnostic angiography (one vessel, 6 mL of contrast), a 4F multipurpose catheter was advanced into the left vertebral artery (VA), with the tip placed at the C3-4 level. A flow-related microcatheter was introduced into the left posterior choroidal branch originating from the left posterior cerebral artery (PCA). The tip was placed against the wall of the arterial feeder with a 1-cm margin to the shunt zone. A control run was done via hand injection through the microcatheter (2 mL) to verify the position. The microcatheter was then flushed with glucose solution, followed by the rapid injection of pure glue to close the fistula and obtain a "mushroom" configuration of the glue cast with only minimal venous penetration. The microcatheter was removed, and a control angiogram performed via the guiding catheter revealed obliteration of the posterior choroidal feeder and significantly reduced flow through the shunt. Visualization of the posterior fossa veins was improved, indicating improvement of the posterior fossa venous drainage (**Fig. 56.2 C,D**). The child had no new neurologic deficits following embolization. He is to be followed with psychomotor neuropediatric assessments every 3 months (including head circumference measurements) and MRI every 6 months. The next embolization session, if no psychomotor retardation occurs, is planned for 1 year after the first embolization.

Discussion

Background

Vein of Galen aneurysmal malformations are arteriovenous malformations of the choroidal system that develop in the early embryonic stage. They account for ~30% of all vascular malformations in the pediatric population. Cardiac failure, the most common presentation in neonates, may progress to multiple-organ failure if left untreated and is probably related to the lower cardiovascular volume of these patients. A clinical presentation with hydrodynamic disorders, such as hydrocephalus and macrocrania, is more commonly seen in older infants. Only rarely is this disorder diagnosed in older children, who are more likely to present with neurologic symptoms such as seizures, neurologic deficits, and even intracranial hemorrhage. These cases are associated with a poor outcome, which is likely related to the degree of brain damage caused by the vein of Galen aneurysmal malformation. Certain angioarchitectural characteristics are specific for vein of Galen aneurysmal malformations. The arterial supply always involves the choroidal arteries, including the anterior choroidal artery, posterior choroidal artery, and subforniceal artery (anterior cerebral artery [ACA] branch). The subependymal arteries and limbic arterial arch (between the PCA and ACA branches) constitute the remainder of the supply. Secondary supply from transcerebral branches of the middle cerebral artery (MCA) typically represents sump effect and arterial steal. Two types of nidi are seen in vein of Galen aneurysmal malformations: a mural type, consisting of direct arteriovenous fistulae within the wall of the median vein of the prosencephalon, and a choroidal type, which corresponds to a more primitive condition. In the choroidal type, a network is interposed between the nidus and the opening into the large venous pouch. Venous drainage is toward the dilated median vein of the prosencephalon, which is the forerunner of the vein of Galen. Although it has been previously reported that no communication between this vein and the deep venous system exists, many case reports have actually documented a connection, typically at the posterior aspect of the dilated venous segment. Several embryonic sinuses often persist in vein of Galen aneurysmal malformations, including a falcine sinus, which may occur with absence of the straight sinus and of the medial occipital and marginal sinuses.

Noninvasive Imaging Workup

CLINICAL EXAMINATION

- The Bicêtre score is used in most centers to evaluate children in whom a vein of Galen malformation is diagnosed (**Table 56.1**). In this system, cardiac, cerebral, respiratory, hepatic, and renal function is evaluated and scored accordingly.
- The following strategy is adopted after scoring: Patients whose score is higher than 12 receive medical treatment (see below) until the age of 4 to 5 months or until a complication occurs; patients whose score is 8 to 11 receive emergency embolization; a score below 8 is an indication for therapeutic abstention. Emergency embolization is also considered if a child has medically refractory heart failure, exhibits an increase in the cranial perimeter, or is not feeding well (no weight gain).
- The Denver scoring system may be employed to evaluate whether developmental milestones have been reached.
- The ocular fundus may be investigated to assess venous congestion.
- Bluish discoloration of the skin is generally a good sign because it means that the brain has "captured" the cavernous sinuses for drainage.

PRENATAL ULTRASOUND

- A dilated median vein of the prosencephalon is seen as an anechoic tubular midline structure located superior to the cerebellum. Increased flow on color Doppler images helps to confirm the diagnosis.
- Prenatal ultrasound is most sensitive for the detection of vein of Galen aneurysmal malformations after the 26th week of gestation.

Table 56.1 Bicêtre Neonatal Evaluation Score

Points	Cardiac Function	Cerebral Function	Respiratory Function	Hepatic Function	Renal Function
5	Normal	Normal	Normal	—	—
4	Overload, no medical treatment	Subclinical isolated EEG abnormalities	Tachypnea, finishes bottle	—	—
3	Failure—stable with medical treatment	Nonconvulsive intermittent neurologic signs	Tachypnea, does not finish bottle	No hepatomegaly, normal hepatic function	Normal
2	Failure—not stable with medical treatment	Isolated convulsion	Assisted ventilation, normal saturation, $FIO_2 < 25\%$	Hepatomegaly, normal hepatic function	Transient anuria
1	Ventilation necessary	Seizures	Assisted ventilation, normal saturation, $FIO_2 > 25\%$	Moderate or transient hepatic insufficiency	Unstable diuresis with treatment
0	Resistant to medical treatment	Permanent neurologic signs	Assisted ventilation, desaturation	Abnormal coagulation, elevated enzymes	Anuria

Abbreviations: EEG, electroencephalographic; FIO_2, fraction of inspired oxygen

Source: Lasjaunias PL, Berenstein A, terBrugge KG. Surgical Neuroangiography. Vol 3: Clinical and Interventional Aspects in Children. 2nd ed. Berlin: Springer; 2006. Reprinted with permission.

CT/MRI

- MRI is the best imaging modality for the evaluation of vein of Galen aneurysmal malformations and can also be done prenatally to assess the brain parenchyma.
- A dilated midline venous pouch, representing a dilated median vein of the prosencephalon, can be seen on CT scan and as a flow-void structure on MRI.
- Parenchymal changes are best seen on FLAIR images and T2-weighted MR sequences and can be classified as focal encephalomalacia or diffuse loss of brain volume.
- Focal encephalomalacia is more likely related to the presence of arterial steal, which is a result of the high-flow sump effect of the vein of Galen aneurysmal malformation. It is characterized by leptomeningeal collateralization of the cortical branches of the MCA or the ACA to the PCA territories, further contributing to the arteriovenous shunt of the vein of Galen aneurysmal malformation, and is best seen on contrast-enhanced CT or as flow-void structures on T2-weighted MRI.
- Diffuse loss of brain volume is usually associated with hydrocephalus and may be reversible following treatment.
- Hydrodynamic disorders caused by vein of Galen aneurysmal malformations include macrocrania, hydrocephalus, and venous congestion.
- Acute venous congestion can result in brain edema, seen as hypodensity on CT or T2 hyperintensity on MRI, and in tonsillar prolapse infratentorially. Chronic venous congestion usually results in parenchymal calcifications, which are better seen on unenhanced CT than on gradient-echo MRI.
- Diffusion-weighted abnormalities tend to indicate a poor prognosis, and therapeutic abstention may be chosen if the diffusion-weighted imaging changes are rapidly progressive.

CTA/MRA

- Early filling of the dilated median vein of the prosencephalon with enlargement of the arterial feeders can be seen on both CTA and MRA. These techniques are able to determine whether a mural or choroidal type of shunt is present.
- CTV and MRV may be helpful in the evaluation of the venous outflow restrictions, usually caused by dysmaturation or stenosis of the jugular bulb, and to evaluate whether cavernous capture has taken place (bulging of the cavernous sinuses).

Invasive Imaging Workup

- Angiography is the gold standard for the detailed evaluation of the angioarchitecture of a vein of Galen aneurysmal malformation and must be done within the same session as the endovascular treatment to avoid multiple punctures to the femoral arteries.
- In neonates, the restricted amount of contrast (maximum, 4 mL/kg) is a major limitation for a complete study.
- One VA and one ICA are evaluated to identify the major feeder and determine how the normal brain drains.

Treatment Options

CONSERVATIVE OR MEDICAL MANAGEMENT

- The therapeutic strategy is to ensure normal development; therefore, the cardiac overload and venous congestion must be reduced, and oral feeding has to be ensured.
- The initial management of a neonate with a vein of Galen aneurysmal malformation and congestive heart failure consists of medical stabilization of the heart failure, typically with digoxin (increase inotropy), diuretics (decrease preload), dopamine (increase cardiac output), mechanical ventilation (less

oxygen needed), or inhaled nitric oxide. These therapies are aimed at allowing the baby to feed orally so that he or she gains weight. If medical therapies fail, endovascular therapies are indicated.

- The best position for the baby is a 20- or 30-degree head-up position in the bed to optimize venous drainage without kinking of the jugular veins.

SURGICAL TREATMENT

- Surgical removal of the lesion is no longer advised because of the hemodynamic instability of these patients and the deep location of the lesion, which result in a high mortality rate.
- Ventricular shunting should be avoided because it does not treat the hydrovenous disorder responsible for the ventricular enlargement. In fact, ventricular shunting frequently worsens the size of a vein of Galen aneurysmal malformation and leads to subcortical calcifications.
- Surgery is reserved for the evacuation of intracranial hematomas in rare cases that bleed and the treatment of severe hydrocephalus that does not decrease after embolization.

ENDOVASCULAR TREATMENT

- Transarterial embolization is the treatment of choice for vein of Galen aneurysmal malformations, and the optimal timing of embolization is at 4 to 5 months of age; this waiting period is not long enough for permanent brain damage to develop yet offers enough benefit concerning arterial access and contrast limitation problems. More urgent treatment may be considered for patients with a Bicêtreneonatal score of 8 to 11, deteriorating or severe congestive heart failure, evidence of arterial steal, and/or progressive occlusion of the venous outflow without permanent brain damage on MRI or CT.
- A femoral arterial access is routinely used in our practice; however, in a newborn up to 3 days of age, an umbilical artery access may be used.
- In the authors' experience, pure glue (2 mL of Histoacryl/0.1 mL of Lipiodol with tantalum powder) is the preferred embolic material for high-flow, mural-type fistulae. The microcatheter is placed against the wall of the feeding artery, and the pure glue is rapidly injected to produce a "mushroom" appearance of the glue cast, which minimally penetrates the proximal venous pouch. A more diluted concentration of glue or other liquid embolic materials, such as Onyx, may be considered with the choroidal type of nidi but tend to be associated with prolonged injection times and radiation exposure, which is a strong concern in pediatric patients.
- Multiple arterial feeders are often encountered; the largest are usually embolized first to allow normal cardiac and neurologic development. Multiple sessions may be required to achieve the desired clinical effect. The goal of the treatment is a child who can develop normally rather than an impaired child who is cured. Progressive thrombosis of a vein of Galen aneurysmal malformation is not infrequent, even after partial treatment with some glue penetration into the venous pouch.
- A transvenous route may also be used but carries a higher risk for complications, including venous perforation and occlusion of the deep venous drainage with fatal brain hemorrhage. It has also proved to be much less efficient than transarterial glue embolization in reversing high-output cardiac failure.

Possible Complications

- Puncture site complications with thrombosis or dissection of the artery and, in the worst case scenario, loss of the lower limb
- Pulmonary emboli
- Migration of the embolic agent into the posterior aspect of the dilated venous pouch, causing occlusion of the deep venous drainage with subsequent venous infarctions/hemorrhage
- Perforation of the arterial feeders
- Reflux of the glue into normal arteries, resulting in ischemic stroke

Published Literature on Treatment Options

Before the advent of embolization, patients with vein of Galen aneurysmal malformations had a dismal prognosis. In the early surgical series, the mortality rate was 99 to 100%. Outcomes improved with advances in endovascular embolization techniques and neonatal care, which led to a 0 to 50% mortality rate (with a 28–68% overall poor outcome). Although the outcome of patients has been improving over the years, the overall outcome was still considered poor in up to 50% of patients in the larger series published by Lasjaunias et al. Approximately 10 to 20% of patients with vein of Galen aneurysmal malformations were considered to be in too poor condition to be treated or expired before treatment. In the largest series reported so far by Lasjaunias et al, in 2006, ~60% of the 233 patients who were treated with endovascular embolization had a good outcome. In their total cohort of 317 patients, spontaneous thrombosis of the shunt occurred in 2.5% (8/317). In a recent series of the Toronto experience by Geibprasert et al, 47% of the patients treated had a good outcome, and 5 of 6 patients in a subgroup of carefully selected patients had a good outcome with conservative management and close follow-up. The criteria for the selection of these patients were as follows: (1) a high neonatal score (> 17); (2) clinical symptoms of only mild congestive heart failure well controlled with medication and no neurologic symptoms; (3) imaging findings indicating no paren-chymal loss, calcifications, hydrocephalus, tonsillar herniation, or evidence of arterial steal; and (4) angioarchitectural findings of low-flow shunts (i.e., two or fewer enlarged arterial feeder groups, lack of deep venous drainage, lack of jugular bulb stenosis). The management of patients with a vein of Galen aneurysmal malformation remains challenging and should be based on an assessment of the individual patient and the operator's personal experience.

PEARLS AND PITFALLS

- Vein of Galen aneurysmal malformations are choroidal arteriovenous malformations that develop during the early embryonic stage and drain into the median vein of the prosencephalon, which is the precursor of the vein of Galen.
- Factors associated with a poor outcome are the following: neurologic symptoms at presentation, a Bicêtre neonatal score of less than 12 of 21, a very poor score of less than 2 of 5 in one (or more) categories, focal parenchymal changes, calcifications, tonsillar herniation, arterial steal, and multiple arterial feeders.
- The management decision is challenging and must be made on an individual basis. The optimal treatment time is at 4 to 5 months of age; however, urgent treatment should be considered for those who have deteriorating congestive heart failure or evidence of arterial steal or progressive occlusion of the venous outflow without evidence of permanent brain damage on CT or MRI.

Further Reading

Alvarez H, Garcia Monaco R, Rodesch G, Sachet M, Krings T, Lasjaunias P. Vein of Galen aneurysmal malformations. Neuroimaging Clin N Am 2007;17(2):189–206

Geibprasert S, Krings T, Armstrong D, Terbrugge KG, Raybaud CA. Predicting factors for the follow-up outcome and management decisions in vein of Galen aneurysmal malformations. Childs Nerv Syst 2010;26(1):35–46

Lasjaunias PL, Berenstein A, terBrugge KG. Surgical Neuroangiography. Vol 3: Clinical and Interventional Aspects in Children. 2nd ed. New York, NY: Springer; 2006

Lasjaunias PL, Chng SM, Sachet M, Alvarez H, Rodesch G, Garcia-Monaco R. The management of vein of Galen aneurysmal malformations. Neurosurgery 2006;59(5 Suppl 3):S184–S194, discussion S3–S13

CASE 57

Case Description

Clinical Presentation

A 7-year-old previously healthy boy has had significant headaches over the past 2 weeks. His parents confirm that he has never had any headaches before. Outside CT has demonstrated dilated vessels, and he is referred to our institution for further workup.

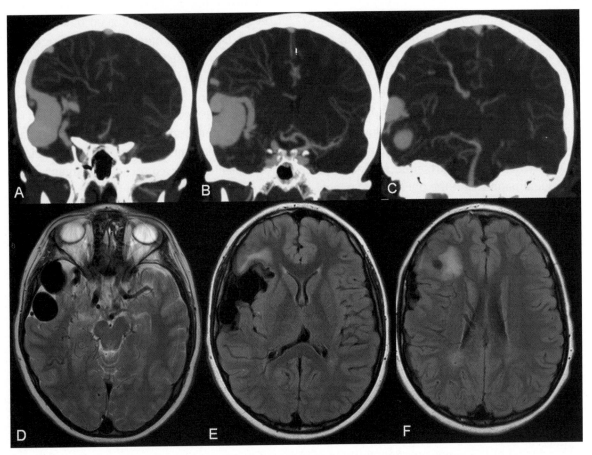

Fig. 57.1 (A–C) Coronal CTA demonstrates a fistula from an MCA branch into multiple, markedly dilated venous pouches with evidence of adjacent skull remodeling. Dilatation of the transmedullary veins was also noted, indicating significant venous congestion. **(D–F)** FLAIR MRI shows the perifocal hyperintense signal of edema surrounding a right frontal venous pouch.

Radiologic Studies

CTA AND MRI

CTA demonstrated massively dilated venous pouches with bony remodeling, the direct fistulous transition of a middle cerebral artery (MCA) branch into a venous pouch, and dilated transmedullary veins as an alternate pathway for the cortical venous drainage, indicating significant venous congestion.

338

Axial FLAIR MRI demonstrated perilesional edema surrounding a right frontal venous pouch. No hydrocephalus was present (**Fig. 57.1**).

DSA

Injection in the right internal carotid artery (ICA) demonstrated a cerebral pial fistula with a high flow rate and significant venous congestion. In addition, distal venous ectases were present, including the one associated with perilesional edema on MRI. There was a direct transition from the MCA into the venous pouch (**Fig. 57.2**).

Diagnosis

Cerebral pial arteriovenous (AV) fistula

Treatment

EQUIPMENT

- Standard 5F access (puncture needle, 5F vascular sheath)
- Standard 5F multipurpose catheter (Guider Soft Tip; Boston Scientific, Natick, MA) with continuous flush and a 0.035-in hydrophilic guidewire (Terumo, Somerset, NJ)
- A 90-degree curved 0.021-in microcatheter (Prowler Select Plus; Cordis, Warren, NJ) with a 0.014-in guidewire (Synchro; Boston Scientific)

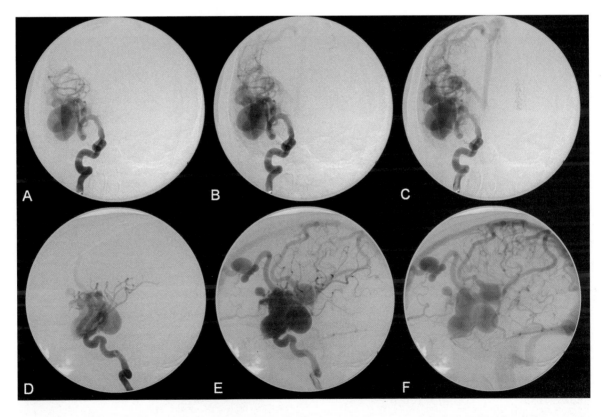

Fig. 57.2 DSA. Right ICA angiogram in **(A–C)** AP and **(D–F)** lateral views reveals a high-flow pial AV fistula from a right MCA branch draining into multiple ectatic venous pouches. There is poor visualization of the right frontal cortical veins, suggestive of significant venous congestion.

- A 10% glucose solution
- Histoacryl/Lipiodol/tantalum powder (2 mL/0.1 mL/1 vial)
- Contrast material
- Steroids

DESCRIPTION

The 5F multipurpose catheter was placed in the distal infrapetrous ICA and continuously flushed. The microcatheter was advanced via the guidewire into the MCA. Injections into the MCA at various points demonstrated the security margin and the single-hole fistulous nature of the malformation. The microcatheter was placed ~5 mm proximal to the fistula, with its tip pointing toward the wall of the artery. After the microcatheter had been flushed with glucose solution, a mixture of 2 mL of glue with a vial of tantalum powder was injected that allowed complete occlusion of the fistula in a mushroom-shaped glue cast **(Fig. 57.3 A,B)**. Follow-up angiography after 6 months verified the stability of the results and complete occlusion of the fistula, as well as normalization of the venous drainage **(Fig. 57.3 C–F)**. No neurologic deficits were noted.

Discussion

Background

Hereditary hemorrhagic telangiectasia (HHT) was first recognized in the 19th century as a familial disorder associated with abnormal vascular structures and bleeding from the nose and gastrointes-

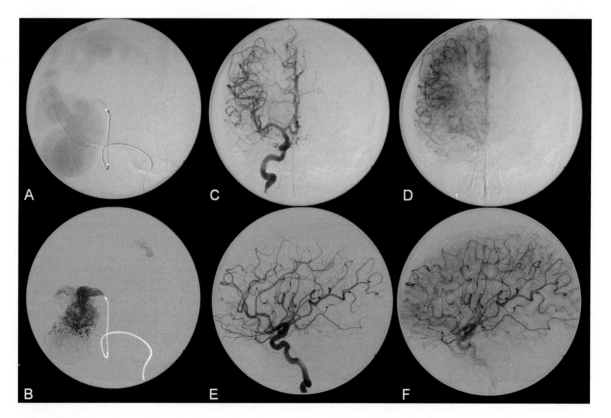

Fig. 57.3 (A) Superselective microcatheter injection and **(B)** the glue cast following embolization demonstrate the mushroom appearance of the glue within the fistula. Right ICA angiography 6 months following embolization in **(C,D)** AP and **(E,F)** lateral views reveals complete occlusion of the fistula with normalization of the venous drainage.

tinal tract. The combination of these clinical findings with iron deficiency anemia and characteristic telangiectasia of the lips, oral mucosa, and fingertips has become firmly established as a medical entity known as Rendu-Weber-Osler disease or HHT. In addition to the previously mentioned microscopic mucocutaneous telangiectases derived from post-capillary venules, abnormal vascular structures may develop at other sites in patients with HHT. AV malformations (AVMs) in the pulmonary, cerebral, and hepatic circulations account for some of the most devastating clinical complications of the disease. The incidence is ~5 in 10,000 persons; 30% of patients with HHT have pulmonary involvement, 30% hepatic involvement, and 10 to 20% cerebral involvement. HHT is inherited as an autosomal-dominant trait; mutations in at least two genes that influence angiogenesis lead to structural abnormalities of the blood vessels, which predispose the patient to the various kinds of AV shunts and telangiectases observed in HHT.

Noninvasive Imaging Workup

PHYSICAL EXAMINATION

- Recurrent spontaneous nosebleeds, mucocutaneous telangiectasia at characteristic sites (lips, oral cavity, fingers, nose), visceral involvement (pulmonary, hepatic, or central nervous system AVMs), and an affected first-degree relative are the diagnostic criteria for HHT. Nosebleeds and telangiectases tend not to occur before the age of 16 years.
- If neurologic symptoms occur, they are more often caused by paradoxical emboli or cerebral abscesses resulting from pulmonary AV fistulae than by primary neurovascular manifestations.

MRI, CT, AND DSA

- Four different neurovascular manifestations of HHT have been reported in the literature: spinal AV fistulae, cerebral pial AV fistulae (as in this case), nidus-type or glomerular brain AVMs, and nonshunting pial capillary vascular malformations.
- Spinal cord AV fistulae in HHT are characterized as perimedullary intradural AV malformations with a high shunting volume and a massively enlarged venous pouch that can be easily identified on MRI. Feeding vessels are dorsolateral or anterior spinal arteries, or both, and multiple feeders converge into the same collector before entering the venous pouch. Younger children are classically affected and become symptomatic because of hemorrhage, venous congestion, or mass effect of the pouches.
- Cerebral pial AV fistulae are macrofistulae of the single-hole type with a high shunting volume and enlarged venous pouches. Signs of venous congestion are often present. Distal venous ectases may be present, and if they are associated with perilesional edema, recent growth of the pouch and instability of the venous outflow must be considered. Associated angiographic abnormalities include venous ectases, venous stenoses, pial reflux, venous ischemia, calcifications, and associated arterial aneurysms. Multiple fistulae can be present in the same patient. Patients become symptomatic at a younger age because of intracerebral hemorrhage, macrocrania, bruit, cognitive deficits, cardiac insufficiency, epilepsy, tonsillar prolapse, or hydrocephalus.
- Cerebral glomerular or nidus-type AVMs can be present that are in our experience nearly always less than 3 cm in maximum diameter and typically located cortically. Their imaging features are indistinguishable from those of sporadic AVMs, and they tend to become symptomatic in older patients when they cause either epilepsy or hemorrhage.
- Pial capillary vascular malformations are lesions without evident early venous drainage; they merely demonstrate an increased capillary blush. They are always found incidentally, are visible only on angiography and MRI at 3T, and in our experience never become symptomatic.

Treatment Options

CONSERVATIVE OR MEDICAL MANAGEMENT

- Conservative management is advocated for pial capillary vascular malformations in HHT. On the other hand, in our opinion treatment should be considered for spinal and cerebral pial AV fistulae, in particular when diagnosed at early age, given their pronounced tendency to cause neurologic complications. Little is known about the natural history of "classic" brain AVMs in HHT, but case series have reported that the annual risk for hemorrhage is likely to be less than 1%, which is lower than the risk associated with classic, sporadic AVMs of the brain. The guidelines discussed in Section II of this book apply.

RADIOSURGERY

- High-flow lesions are thought to be less likely to become obliterated following radiosurgery. Definition of the target may be difficult because of the massively enlarged venous pouches, and the longer time required for obliteration following radiosurgery is not desirable. Finally, radiosurgery in children may put the developing brain at risk.

SURGICAL TREATMENT

- For high-flow lesions, surgical accessibility and success rates are considered inferior to those of endovascular approaches.

ENDOVASCULAR TREATMENT

- For cerebral pial AV fistulae, endovascular therapies are the method of choice.
- Because of the high flow through the shunt compared with that in "classic" AVMs, a liquid embolic agent that polymerizes very fast is required, which is why we use pure N-butyl cyanoacrylate (Histoacryl) mixed with tantalum powder in these cases.
- A high rate of injection is necessary to avoid prolonged venous penetration; therefore, larger-bore microcatheters must be used ($\geq$ 0.014 in) These catheters have the additional benefit of being stiffer and are therefore less likely to enter the venous site, spring backward during injections, or dislodge proximally because of jet effects.
- We employ catheters with a short, sharp bend to direct the flow primarily against the wall, where the laminar flow is slower than the flow in the central part of the feeding vessel. This technique allows a more controlled, "mushroom-like" embolization, similar to the embolization of a vein of Galen malformation (see Case 56).
- In our practice, steroids are given following Histoacryl embolization to compensate for the exothermic effect of the glue.

Possible Complications

- Standard angiographic complications (at the puncture site: bleeding, false aneurysms, fistula; in catheterized vessels: emboli, dissections; systemically: contrast reaction, renal failure)
- Migration of the embolic agent into the draining vein with potential occlusion, proximal occlusion with delayed reopening, and arterial ischemia due to reflux of the embolic agent into brain-supplying arteries
- Seizures following successful treatment due to significant alterations in cerebral hemodynamics
- Delayed venous thrombosis due to significant flow reduction

Published Literature on Treatment Options

Cerebral pial AV shunts in children should raise suspicion of the possibility of an HHT disorder; the diagnosis is nearly certain to be HHT if multiple AV shunts are demonstrated. Fifty percent of patients with HHT have multiple AV shunts. When detected, we tend to treat the children because bleeding is not the only serious risk associated with these vascular malformations. Others include the following: neurologic deficits due to venous congestion, venous ischemia, spontaneous partial thrombosis with acute neurologic deficits, subarachnoid hemorrhage, congestive cardiac failure, hydrocephalus, macrocrania, and brain atrophy. New neurologic symptoms (including new, atypical headaches), edema surrounding a lesion, or changes in the size of the venous pouches are in our experience signs of an unstable situation and warrant expedited treatment. Likewise, AV fistulae of the spinal cord tend have a poor prognosis and once detected should in our opinion be treated.

Given the risks associated with surgery or radiosurgery, an endovascular treatment is chosen in most centers, with the aim of obliterating the fistulous zone. This may be achieved by pushing glue via the artery into the venous pouch to establish a mushroom-shaped glue cast that occludes the single-hole fistula. Because a major problem of glue embolization is the uncontrollable propagation of glue into veins, with secondary venous occlusion and hemorrhage, we try to minimize this risk by using undiluted glue with tantalum powder at a position close to the shunting zone with the catheter tip pointed against the arterial vessel wall. Alternatively, or in conjunction with the glue injection, coils may be used to selectively occlude the fistulous site; however, the high flow may necessitate the use of double catheterization techniques (with the first coil not detached until a stable cage is established) or more thrombogenic (fibered) coils. In selected patients, flow may be reduced with coils before glue embolization.

PEARLS AND PITFALLS

- In children with pial AV fistulae, HHT should be suspected. Because children rarely exhibit classic telangiectases and do not yet present with epistaxis, first-degree relatives must be asked about these classic manifestations of HHT.
- If HHT is suspected, screening of the lungs is recommended to rule out pulmonary AV fistulae that may lead to paradoxical infarctions.
- Four different neurovascular manifestations of HHT have been described: spinal and cerebral AV fistulae, glomerular AVMs, and capillary vascular malformations without shunting. About 50% of patients with HHT who have neurovascular brain involvement will have more than one AV shunt.
- Following embolization, headaches and seizures may develop transiently. If new neurologic symptoms occur, follow-up imaging is necessary to rule out excessive venous thrombosis.

Further Reading

Faughnan ME, Palda VA, Garcia-Tsao G, et al. International guidelines for the diagnosis and management of hereditary hemorrhagic telangiectasia. J Med Genet 2009 Jun 29. [Epub ahead of print]

Krings T, Chng SM, Ozanne A, Alvarez H, Rodesch G, Lasjaunias PL. Hereditary hemorrhagic telangiectasia in children: endovascular treatment of neurovascular malformations: results in 31 patients. Neuroradiology 2005;47(12):946–954

Krings T, Ozanne A, Chng SM, Alvarez H, Rodesch G, Lasjaunias PL. Neurovascular phenotypes in hereditary haemorrhagic telangiectasia patients according to age. Review of 50 consecutive patients aged 1 day-60 years. Neuroradiology 2005;47(10):711–720

Matsubara S, Mandzia JL, ter Brugge K, Willinsky RA, Faughnan ME. Angiographic and clinical characteristics of patients with cerebral arteriovenous malformations associated with hereditary hemorrhagic telangiectasia [published correction appears in AJNR Am J Neuroradiol 2001;22(7):1446]. AJNR Am J Neuroradiol 2000;21(6):1016–1020

Shovlin CL, Guttmacher AE, Buscarini E, et al. Diagnostic criteria for hereditary hemorrhagic telangiectasia (Rendu-Osler-Weber syndrome). Am J Med Genet 2000;91(1):66–67

CASE 58

Case Description

Clinical Presentation

A 7-month-old previously healthy infant loses consciousness and is brought to the emergency department. The mother reports that approximately 2 weeks earlier, the child sustained a moderate head injury. Emergency CT is performed, followed by angiography.

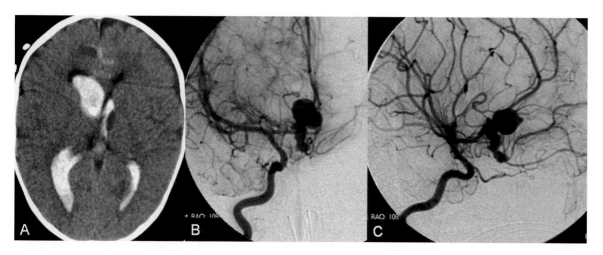

Fig. 58.1 **(A)** Unenhanced axial CT demonstrates a large amount of intraventricular hemorrhage and minimal subarachnoid hemorrhage with mild ventricular dilatation. DSA. Right ICA angiogram in **(B)** AP and **(C)** oblique views shows a multilobulated, irregularly shaped aneurysm at the right A1-anterior communicating artery junction.

Radiologic Studies

CT

CT demonstrated intraventricular and subarachnoid hemorrhage with mild ventricular dilatation (**Fig. 58.1A**).

DSA

Injection in the right internal carotid artery (ICA) demonstrated a multilobulated, irregularly shaped, large aneurysm arising from the junction of the right A1 with the anterior communicating artery (**Fig. 58.1 B,C**).

Diagnosis

False or dissecting post-traumatic pediatric aneurysm

Treatment

EQUIPMENT

- Standard 5F access (puncture needle, 5F vascular sheath)

344

- 5F multipurpose catheter (Guider Soft Tip; Boston Scientific, Natick, MA) with continuous flush and a 0.035-in hydrophilic guidewire (Terumo, Somerset, NJ)
- Straight microcatheter with a 1.7F tip and a 0.0165-in inner lumen (Excelsior SL 10; Boston Scientific) with a 0.014-in guidewire (Synchro 14; Boston Scientific)
- Coil selection: GDC 360-degree coil 3 mm × 6 cm; for subsequent filling, two GDC HyperSoft coils 2 mm × 4 cm (Boston Scientific)
- Contrast material
- Heparin

DESCRIPTION

A 5F multipurpose catheter was placed in the distal right ICA. Under roadmap conditions, the microcatheter was advanced over the wire into the anterior communicating artery, which was subsequently occluded with a dense coil mesh that extended over the aneurysm neck into the right A1 portion. Control from the right ICA immediately after coiling demonstrated leptomeningeal retrograde filling of the anterior cerebral artery (ACA) territory via the middle cerebral artery (MCA; **Fig. 58.2**). Follow-up control after 6 months demonstrated no aneurysm recurrence and sufficient filling of the entire ACA territory via leptomeningeal collaterals from the MCA. The child had no neurologic deficit (**Fig. 58.3**).

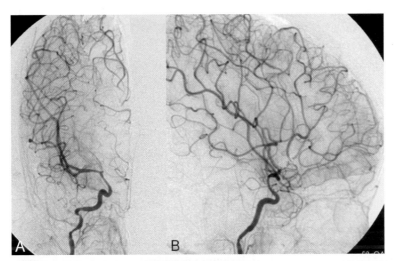

Fig. 58.2 Right ICA angiogram in **(A)** AP and **(B)** lateral views immediately after coiling reveals complete occlusion of the aneurysm with leptomeningeal filling of the right ACA territory from the MCA branches.

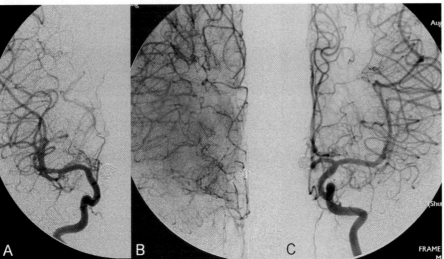

Fig. 58.3 (A,B) Right and **(C)** left ICA angiograms at 6 months after embolization show no evidence of aneurysm recurrence. **(B)** Note that the entire right ACA territory is filled by leptomeningeal collaterals from the MCA branches in the late arterial phase.

Discussion

Background

Children with intracranial aneurysms account for fewer than 5% of the total number of patients with aneurysms. There are no reports of incidentally discovered aneurysms during routine autopsy studies in children, which indicates that the vast majority (if not all) aneurysms in the pediatric age group are symptomatic. There is an overall male predominance. Nearly five times as many aneurysms involve the ICA termination (25% vs. 5%), and the incidence of aneurysms of the posterior circulation is nearly threefold higher in the pediatric age group than in adults (15% vs. 5%). Distal and "atypical" locations are more common in children than in adults. "Classic" saccular aneurysms are found in only 30% of cases and tend to occur in older children. The most commonly seen aneurysms in childhood are dissecting aneurysms (50%), infectious aneurysms (10–15%), and traumatic aneurysms (5–10%).

Noninvasive Imaging Workup

PHYSICAL EXAMINATION

- Although subarachnoid, intraparenchymal, or intraventricular hemorrhage is the most common presenting symptom, nonhemorrhagic aneurysms may also be present and are more common in children than in adults, with mass effect, headaches, neurologic deficits, and epilepsy as potential primary symptoms.
- Post-traumatic aneurysms classically occur 2 to 4 weeks following trauma (which can be minor).

CT/CTA AND MRI/MRA

- Noninvasive imaging should try to elucidate the underlying pathologic mechanism of a pediatric aneurysm, given the diverse array of possible causes previously discussed.
- MRI can better visualize whether mural pathology is present.

Invasive Imaging Workup

- Pediatric aneurysms may be multifocal; dissections can be bilateral, infectious aneurysms are often present in different arterial territories, and an underlying vessel wall disease may be present. Therefore, if there are no restrictions concerning the amount of contrast material that can be administered given the body weight of the patient (maximum of amount of contrast [mL] = 4 × body weight [kg]), the angiographic evaluation should cover all four brain-supplying arteries.

Treatment Options

The treatment options depend on the underlying pathologic mechanism and are described in the next section.

Published Literature on Treatment Options

Traumatic pediatric aneurysms involve the distal ACA adjacent to the falx in ~40% of cases, the major vessels along the skull base in 35%, and the distal cortical vessels in 25%. The classic clinical presentation following trauma is a hemorrhagic episode ~2 to 4 weeks after the original injury. The majority of children have sustained a closed head injury; penetrating or surgical injuries are less common. These injuries result in the formation of a false sac, or pseudoaneurysm, which is produced by disruption of the entire arterial wall. An extravascular hematoma communicates with the arterial lumen.

The fibrotic reaction in the surrounding tissues forms the "wall" of the false aneurysm; therefore, endovascular filling of the ruptured pouch should not be attempted. Occlusion of the parent vessel wall directly proximal to the aneurysm, with either coils or liquid embolic materials, is instead the treatment of choice. In neonates and very young infants, this therapeutic strategy is usually well tolerated because of the presence of sufficient leptomeningeal collaterals; in older children, however, the collaterals may not always be sufficient to prevent downstream ischemia in the case of a large parent vessel sacrifice. Therefore, in the older age group, surgical exploration with an attempt to reconstruct the vessel or a combined approach of parent vessel occlusion following bypass surgery may be contemplated. "Healed" false aneurysms (i.e., those that reach a chronic phase without having led to hemorrhage) classically do not rupture, and these dolichosegments may persist into adulthood.

Infectious pediatric aneurysms are discussed in detail in Case 14. "Classic" saccular or berry-type aneurysms are rarely seen in neonates, infants, and children younger than 8 years of age; their incidence increases with age. Despite their location at the bifurcation of various vessels, intrinsic hemodynamic factors almost certainly play less of a role than in adults, and other factors, such as an underlying vessel wall disease, may play a more important role. In our opinion, the treatment and natural history of these aneurysms do not differ from those of adult aneurysms, so that a multidisciplinary approach with both surgery and endovascular coil occlusion as the two standard treatments is necessary, as discussed in Cases 1 through 5.

Dissections are the most often encountered pathologic mechanism in pediatric aneurysms and are at least four times more common than in adults. Dissections can lead to hemorrhagic or ischemic symptoms, or both. If blood enters the subintimal space as the consequence of a subintimal vessel wall tear, several pathologically distinct fates are possible. (1) If the hematoma disrupts the entire vessel wall, a transmural dissection is present, and the clinical symptoms will depend on the surroundings of the vessel wall. (a) An intradural transmural dissection will lead to a subarachnoid hemorrhage. (b) If the transmural dissection occurs in a vessel segment that is surrounded by a venous plexus (i.e., the cavernous sinus or the vertebral venous plexus at the atlantal loop), an arteriovenous fistula will develop. (c) If the transmural dissection occurs in soft tissues, a false aneurysm (i.e., extramural hematoma) will occur that may lead to mass effect, stenosis, or occlusion of the parent vessel. (2) If the dissection remains subintimal, a subadventitial hematoma will develop in the vessel wall, and the clinical symptoms will again depend on the fate of the subadventitial hematoma. (a) If the true vessel lumen reopens, the hematoma (having clotted in the false lumen) can be washed out, leading to distal embolization. This is the pathologic mechanism most commonly seen in adults with extradural ICA dissections. (b) If the hematoma grows inside the vessel wall, the wall itself enlarges; this can result in progressive stenosis of the true lumen (leading to hemodynamic infarctions or embolic events due to critical narrowing and turbulent flow). In the intradural portion, a growing hematoma can occlude perforating branches coming off the dissected parent vessel, leading to local ischemia. (c) Finally, if chronic, the intramural hematoma can organize in the vessel wall, vasa vasorum may sprout in the organizing hematoma, and a growing intramural hematoma (due to repetitive dissections) can develop, leading to a "giant partially thrombosed aneurysm." Consequently, in dissecting aneurysms in the pediatric population, the symptoms can be related to mass effect, ischemia, or subarachnoid hemorrhage. In rare cases, a combination of different symptoms may be present. Treatment strategies depend on these pathologic mechanisms and are discussed in Cases 11 through 13.

PEARLS AND PITFALLS _____

- Pediatric aneurysms are rare and nearly always symptomatic.
- There is a male predominance, and the posterior circulation, ICA termination, and distal arteries are more often involved than in adults.

- The clinical findings are hemorrhage, mass effect, headaches, and neurologic deficits.
- Causes include dissections, trauma, and infections, and saccular aneurysms are much rarer than in adults.

Further Reading

Agid R, Souza MP, Reintamm G, Armstrong D, Dirks P, TerBrugge KG. The role of endovascular treatment for pediatric aneurysms. Childs Nerv Syst 2005;21(12):1030–1036

Herman JM, Rekate HL, Spetzler RF. Pediatric intracranial aneurysms: simple and complex cases. Pediatr Neurosurg 1991-1992;17(2):66–72, discussion 73

Krings T, Geibprasert S, Terbrugge K. Pathomechanisms and treatment of pediatric aneurysms. Childs Nerv Syst 2009 Dec 24. [Epub ahead of print]

Lasjaunias P, Wuppalapati S, Alvarez H, Rodesch G, Ozanne A. Intracranial aneurysms in children aged under 15 years: review of 59 consecutive children with 75 aneurysms. Childs Nerv Syst 2005;21(6):437–450

Ostergaard JR. Aetiology of intracranial saccular aneurysms in childhood. Br J Neurosurg 1991;5(6):575–580

Songsaeng D, Srivatanakul K, Krings T, Geibprasert S, Ozanne A, Lasjaunias PL. Symptomatic spontaneous dissecting arterial diseases of the vertebrobasilar system in children less than 16 years old: review of 29 consecutive patients. J Neurosurg Pediatrics 2010. In press

Ventureyra EC, Higgins MJ. Traumatic intracranial aneurysms in childhood and adolescence. Case reports and review of the literature. Childs Nerv Syst 1994;10(6):361–379

CASE 59

Case Description

Clinical Presentation

A 1-day-old baby boy has had cardiac failure since birth. Physical examination reveals mild respiratory distress with mild hepatomegaly. The neurologic examination is within normal limits. MRI is performed. His condition worsens despite medical treatment during the next week, and therefore further angiography and treatment are undertaken.

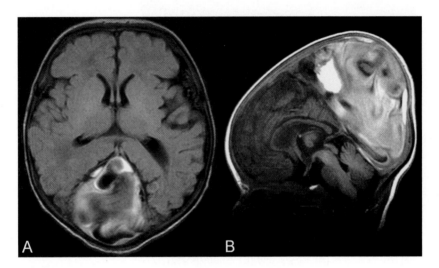

Fig. 59.1 **(A)** Axial FLAIR and **(B)** sagittal T1-weighted MR images.

Radiologic Studies

MRI

MRI showed a huge extra-axial dilated vascular structure at the level of the posterior superior sagittal sinus involving the torcular. There was internal heterogeneous hyperintense T1 and T2 signal, suggestive of thrombosis and turbulent flow. Mass effect on the parieto-occipital lobe was noted. The brain parenchymal signal appeared normal. There was no evidence of tonsillar herniation (**Fig. 59.1**).

DSA

Bilateral common carotid artery (CCA) angiograms revealed dural arteriovenous (AV) shunts, supplied by enlarged branches from both middle meningeal arteries (MMAs) and the left anterior falcine artery from the left ophthalmic artery, draining into the hugely dilated posterior superior sagittal sinus, and also involving the torcular. There was evidence of contrast stagnation within the dural lakes before further drainage through the transverse-sigmoid sinuses and jugular bulbs, which were patent, likely related to partial thrombosis and turbulent flow (**Fig. 59.2**). Although no cortical venous reflux was seen, there was delayed venous drainage of both cerebral hemispheres, worse on the left side.

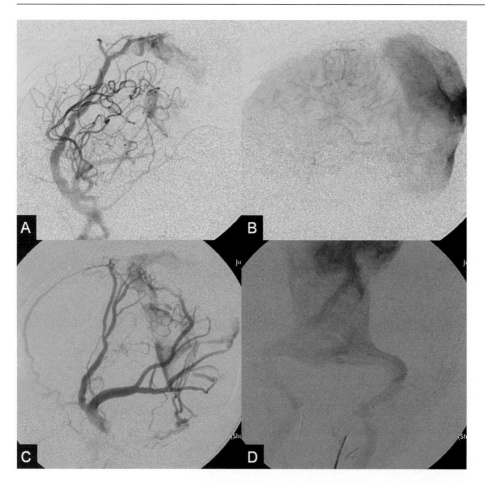

Fig. 59.2 DSA. Right CCA angiogram in lateral view in **(A)** arterial and **(B)** venous phases. Left CCA angiogram in **(C)** lateral view in arterial phase and **(D)** AP view in venous phase.

Diagnosis

Dural sinus malformation (DSM) with secondary dural arteriovenous fistulae (DAVFs)

Treatment

EQUIPMENT

- Standard 4F access (puncture needle, 4F vascular sheath)
- Standard 4F multipurpose catheter with continuous flush and a 0.035-in hydrophilic guidewire (Terumo, Somerset, NJ)
- A 0.012-in flow-directed microcatheter (Magic; Balt International, Montmorency, France) with a 0.008-in micro-guidewire (Mirage; ev3, Plymouth, MN)
- A 10% glucose solution
- Histoacryl/Lipiodol (1 mL/1 mL)
- Contrast material

DESCRIPTION

Following diagnostic angiography, a 4F multipurpose catheter was advanced into the right internal maxillary artery (IMA). A flow-directed microcatheter was introduced over a micro-guidewire into the dural branches originating from the right MMA, with the catheter tip positioned as close to the shunt zone as possible. Control runs were done via hand injection through the microcatheter to verify the position. The microcatheter was flushed with glucose solution, followed by the injection of glue at 50% concentration to close the shunt zone with only minimal venous penetration. The 4F multipurpose catheter was moved to the left IMA. The same procedure was repeated in two branches of the left MMA. Control angiograms of both CCAs still revealed minimal AV shunting from branches of the right meningohypophyseal trunk, left anterior falcine artery, and left stylomastoid branches; however, there was marked improvement in the venous drainage of the left cerebral hemisphere, with evidence of cavernous capture (**Fig. 59.3**). Follow-up MRI studies at 1, 3, and 5 years after embolization showed progressively decreased size and remodeling of the previously dilated posterior third of the superior sagittal sinus (**Fig. 59.4**).

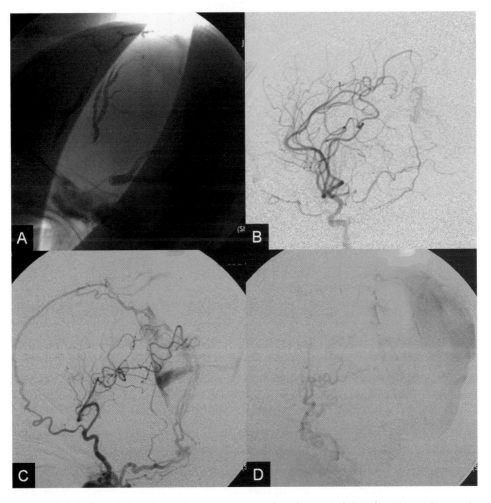

Fig. 59.3 (A) Plain skull radiography demonstrates the glue cast. **(B)** Right CCA angiogram in arterial view and left CCA angiogram in lateral view in **(C)** arterial and **(D)** venous phases after embolization.

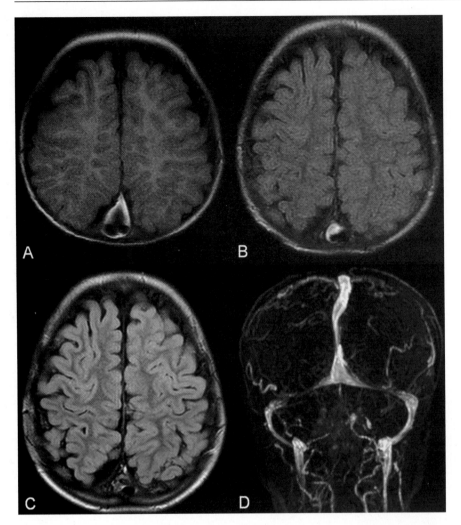

Fig. 59.4 Follow-up FLAIR MRI sequences at **(A)** 1 year, **(B)** 3 years, and **(C)** 5 years after embolization show progressive decrease in size of the partially thrombosed venous lakes. **(D)** MRV at 5 years after embolization shows remodeling with nearly normal size of the dural sinuses.

Discussion

Background

Pediatric DAVFs are a rare entity, accounting for ~10% of all intracranial AV shunts in children. Adult DAVFs are considered to be acquired lesions, but the etiology of pediatric DAVFs is still unclear. There are three major subgroups: DSMs, infantile DAVFs, and adult-type DAVFs. DSMs are characterized by giant, partially thrombosed epidural venous lakes with moderate cardiac failure. Infantile DAVFs are multifocal, frequently are associated with high flow, and typically present in early childhood, whereas adult-type DAVFs are usually located at the cavernous sinus or sigmoid sinus regions and are similar to adult DAVFs. DSMs are believed to correspond to the abnormal perinatal persistence of sinus ballooning with the associated uncontrolled development of venous channels and the formation of segmental giant dural lakes. This is followed by thrombosis due to turbulent and slow flow and the secondary development of AV shunts within the wall of the malformed sinus. Neonates commonly present with cardiac failure related to the secondary shunts, whereas macrocrania and symptoms of increased intracranial pressure are usually seen in infants. Restriction of venous outflow is the underlying pathologic mechanism of the macrocrania and the raised intracranial pressure and can be due to extensive thrombosis, endothelial proliferation, and/or jugular bulb dysmaturation. The development of collateral drainage pathways through the cavernous sinuses (cavernous capture) will prevent progression to acute hydrocephalus, venous infarctions, or even intraparenchymal hemorrhage. Cases without torcular involvement (transverse sinus locations) tend to have a better prognosis than those with torcular involvement because the chances of alternative drainage pathways of the brain are increased. Associated vascular anomalies, such as scalp hemangiomatous lesions, maxillofacial venolymphatic malformations, developmental venous anomalies, and midline vascular anomalies, have been reported.

Noninvasive Imaging Workup

CT/MRI

- MRI is the best imaging modality for the evaluation of these lesions. Both CT and MRI will demonstrate the markedly dilated dural sinus. Turbulent, slow flow and thrombosis can be seen as heterogeneous signal on both T1- and T2-weighted sequences.
- T2-weighted and FLAIR sequences are necessary for evaluation of the brain parenchyma.
- Brain calcifications, encephalomalacic change (melting brain), venous infarctions, and hemorrhage are associated with a poor neurologic outcome.
- Associated developmental venous anomalies in the posterior fossa, seen as tubular structures with a caput medusae appearance, are best visualized on post-contrast CT and post-gadolinium T1-weighted MRI. The connection between the developmental venous anomaly and the transverse sinus or involved DSM must be evaluated and preserved during treatment.
- Early filling of the involved malformed sinus with enlargement of the dural arterial feeders can be seen on both CTA and MRA.

Invasive Imaging Workup

- Angiography is required for evaluation of the brain parenchymal drainage, and selective injection of the internal carotid arteries should be done whenever the contrast load permits.
- Angiography is usually performed in the same session as the endovascular treatment to avoid multiple punctures to the femoral arteries.

Treatment Options

SURGICAL TREATMENT

- Hydrocephalus is typically related to hydrovenous disorders caused by restriction of the venous outflow and superimposed secondary AV shunts; it can therefore usually be managed by endovascular occlusion of the AV shunts. Ventriculoperitoneal shunts or extraventricular drainage is rarely required and is reserved for patients with severe hydrocephalus that does not decrease after embolization.
- Surgical sinus disconnection and resection have been reported; however, because these major sinuses play a role in drainage of the normal brain, the surgical procedure can result in extensive venous infarctions and eventual death and should therefore be reserved for severe cases in which other treatment modalities have failed. In these cases, preoperative embolization may help to reduce surgical blood loss.

ENDOVASCULAR TREATMENT

- Transarterial embolization is the treatment of choice for the secondary AV shunts; the aim is to close the shunt within the wall of the malformed sinus without occluding the sinus itself.
- Therefore, the complete obliteration of all shunts during the same embolization session is not only unnecessary but also dangerous because it may lead to (fatal) complete thrombosis of the superior sagittal sinus.
- In our experience, glue is the preferred embolic material.
- Cases with evidence of brain damage and/or those with DSMs involving the torcular often have a poorer prognosis.
- Anticoagulants, such as heparin or low-molecular weight heparin, may be indicated if extensive thrombosis of the venous outflow pathways occurs.
- In some cases with compartmentalization of the DSM, coils or liquid embolic agents may be used for selective transvenous occlusion of the compartment with cortical venous reflux.

Possible Complications

- Extensive occlusion of the venous outflow pathways with subsequent venous infarctions and/or hemorrhage

Published Literature on Treatment Options

The true incidence of DSMs is still unknown. Treatment is not always necessary because cases have been reported in which a prenatally diagnosed DSM completely regressed spontaneously during follow-up, either before or after birth. This, of course, raises questions about the expected evolution and management and about counseling when a DSM is diagnosed prenatally. After birth, re-treatment is necessary only in symptomatic patients in whom the induced dural AV shunt leads to cardiac insufficiency or dural sinus hyperpressure leads to a delay in brain maturation. Aggressive therapy may be dangerous because it may lead to excessive thrombosis of the venous outlets required to drain the brain. The treatment of DSMs is therefore a balancing act and requires close clinical observation. Still, the mortality rate of DSMs persisting in childhood is high and reported to be between 38% and 67%. In the largest series (involving 30 patients with DSMs), all treated with embolization, Barbosa et al described an overall favorable clinical evolution in 58% of the cases. Interestingly, to achieve this good result, complete closure of the DSM was necessary in only 60%. DSMs that do not involve the torcular or that have cavernous capture tend to have a better neurologic outcome, given the potential for drainage of the brain via alternate pathways. This is similar to the situation in patients with vein of Galen malformations, in whom the clinical outcome is positively influenced by a combination of early capture of the cortical venous system of the brain (alternate venous outlet for the brain) and normal maturation of the jugular bulbs (dysmaturation leads to stenosis and venous outlet obstruction).

PEARLS AND PITFALLS

- The management of DSMs is geared toward preserving flow in the dural sinuses while diminishing the amount of shunting responsible for cardiac symptoms.
- Midline DSMs tend to have a worse outcome than DSMs with a transverse sinus location.
- Cavernous sinus capture and jugular bulb maturation will influence the clinical outcome.
- Multifocal, high-flow dural AV shunts are often associated with jugular bulb dysmaturation and a poor outcome.

Further Reading

Barbosa M, Mahadevan J, Weon YC, et al. Dural sinus malformations (DSM) with giant lakes, in neonates and infants: review of 30 consecutive cases. Interv Neuroradiol 2003;9:407–417

Kincaid PK, Duckwiler GR, Gobin YP, Viñuela F. Dural arteriovenous fistula in children: endovascular treatment and outcomes in seven cases. AJNR Am J Neuroradiol 2001;22(6):1217–1225

Lasjaunias P, Berenstein A, terBrugge KG. Surgical Neuroangiography. Vol 3: Clinical and Interventional Aspects in Children. 2nd ed. New York, NY: Springer; 2006

CASE 60

Case Description

Clinical Presentation

A 63-year-old man presents with a 6-month history of progressive gait disturbance, weakness and diffuse paresthesias in his legs, and low back pain. MRI is performed.

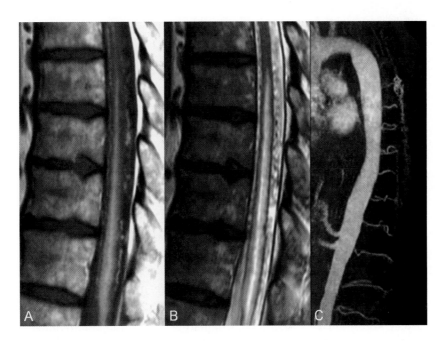

Fig. 60.1 (A) Sagittal T1-weighted contrast-enhanced and **(B)** T2-weighted MRI demonstrates dilated perimedullary vessels along the posterior surface of the cord. Evidence of cord edema with contrast enhancement is noted, suggestive of venous congestion. **(C)** Contrast-enhanced MRA during the arterial phase shows early filling of venous structures corresponding to an AV shunt.

Radiologic Studies

MRI

MRI demonstrated pathologically dilated perimedullary vessels along the posterior and, to a lesser degree, anterior surfaces of the cord on T2-weighted scans. In addition, evidence of cord edema was noted on T2-weighted scans. Following contrast enhancement, the pathologic vessels were detected again, and there was evidence of contrast enhancement within the cord. Contrast-enhanced MRA demonstrated filling of venous structures in the early arterial phase, indicating an arteriovenous (AV) shunt. No pathologic vessels were seen within the cord parenchyma (**Fig. 60.1**).

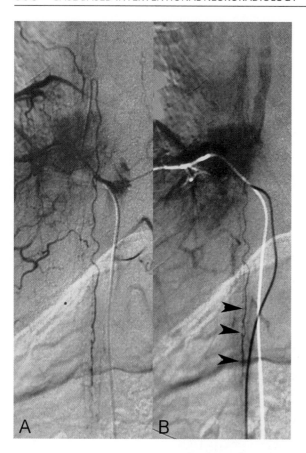

Fig. 60.2 DSA. Injection into the segmental artery from which the ASA originates in AP view in **(A)** arterial and **(B)** venous phases demonstrates stagnation of contrast within the ASA (arrowheads).

DSA

After injection into the segmental artery from which the anterior spinal artery (ASA) originated, stagnation of contrast in the ASA was observed until late in the venous phase, indicating interference with the circulation that was likely caused by venous hyperpressure (**Fig. 60.2**). Following injection into the right T10 segmental artery, the shunt was identified, originating from a radiculomeningeal artery and filling in retrograde fashion a radicular vein that ascended toward the perimedullary veins (**Fig. 60.3**).

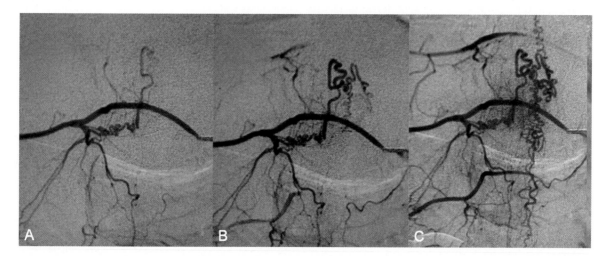

Fig. 60.3 DSA. Right T10 segmental artery angiogram in AP view reveals a DAV shunt from a radiculomeningeal artery to perimedullary veins in the **(A,B)** early and **(C)** late arterial phases.

Diagnosis

Spinal dural arteriovenous fistula (DAVF) with venous congestion

Treatment

EQUIPMENT

- Standard 5F access (puncture needle, 5F vascular sheath)
- 5F Cobra catheter with continuous flush and a 0.035-in hydrophilic guidewire
- A 0.012-in flow-directed microcatheter (Magic; Balt International, Montmorency, France) with a 0.008-in guidewire (Mirage; ev3, Plymouth, MN)
- A 10% glucose solution
- Histoacryl/Lipiodol (0.5 mL/1.5 mL)
- Contrast material

DESCRIPTION

A 5F Cobra catheter was placed distally into the segmental artery with the aid of a guidewire, which was placed far distally to ensure stability when the guiding catheter was pushed. Once stable access was achieved, a roadmap was performed, and a flow-directed microcatheter with a steam-shaped 45-degree curve was introduced into the segmental artery and advanced as far distally toward the shunting zone as possible with the aid of a micro-guidewire. Here, microcatheter injections demonstrated a shunting zone underneath the pedicle of the T10 vertebral body. After the microcatheter had been flushed with glucose solution, a mixture of 0.5 mL of glue with 1.5 mL of Lipiodol was slowly injected that penetrated through the fistulous zone into the vein, thereby occluding the distal arterial segment, the proximal vein, and the intervening shunting zone (**Fig. 60.4**).

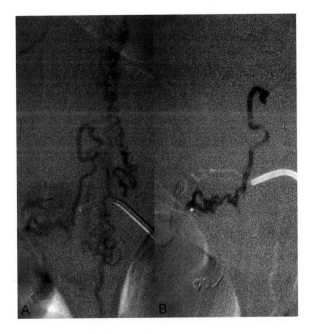

Fig. 60.4 (A) Superselective microcatheter injection and **(B)** glue cast following embolization show penetration of the glue through the fistulous zone into the proximal vein.

Discussion

Background

Spinal DAVFs are the most frequent vascular malformation of the spine, accounting for ~70% of all vascular malformations of the spine. Spinal DAVFs tend to affect elderly men. Most fistulae are solitary lesions and found in the thoracolumbar region. Spinal DAVFs are acquired, although the exact etiology is not known. The AV shunt is usually located at the level of the dura close to the spinal nerve root, where blood from the radiculomeningeal artery (i.e., the artery that supplies the nerve root and meninges but not necessarily the spinal cord!) enters a radicular vein; the latter passes the dura at the dorsal surface of the dural root sleeve in the intervertebral foramen. The transition is classically located directly underneath the pedicle of the vertebral body supplied by the injected segmental artery. This location is the most frequent, but shunts may occur in other locations along the dura between the nerve roots. Supply to shunts in these locations is from the adjacent segmental levels, so that dual supply is common. The increase in spinal venous pressure due to arterialization diminishes the AV pressure gradient and leads to decreased drainage of the normal spinal cord veins with venous congestion, which results in intramedullary edema. This in turn causes chronic hypoxia and progressive myelopathy.

Noninvasive Imaging Workup

PHYSICAL EXAMINATION

- Initial symptoms of venous congestion of the cord are nonspecific and include difficulty climbing stairs and gait disturbances. More often, sensory symptoms such as paresthesias, diffuse or patchy areas of sensory loss, and radicular pain may affect both lower limbs or, initially, one limb. Lower back pain without a radicular distribution is also frequently encountered. These neurologic symptoms are progressive and often ascending. Bowel and bladder incontinence, erectile dysfunction, and urinary retention are more often seen late in the course of the disease. These symptoms are invariably progressive.

CT/CTA

- The initial diagnosis of a dural AV shunt cannot be made on unenhanced CT. Spinal CTA may demonstrate enlarged vessels but is rarely used for screening. Because DAVFs can be present from the level of the foramen magnum to the sacral region, the radiation burden for CTA is unnecessarily high, given the better MRA options for visualizing the origin of a shunt.

MRI/MRA

- In our experience, the diagnosis is often strongly suspected by MRI and confirmed by contrast-enhanced MRI. On T2-weighted sequences, cord edema is depicted over multiple segments; this is often accompanied by a hypointense rim, most likely representing deoxygenated blood within the dilated capillary vessels surrounding the region of congestive edema. Further in the course of the disease, the cord will become atrophic.
- The perimedullary vessels are dilated and can be observed on T2-weighted images as flow voids, which are often more pronounced on the dorsal surface than on the ventral surface. However, if the shunt volume is small, they may be seen only after contrast enhancement. The serpiginous vascular structures may be better appreciated on heavily T2-weighted sequences (CISS [constructive interference in steady state], FIESTA [fast imaging employing steady-state acquisition], or 3D TSE [turbo spin echo]) than on standard T2 TSE sequences. In addition, these sequences may be useful to differentiate pulsation artifacts, which are sometimes mistaken for flow voids, from true vascular structures.

- Neither the location of the pathologic vessels nor the intramedullary imaging findings seem to be related to the actual level of the fistula.
- On T1-weighted scans, the swollen cord is slightly hypointense and enlarged. Following the administration of contrast, diffuse enhancement may be seen within the cord as a sign of chronic venous congestion with breakdown of the blood–spinal cord barrier.
- Spinal DAVFs may occur anywhere from the level of the foramen magnum to the sacrum, and the localization of these lesions can be difficult and challenging, especially in cases in which the cord edema is distant from the AV shunt. Thus, a noninvasive evaluation of the shunt location is extremely helpful to guide invasive catheter angiography.
- Contrast-enhanced MRA of the spine has greatly contributed to the localization of these lesions and helps avoid unnecessary superselective injections of all possible arterial feeders. The technique of first-pass gadolinium-enhanced MRA can clearly demonstrate early venous filling, thereby confirming the presence of a shunt. In most cases, it can also demonstrate the level of the shunt.

Invasive Imaging Workup

- On selective angiography, stasis of contrast material in the radiculomedullary arteries, especially the ASA, can be seen. Delayed venous return following an ASA injection indicates venous congestion and the need to search for a shunting lesion, whereas normal venous return following injection of the ASA will in most cases exclude the possibility of a spinal DAVF.
- After injection into the segmental artery harboring an AVF, early venous filling and the retrograde uptake of contrast in the radiculomedullary veins are visualized. Often, an extensive network of dilated perimedullary veins is visible. This network may even recruit supply from dural arteries that ascend or descend from neighboring radiculomeningeal arteries.
- The shunting zone is frequently located underneath the pedicle of the injected segmental artery where the radiculomeningeal artery pierces the dura.
- In rare cases, the flow from the radiculomeningeal artery into the radicular vein may be slow; therefore, we classically perform spinal angiography to search for DAVFs with a slow frame rate (one image per second) and wait for at least 4 seconds to exclude delayed retrograde filling of the radicular veins.

Differential Diagnosis

- The clinical differential diagnosis of entities with the rather unspecific neurologic symptoms is manifold and includes polyneuropathy, tumor, and degenerative disk disease. Urinary retention may be misinterpreted as related to prostrate hypertrophy.
- The dual MRI findings of cord edema and dilated perimedullary vessels without any intramedullary nidus of vessels are typical of spinal DAVF. However, the findings in reality are nonspecific and can also be seen with epidural and paraspinal AV shunts, which are characterized by retrograde drainage toward the perimedullary venous system of the cord as well as vascular lesions of the spinal cord, such as multiple hemangioblastomas.
- A spinal DAVF that drains solely into the anterior spinal veins may only demonstrate cord hypersignal on T2-weighted images because the anterior spinal veins have a subpial location and may therefore not be visualized as dilated. In these cases, a glioma (especially when contrast uptake is present), an inflammatory lesion, or spinal ischemia must be included in the differential diagnosis.
- On DSA, radicular arteriovenous malformations (rAVMs), epidural AV shunts, and perimedullary AVFs must be differentiated; rAVMs or AVMs of the nerves usually have abnormal vessels that

form a nidus surrounding the nerve root, whereas spinal DAVFs have an apparent shunt zone with radicular feeders converging into the same draining vein. These patients often present with radicular pain, not direct symptoms of congestive venous myelopathy. Epidural AV shunts are located in the epidural space and normally recruit supply from the vertebral body and surrounding structures, with drainage directly into the epidural plexus and not necessarily a perimedullary vein. Symptoms are related to compression of the adjacent nerve root or cord rather than venous congestion, unless unusual cases of perimedullary reflux occur. Perimedullary AVFs, including fistulae of the filum terminale, are flow shunts at the surface of the cord (or the filum) that are invariably supplied by arteries that in normal circumstances would supply the cord (i.e., the radiculomedullary arteries forming the ASA or the radiculopial arteries via the posterior spinal artery).

Treatment Options

SURGICAL TREATMENT

- Surgery is aimed at identifying and obliterating the fistulous point, which most of the time is underneath the pedicle of the injected segmental artery from which the supply to the fistula was visualized.
- Infrequently, the dural shunt is located between segmental levels, and the leptomeningeal vein enters the dura by itself between levels.
- A hypervascularized network can be present within the dura that opens into the (intradural) radicular vein. Disconnection of the vein with or without coagulation of the arterialized network within the dura can be performed to treat the condition surgically.

ENDOVASCULAR TREATMENT

- In our practice, embolization with liquid material (diluted glue) is the therapy of choice.
- The embolic material must reach the proximal part of the vein.
- If the supply to the spinal cord is seen to arise from the same segmental level, endovascular therapies will be associated with a higher risk for neurologic deterioration if the spinal cord supply is inadvertently occluded, and surgical treatment strategies will be preferable.
- Postprocedural heparin to prevent excessive venous thrombosis may be recommended if significant passage of the liquid embolic agent occurs.

Possible Complications

- Failure to penetrate the proximal vein will likely result in delayed reopening of the fistula (see Case 61).
- To avoid reflux into an artery supplying the spinal cord, a careful evaluation is necessary to determine the presence of vessels supplying the spinal cord from the segmental artery to be injected, from the same level on the opposite side, and from the segmental arteries above and below the injected pedicle.
- Far distal migration of the embolic agent into the draining vein can cause symptoms to worsen and must be avoided.

Published Literature on Treatment Options

There are two options in the treatment of spinal DAVFs: surgical disconnection of the leptomenigeal vein that receives the blood from the shunt zone (a relatively simple and safe intervention) and endovascular therapy with a liquid embolic agent after superselective catheterization of the feeding radiculomeningeal artery. The embolic agent must reach the nidus and occlude the proximal segment of the draining vein to prevent recurrence of the fistula. The success rates of endovascular therapy have been reported to vary between 25 and 75%, whereas a recent meta-analysis suggested that the rate of complete occlusion of a fistula following surgery is 98%. Because DSA is necessary to confirm the diagnosis, the treatment strategy that is adopted by most centers nowadays includes a tentative embolization if this is felt to be a safe (i.e., no artery supplying the spinal cord arises from the same pedicle as the shunt feeder). If the liquid embolic agent penetrates the vein, long-term clinical follow-up has shown that this results in complete obliteration of the fistula and a good clinical outcome. If the glue remains in an intra-arterial location, the liquid embolic agent may at least be used to identify the feeding artery and so facilitate the intraoperative fluoroscopic localization of the exact level of the fistula.

PEARLS AND PITFALLS

- Spinal DAVFs are a rare but treatable cause of otherwise progressive paraplegia. The neuroradiologist plays a major role in the detection of these lesions, as well as their treatment.
- The neurologic symptoms are nonspecific, but the MRI triad of cord edema, prominent perimedullary vessels, and contrast enhancement of the cord in elderly men should lead to the diagnosis of a DAV shunt. The exact level of the shunt can be predicted by contrast-enhanced MRI, then confirmed by selective DSA.
- Treatment must be aimed at occluding the proximal portion of the leptomeningeal vein in which reflux is occurring.

Further Reading

Farb RI, Kim JK, Willinsky RA, et al. Spinal dural arteriovenous fistula localization with a technique of first-pass gadolinium-enhanced MR angiography: initial experience. Radiology 2002;222(3):843–850

Krings T, Geibprasert S. Spinal dural arteriovenous fistulas. AJNR Am J Neuroradiol 2009;30(4):639–648

Van Dijk JM, TerBrugge KG, Willinsky RA, Farb RI, Wallace MC. Multidisciplinary management of spinal dural arteriovenous fistulas: clinical presentation and long-term follow-up in 49 patients. Stroke 2002;33(6):1578–1583

CASE 61

Case Description

Clinical Presentation

A 41-year-old man presents with a 3-month history of paresthesias and weakness when climbing stairs, and he has been experiencing erectile dysfunction during the past few weeks. MRI demonstrates the classic findings of a spinal dural arteriovenous shunt with dilated perimedullary vessels on T2-weighted images, and MRA shows cord edema and evidence of early vein filling. Angiography with possible embolization is performed.

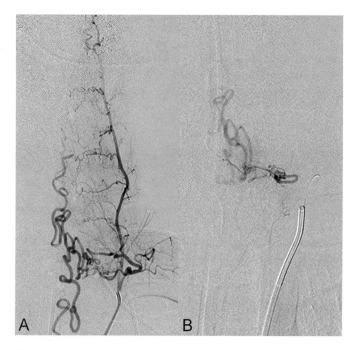

Fig. 61.1 DSA. **(A)** Left T2 segmental artery angiogram in AP view and **(B)** superselective microcatheter injection demonstrate a shunt from a radiculomeningeal artery draining into perimedullary veins.

Radiologic Studies

DSA

Injection of the left deep cervical artery demonstrated the T2 segmental artery to be opacifying a shunting zone underneath the pedicle of the left T2 vertebral body. The shunt was fed by the radiculomeningeal artery and drained both cranially and caudally via the radicular vein into the perimedullary veins (**Fig. 61.1**).

Diagnosis

Spinal dural arteriovenous fistula (DAVF) at T2 with venous congestion

Treatment

EQUIPMENT

- Standard 5F access (puncture needle, 5F vascular sheath)
- 5F Cobra catheter with continuous flush and a 0.035-in hydrophilic guidewire
- A 0.012-in flow-directed microcatheter (Magic; Balt International, Montmorency, France) with a 0.008-in guidewire (Mirage; ev3, Plymouth, MN)
- A 10% glucose solution
- Histoacryl/Lipiodol (0.5 mL/1.5 mL)
- Contrast material

DESCRIPTION

The 5F Cobra catheter was placed distally into the segmental artery, and a flow-directed microcatheter with a steam-shaped 45-degree curve was introduced into the segmental artery and advanced as far distally toward the shunting zone as possible with the aid of a micro-guidewire. Here, microcatheter injections demonstrated the shunt to be in close proximity to the tip of the microcatheter. After the microcatheter had been flushed with glucose solution, a mixture of 0.5 mL of glue with 1.5 mL of Lipiodol was injected that precipitated before entering the proximal vein and remained at the level of the dura. Follow-up angiography demonstrated no filling in the veins; however, given the incomplete venous penetration, which was verified by axial CT scans through the embolized region, the patient was forewarned that his symptoms would likely recur and that surgical intervention would then be necessary (**Fig. 61.2**). After an initial decrease in his symptoms, the patient again noticed increasing weakness 4 weeks after the embolization procedure. Follow-up angiography demonstrated the predicted reconstitution of the fistula (**Fig. 61.3**). Subsequent uneventful surgery resulted in complete obliteration of the fistula.

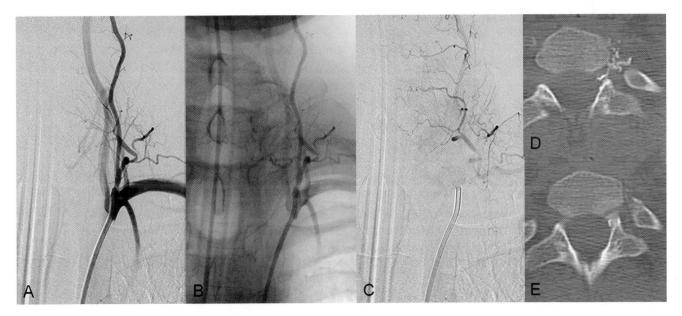

Fig. 61.2 (A) Left deep cervical artery angiogram in AP view after embolization in arterial phase, **(B)** unsubtracted image, and **(C)** angiogram in capillary phase following embolization reveal no filling of the veins; however, there is incomplete penetration of the glue cast into the proximal vein, which is also demonstrated on **(D,E)** unenhanced axial CTs in bone window.

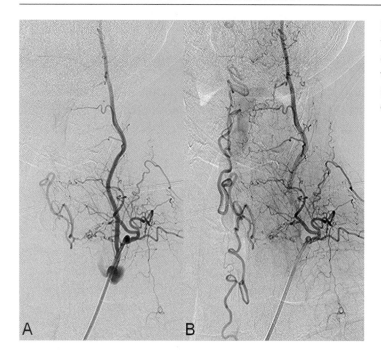

Fig. 61.3 (A,B) Follow-up angiography in the left deep cervical artery after 4 weeks demonstrates reconstitution of the shunt via a different dural branch (early and late phases in AP view). Surgery resulted in obliteration of the shunt.

Discussion

Background

Incomplete occlusion of a shunt because of the failure of venous penetration occurs in 25 to 75% of cases and is typically due to early polymerization of the embolic agent before it reaches the venous site. It is the task of the neurointerventionalist to recognize this rather common technical failure and to arrange for the patient to undergo surgery when clinical symptoms recur. The patient generally experiences a short decrease in symptoms; however, because of good collateralization within the dura, the fistula invariably reopens at some time in the subsequent weeks or months.

Noninvasive Imaging Workup

PHYSICAL EXAMINATION

- Symptoms may decrease initially because the immediate pressure in the venous system is reduced. This is classically followed after weeks or months by a slow deterioration of the clinical status.

CT/CTA

- If it is questionable whether the liquid embolic material has penetrated the proximal (intradural) vein, unenhanced CT may help to detect the glue cast and its extension toward the vein.
- Because the location of the shunt is known, CTA may prove helpful to evaluate filling of the shunting zone in the arterial phase and reconstitution of the fistula.

MRI/MRA

- Following incomplete embolization of a shunt, MRI may initially demonstrate a reduction in flow voids and even cord edema; however, with reconstitution of the shunt via collaterals (this will invariably happen), findings similar to those on the pre-embolization MR images will be seen, with reappearance of the flow voids and cord edema.
- Contrast-enhanced MRA will visualize reconstitution of the fistula; however, the spatial resolution may not be sufficient to answer the question of whether the same or adjacent feeders are involved in reconstitution of the fistula.

Invasive Imaging Workup

- Immediately after unsuccessful embolization, injection into the segmental artery that harbored the shunt will not demonstrate any residual filling; however, because of the dense collateralization in the dura, a delayed reopening of the shunt will occur.
- Therefore, following incomplete (i.e., proximal) embolization of a spinal dural AV shunt, follow-up angiography must include not only the segmental artery that previously harbored the shunt but also adjacent and contralateral segmental arteries because they may reconstitute the shunting zone via intersegmental dural or paravertebral anastomoses.

Differential Diagnosis

- Clinical deterioration following embolization of a spinal DAVF is in most cases related to insufficient venous penetration and reopening of the fistula. However, in patients with long-standing symptoms, these may worsen progressively despite complete occlusion of the fistula because of progressive cord atrophy. However, the metachronous appearance of a secondary DAVF must also be considered.
- MRA may help to identify a shunt (either residual or de novo).

Treatment Options

SURGICAL TREATMENT

- Surgery is the method of choice once endovascular treatment options have proved unsuccessful.
- The (proximal) glue cast can help the neurosurgeon identify the correct level before opening the dura and occluding the radicular vein.

ENDOVASCULAR TREATMENT

- Following proximal embolization and reconstitution of the fistula via dural collaterals, a more diffuse dural network is classically present. In addition, supply from adjacent segmental arteries is often seen. In these cases, endovascular treatment options are limited, and surgery should be performed.

Possible Complications

- The likelihood of failure to penetrate the proximal vein is significantly increased in reconstituted DAVFs (i.e., shunts that were unsuccessfully treated in the first session).
- To avoid further neurologic deterioration, surgery should be performed without delay.

Published Literature on Treatment Options

The aim of treatment in spinal DAVFs is to occlude the shunting zone (i.e., the most distal part of the artery together with the most proximal part of the draining vein). A proximal arterial occlusion will lead to a transient decrease in symptoms. Because of the good collateralization of the dura, however, the fistula tends to recur within the following months. Therefore, proximal occlusions with coils or Gelfoam are contraindicated. Embolization with particles is also likely to lead to early recanalization and is therefore not indicated. Liquid agents are the embolic materials of choice, and both Onyx and glue can be used. The only caveat is that because of the rich anastomotic network, caution must be taken that the liquid embolic material does not penetrate adjacent segmental arteries, which may be supplying the spinal cord. It is therefore our policy to check the adjacent levels for spinal cord supply before performing liquid embolic material embolization and to stop the injection when the embolic material reaches the adjacent segmental arteries if supply to the cord from these vessels has been visualized. If the embolic agent does not reach the venous site, we strongly advocate early surgical intervention because a recent study has shown that patients with an incomplete endovascular occlusion who subsequently required surgical intervention had a poor clinical outcome, which was likely at least in part due to delay of the secondary intervention.

Treatment is aimed at halting the progression of the disease, and the prognosis depends on the duration of symptoms and degree of disability before treatment. Following complete occlusion of the fistula, the progression of the disease can be stopped in most instances; however, only two-thirds of all patients experience a regression of their motor symptoms (including impaired gait and weakness), and only one-third experience a regression of their sensory disturbances. Impotence and sphincter disturbances are seldom reversible, and pain may persist. In rare cases of long-standing spinal DAVF, symptoms may worsen despite complete occlusion. Still, a recurrence of symptoms after initial relief should alert the clinician to recanalization of the shunt or the development of a secondary shunt.

PEARLS AND PITFALLS

- A proximal vessel occlusion is not sufficient, despite initial angiographic occlusion, because the DAVF will recruit meningeal collaterals and will be reconstituted within the following weeks or months.
- If it is uncertain that glue has reached the vein, CT may be helpful to demonstrate penetration distal to the dura.
- Neurologic deterioration following embolization of a DAVF may be due to (1) reopening of the fistula, (2) development of a secondary fistula at a different location, or (3) progressive cord atrophy in a patient with long-standing symptoms despite complete occlusion.

Further Reading

Krings T, Geibprasert S. Spinal dural arteriovenous fistulas. AJNR Am J Neuroradiol 2009;30(4):639–648

Ling JCM, Agid R, Nakano S, et al. Metachronous multiplicity of spinal cord arteriovenous fistula and spinal dural AVF in a a patient with hereditary haemorrhagic telangiectasia. Interv Neuroradiol 2005;11(1):79–82

Van Dijk JM, TerBrugge KG, Willinsky RA, Farb RI, Wallace MC. Multidisciplinary management of spinal dural arteriovenous fistulas: clinical presentation and long-term follow-up in 49 patients. Stroke 2002;33(6):1578–1583

Willinsky RA, terBrugge K, Montanera W, Mikulis D, Wallace MC. Posttreatment MR findings in spinal dural arteriovenous malformations. AJNR Am J Neuroradiol 1995;16(10):2063–2071

CASE 62

Case Description

Clinical Presentation

A 54-year-old woman presents with weakness of her lower legs, paresthesias, and hypoesthesias ascending from her feet to her legs without a dermatomal distribution. The symptoms started 6 weeks earlier and are slowly progressive.

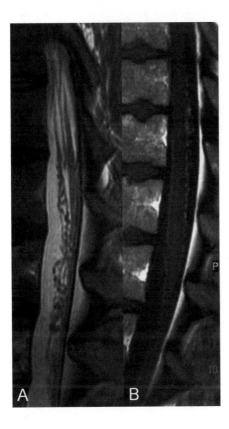

Fig. 62.1 (A) Sagittal T2-weighted and **(B)** T1-weighted post-contrast MR images demonstrate dilated perimedullary vessels, predominantly at the dorsal aspect, with evidence of cord edema.

Radiologic Studies

MRI

Spinal MRI demonstrated perimedullary flow voids, more on the dorsal than on the ventral surface of the cord, as well as cord edema. Flow voids were also visible below the conus. No abnormal intramedullary vessels were seen (**Fig. 62.1**). The images suggested a vascular malformation of the spine, and further angiographic workup was performed.

DSA

The left T10 segmental artery opacified the anterior spinal artery (ASA). The ASA was not abnormally dilated. The contrast material filled the "basket" anastomosis, and both posterior spinal arteries (PSAs) were visualized. Retrograde flow via both the basket and a segmental vasa corona anastomosis to a dilated PSA was seen. This vessel fed a deep-seated shunt close to the conus that had descending and ascending veins. Injection into the left L2 segmental artery, from which the aforementioned PSA origi-

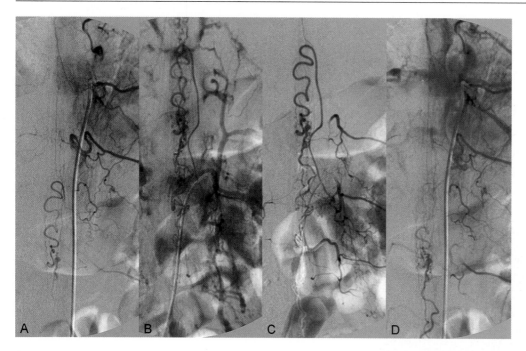

Fig. 62.2 DSA. Left T10 segmental artery angiogram in AP view in **(A)** arterial and **(B)** venous phase shows visualization of a normal-size ASA and filling of both PSAs via a "basket" anastomosis. Retrograde flow through both the basket and a segmental vasa corona anastomosis to a dilated PSA was noted, which supplied a shunt close to the conus draining into descending and ascending veins. Left L2 segmental artery angiogram in AP view in **(C)** early arterial and **(D)** venous phases shows a radiculopial supply to the PSA supplying the shunt.

nated, demonstrated dilatation and a tortuous course of the PSA and a fistulous transition without associated venous pouches into the perimedullary veins, which had both an ascending and descending course (**Fig. 62.2**). No other feeding vessels were identified on a complete spinal angiogram.

Diagnosis

Spinal pial arteriovenous (AV) shunt of the fistulous type associated with venous congestion

Treatment

EQUIPMENT

- Standard 5F access (puncture needle, 5F vascular sheath)
- 5F Cobra catheter with continuous flush and a 0.035-in hydrophilic guidewire
- A 0.012-in flow-directed microcatheter (Magic; Balt International, Montmorency, France) with a 0.008-in guidewire (Mirage; ev3, Plymouth, MN)
- A 10% glucose solution
- Histoacryl/Lipiodol (1 mL/1.2 mL)
- Contrast material

DESCRIPTION

The 5F Cobra catheter was placed distally into the L2 segmental artery. The flow-directed microcatheter was introduced into the segmental artery, advanced via the micro-guidewire into the dilated PSA, and slowly advanced through the tortuous anatomy just proximal to the fistula. Injections with the microcatheter confirmed the position of the catheter distal to any cord-supplying branches. After

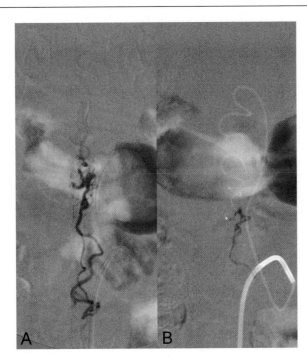

Fig. 62.3 (A) Superselective microcatheter injection and **(B)** glue cast demonstrate penetration of the glue into the proximal vein, completely occluding the shunt zone.

the catheter had been flushed with glucose solution, a mixture of 1 mL of Histoacryl and 1.2 mL of Lipiodol was injected. Glue penetrated from the arterial site into the venous site and completely excluded the shunting zone (**Fig. 62.3**). Verification via both the L2 segmental artery and the ASA axis (**Fig. 62.4**) demonstrated complete exclusion of the shunt. The dorsolateral artery was still patent

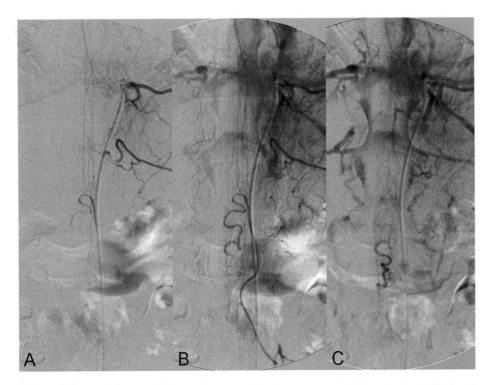

Fig. 62.4 DSA. Left T10 segmental artery angiogram in AP view in **(A)** early arterial, **(B)** capillary, and **(C)** venous phases shows patency of the ASA anastomosis to the dorsolateral spinal artery that harbored the shunt with no residual venous filling, verifying complete occlusion of the shunt.

and demonstrated residual anastomotic flow via the ASA, but the fistula was no longer visualized. The patient did not experience any new neurologic symptoms and at 3-month clinical follow-up was noted to be free of neurologic deficits.

Discussion

BACKGROUND

Spinal AV shunting lesions can be categorized as follows: (1) those supplied by dural (or radiculomeningeal) arteries that do not supply the spinal cord under normal circumstances and (2) those supplied by arteries that under normal circumstances also supply the spinal cord. According to their nidal configuration, these spinal pial AV malformations (AVMs) are either glomerular or fistulous in nature. Fistulous pial AVMs can be further differentiated into macrofistulae, with a high fistula volume, and microfistulae, with a small fistula volume. Glomerular (nidus-type, or plexiform) AVMs may be further divided into focal and diffuse lesions. Fistulous AVMs are located superficially on the spinal cord and are characterized by a direct transition from an artery to a vein without an intervening network of abnormal vessels. Given their perimedullary location, they may cause subarachnoid hemorrhage or (less likely) intramedullary hemorrhage. Because they arterialize the spinal cord veins, symptoms of venous congestion may be present that cannot be distinguished from the symptoms of spinal dural AV fistulae.

Noninvasive Imaging Workup

PHYSICAL EXAMINATION

- Pathophysiologic mechanisms in spinal cord AVMs include venous congestion, hemorrhage, and space-occupying effects.
- If the AVM does not present initially with an acute hemorrhage, the symptomatology is non-specific. Patients may experience hypoesthesia or paresthesia, weakness, and diffuse back and muscle pain. Sensorimotor symptoms can develop slowly and progressively or worsen acutely, then regress in time.

MRI/MRA

- If these shunts present with venous congestion rather than with hemorrhage, they may be difficult to differentiate from dural AV shunts both clinically and on MRI. Given their perimedullary location, intramedullary vessels may not be present, and only perimedullary dilated vascular structures are seen, together with cord edema.
- Early visualization of veins on MRA will indicate a shunt, but in most instances the spatial resolution of the MRA sequence will not be sufficient to differentiate dural from pial AVFs.
- Imaging features that point toward pial rather than dural fistulae are venous pouches, relatively prominent flow voids due to a higher shunting volume, and blood degradation products.

INVASIVE IMAGING WORKUP

- In spinal cord AVMs of both the fistulous and glomerular types, a complete angiographic workup is necessary, not only to identify all arteries that supply the AVM but also to identify the normal supply to the cord.
- If stasis of contrast material in cord-supplying arteries that do not feed the shunt is noted, venous congestion can be assumed to be present.
- Injection into different arteries supplying an AVM will identify the number of compartments and whether they are interconnected. Fistulous AVMs, however, classically have only a single compartment, and filling of the same fistula from different arteries favors either a single-hole fistula or, as in this case, a proximal anastomosis to the artery supplying the shunt.

Differential Diagnosis

- The size of the feeding vessels and draining veins is classically larger in fistulae of the perimedullary type than in dural AV shunts; still, in some fistulous AVMS (especially those of the filum terminale), differentiation between a dural AV shunt and a fistulous AVM is possible only with analysis of the feeding artery if the only presenting symptoms are those of venous congestion.

Treatment Options

SURGICAL TREATMENT

- Surgery is aimed at identifying and obliterating the fistulous point, which may be difficult depending on the location of the shunt (subpial space or even a central sulcus location in anterior spinal cord lesions), the flow volume, and the number of dilated vessels. Because all vessels are arterialized, identification of the feeding artery and draining vein may be a challenge.

ENDOVASCULAR TREATMENT

- In fistulous AVMs in which the feeding vessel has a very tortuous course and the fistula volume is small, the only catheters that are likely to reach the fistulous site are flow-directed 0.012-in microcatheters.
- If distal placement close to the fistulous site is not possible, alternative treatment strategies must be employed.
- In our practice, embolization with liquid material is the therapy of first choice. The concentration of the glue must be adjusted depending on the flow volume of the shunt and the distance between the tip of the catheter and the shunting zone.
- The embolic material must penetrate from the distal arterial segment into the proximal part of the vein.
- Postprocedural heparin may be recommended if the passage of liquid embolic agent has been significant to prevent excessive venous thrombosis.

Possible Complications

- Incomplete embolization with residual shunting or delayed reopening of the fistula due to failure to penetrate the proximal vein
- Reflux into arteries supplying the spinal cord with associated spinal cord ischemia
- Far distal migration of the embolic agent into the draining vein, with a worsening of venous congestion

Published Literature on Treatment Options

Before embolization of a fistulous spinal AVM, great care must be taken to identify the normal spinal cord arteries, which may be difficult to demonstrate because flow is being directed primarily into the fistula. Therefore, before therapy is contemplated, complete spinal angiography is done to evaluate potential collaterals to the anterior and posterior spinal arteries. As shown in this case, injection in a different artery feeding the spinal cord may be able to demonstrate the fistula and, following therapy, its complete occlusion. Before therapy with a liquid embolic agent is contemplated, the security margin must be defined because reflux of the embolic agent may occur (especially in small fistulae). A distance between the microcatheter tip and the adjacent spinal arterial system that is too short may therefore carry a large risk. On the other hand, a position of the microcatheter tip that is too proximal may prevent the embolic agent from reaching the vein, resulting in a proximal arterial occlusion. In the present case, the excellent supply of the entire basket via the ASA with retrograde filling toward the fistula-carrying PSA allowed a long security margin. In addition, the microcatheter could be advanced far distally toward the shunting zone. Embolization with a liquid embolic agent was therefore deemed safe. Although in our opinion endovascular therapies are the method of choice, depending on the location of the shunt and the clinical presentation, surgery may be considered as an option, especially for fistulous perimedullary lesions that are fed primarily by dorsolateral arteries (i.e., those located on the dorsal surface of the cord).

PEARLS AND PITFALLS

- Spinal cord fistulous AVMs can cause the same symptoms and imaging findings as spinal dural AV fistulae (i.e., venous congestion). Differentiation is possible only by evaluation of the feeding arteries.
- In our experience, flow voids below the conus favor (1) a caudally located (sacral or lower lumbar) dural AV fistula, (2) a fistula of the filum terminale, or (3) a perimedullary fistulous AVM, as in this case.

Further Reading

Krings T, Lasjaunias PL, Hans FJ, et al. Imaging in spinal vascular disease. Neuroimaging Clin N Am 2007;17(1):57–72

Mourier KL, Gobin YP, George B, Lot G, Merland JJ. Intradural perimedullary arteriovenous fistulae: results of surgical and endovascular treatment in a series of 35 cases. Neurosurgery 1993;32(6):885–891, discussion 891

Rodesch G, Hurth M, Alvarez H, Tadie M, Lasjaunias PL. Spinal cord intradural arteriovenous fistulae: anatomic, clinical, and therapeutic considerations in a series of 32 consecutive patients seen between 1981 and 2000 with emphasis on endovascular therapy. Neurosurgery 2005;57(5):973–983, discussion 973–983

CASE 63

Case Presentation

Clinical Presentation

A 23-year-old man presents with the sudden onset of back and neck pain, followed by bilateral leg weakness and hypoesthesias. A spinal MRI is performed.

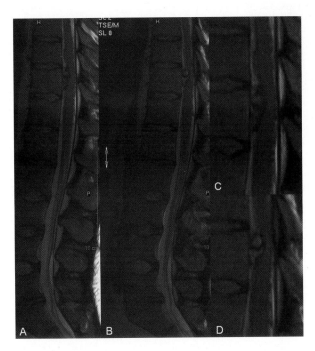

Fig. 63.1 (A,B) Sagittal T2-weighted MRI and **(C,D)** magnification views before treatment demonstrate a vessel outpouching anterior to the spinal cord, dilated perimedullary vessels, and slight edema in the cord.

Radiologic Studies

MRI

Initial MRI demonstrated evidence of a spinal subarachnoid hemorrhage, with edema involving the lower thoracic cord and conus region as well as prominent perimedullary vessels. A large outpouching of one of these vessels was visualized ventral to the spinal cord within the anterior central sulcus. No pathologic vessels were seen within the cord parenchyma (**Fig. 63.1**).

DSA

Injection in the right L2 segmental artery revealed the anterior spinal artery (ASA) with a classic ascending course along the nerve root to the anterior midline, where it formed a hairpin curve with a large descending and a smaller ascending branch. The descending branch had a fistulous connection to a venous outpouching. This fistulous connection seemed to be "en passage," with the normal ASA descending toward the conus and no evidence of a sulcocommissural or vasa corona branch feeding

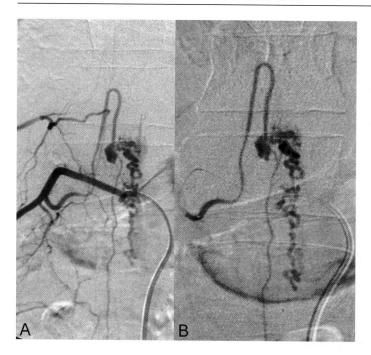

Fig. 63.2 DSA. **(A)** Right L2 segmental artery angiogram in AP view in the acute phase and **(B)** superselective microcatheter injection 2 weeks after the acute event reveal the pial AV fistula and vasospasm of the anterior spinal artery in **(A)** the acute stage, which resolved on **(B)** the study 2 weeks later.

the fistula (**Fig. 63.2**). No other feeding vessels were demonstrated at complete spinal angiography, and no further flow to the conus was visualized other than the supply from the ASA. In the acute stage, significant vasospasm was present in the ASA, and treatment was postponed for 2 weeks.

Diagnosis

Spinal pial arteriovenous malformation (AVM) of the fistulous type with a venous outpouching

Treatment

EQUIPMENT

- Standard 5F access (puncture needle, 5F vascular sheath)
- 5F Cobra catheter with continuous flush and a 0.035-in hydrophilic guidewire
- Straight microcatheter (Excelsior SL 10; Boston Scientific, Natick, MA) with a guidewire (Synchro 14; Boston Scientific)
- Various GDC HyperSoft stretch-resistant coils: 3 mm × 4 cm, 2 mm × 4 cm, 2 mm × 3 cm, 2 mm × 2 cm (Boston Scientific)
- Contrast material

DESCRIPTION

The 5F Cobra catheter was placed distally into the L2 segmental artery, and the microcatheter was introduced into the segmental artery and advanced via the micro-guidewire into the ASA, then slowly advanced via the hairpin curve downward and into the venous pouch. Once it was in the venous pouch, a complex coil was carefully introduced, and the venous pouch was filled with platinum coils in a fashion similar to that used to coil an arterial intracranial aneurysm (framing and subsequent filling). Because it was feared that the microcatheter, given its considerable size, was obstructing the flow through the ASA and because there was a lack of collateral flow, the procedure was stopped after three coils had been introduced into the venous pouch. The control run via the segmental artery after careful and slow removal of the microcatheter demonstrated reduced flow through the fistula and persistent distal flow to the cone (**Fig. 63.3**). Follow-up after 4 weeks demonstrated no further

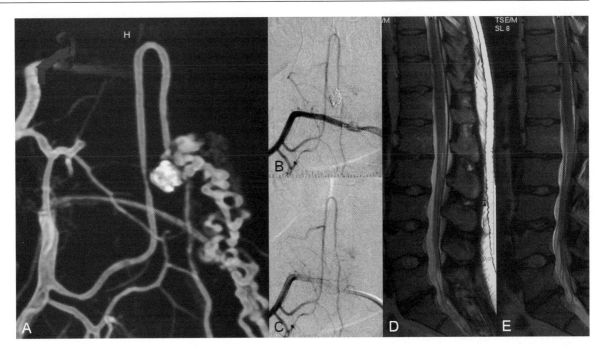

Fig. 63.3 (A) Right L2 segmental artery angiogram in 3D reconstruction 4 weeks after the first embolization session demonstrates decreased but persistent shunting through the coil mesh in the venous pouch. **(B,C)** Follow-up right L2 segmental artery angiogram 4 weeks after the second session of embolization demonstrates complete occlusion of the shunt and normal flow in the distal ASA. **(D,E)** Follow-up sagittal T2-weighted MRI reveals no evidence of recurrence, with disappearance of the venous pouch and cord edema.

occlusion of the shunt (which had been hoped for), and the procedure was repeated with the use of small GDC HyperSoft coils for dense packing of the venous pouch. Following the procedure, there was residual slow flow through the shunt and another session was scheduled, but at that time, complete occlusion of the shunt was demonstrated. MRI follow-up demonstrated stable occlusion, regression of the cord edema, and the absence of dilated veins. The patient had no neurologic deficits.

Discussion

Background

Spinal cord AVMs are fed by radiculomedullary and/or radiculopial arteries (i.e., arteries that feed the spinal cord) and drained by spinal cord veins. These shunts may have an intramedullary and/or perimedullary location and can be differentiated according to the transition from artery into vein as fistulous or glomerular AVMs. Fistulous AVMs (which are also called AVMs of the perimedullary fistula type or intradural AV fistulae) are direct AV shunts located superficially on the surface of the spinal cord and only rarely possess intramedullary compartments. Depending on the size of the feeding vessels, shunt volume, and size of the draining veins, these fistulae can be further categorized into (1) those with a low shunt volume and only moderately enlarged feeding arteries and draining veins (microfistulae) and (2) those with a high shunt volume that leads to massive remodeling of the blood vessels, with enlarged arteries and dilated venous pouches (macrofistulae). The latter type is typically encountered in children with a history of hereditary hemorrhagic telangiectasia (HHT). Fistulous AVMs are found in the subpial space in ventral locations and in the subarachnoid space in dorsal locations. They are more often encountered in younger patients, with the exception of AVMs of the filum terminale, which are classically encountered in elderly patients.

Noninvasive Imaging Workup

CT/CTA

- It is only in high-flow fistulae that CT may play a role by demonstrating bony remodeling surrounding ectatic venous pouches. Otherwise, CT does not have a role in the diagnosis or management of fistulous spinal pial AVMs.

MRI/MRA

- MRI can detect the dilated vessels, blood products, and extent of intramedullary edema. Because intramedullary components are rarely present in fistulous AVMs, the pathologically dilated vessels will surround the cord.
- A dilated pouch together with perimedullary flow voids in a young patient with a history of spinal hemorrhage is classic for a fistulous AVM.
- The location of the venous pouches can sometimes be helpful in identifying the presumed nature of the feeding artery (i.e., ASA axis or posterolateral spinal arteries).
- Massively dilated venous pouches in young children strongly suggest an underlying disease (HHT).

Invasive Imaging Workup

- To identify the transition from artery to vein, 3D angiography of the fistula may be helpful; classically, a change in caliber is seen at the transition point, and in some instances a venous pouch is present.
- It is necessary to search for the course of the distal (normal) vessel and its potential anastomoses from above or below, and for anastomoses between the anterior and dorsolateral spinal artery axes.
- If multiple feeders converge toward the same pouch, a "single-hole" fistula is likely to be present, which strongly favors the diagnosis of HHT.

Differential Diagnosis

- In acute spinal cord hemorrhage, cavernomas and metastases must be ruled out. Classically, the presence of flow voids will point toward a shunting lesion.
- Spinal arterial aneurysms without associated shunting lesions are exceedingly rare and often associated with an underlying vessel wall disease that makes the arteries more prone to dissection.
- Given these entities in the differential diagnosis, it is our policy to perform complete invasive angiography in a patient with spinal cord hemorrhage (subarachnoidal or intramedullary) without a visible cause (i.e., cavernoma).

Treatment Options

SURGICAL TREATMENT

- Depending on the location and flow volume of the shunt, surgery may be an alternative to endovascular therapies. However, lesions with a high flow rate or an ASA supply may cause problems, as may the presence of multiple dilated vessels.

ENDOVASCULAR TREATMENT

- In fistulous AVMs, the treatment can be with either liquid embolic agents or coils. If no safe position for injecting the liquid embolic agent is found, as in the present case, detachable coils may be a more controlled and safer embolic material.

- A staged approach to promote thrombotic occlusion of the venous pouch may be warranted in selected cases.

Possible Complications

- Failure of the embolic material to penetrate the proximal vein will lead to collateral filling and secondary reopening of the fistula.
- Occlusion of the ASA leads in most instances to significant morbidity.
- A liquid embolic material can penetrate the ASA following injection into the posterior spinal artery because of the presence of transmedullary and vasa corona anastomoses.

Published Literature on Treatment Options

In fistulous spinal AVMs, the aim is to obliterate the point of fistulization by embolizing the most proximal venous segment together with the most distal arterial segment. This can be accomplished with liquid embolic agents (see Case 62) or coils. Before the choice of embolization material is contemplated, the most important (and difficult) step is to determine the shunting zone (i.e., the point where the artery stops and the vein starts). A proximal occlusion of the artery will lead to collateral filling and secondary reopening due to the vast network of anastomoses within the spinal cord and may carry a risk for inadvertent occlusion of the spinal cord supply. A purely venous occlusion that leaves the fistula open may, on the other hand, result in hemorrhage. The transition from artery to vein may be marked by a venous (pseudo)aneurysm (which is often the site of rupture, as in our case), by an enlarged venous pouch (typically present in high-flow, single-hole fistulae), or by a slight change (enlargement) in vessel caliber. A 3D reconstruction of the angiogram is in our opinion particularly helpful to define the fistulous point.

When an embolic agent is chosen, several specific features of the AVM must be kept in mind. In the present case, there was no point of security, given the "en passage" supply from the ASA directly into the venous pouch. In addition, it was unlikely that collateralization via the basket anastomosis surrounding the conus was possible because no dorsolateral feeders could be identified during complete angiography. Under such conditions, controlled occlusion of the fistula with detachable coils is in our opinion the treatment of choice; it will reduce flow through the shunt, induce thrombosis within the vein, and remodel the normal ASA supply. Alternatively, especially in dorsally located shunts, one may opt for surgical treatment of the fistula.

In high-flow macrofistulae (which can be indicative of an underlying genetic disorder, such as HHT), a strategy similar to that used in the management of a single-hole brain AV fistulae must be adopted. In these types of fistulous AVMs, the dilated feeding vessels will allow superselective catheterization close to the fistula. Closure with highly concentrated glue is therefore possible, with the aim of obliterating the fistulous area by pushing the glue via the distal artery into the proximal venous pouch and establishing a mushroom-shaped glue cast that occludes the fistula. This is preferably done via a posterior spinal arterial feeder, with occlusion of the fistula confirmed when the other, previous feeders are injected. Because the volume of the venous pouch is typically large and may further enlarge following thrombosis (which will happen within the first 24 hours after occlusion), compression of the cord may occur. This rare evolution may require surgical decompression. Given these assumptions, a stepwise approach in several sessions, in which the flow (and subsequently the size of the venous pouch) is reduced with coils at the site of the fistula, may be a reasonable alternative treatment strategy.

PEARLS AND PITFALLS _____

- Early rebleeding in spinal cord AVMs is rare; a staged treatment approach may therefore be employed.
- Endovascular therapy is the method of choice; however, depending on the location of the shunt (dorsal vs. ventral), surgery is also an option.
- High-flow, "single-hole" spinal AV fistulae in young children strongly suggest an underlying disease such as HHT, and screening of the lungs may therefore be indicated.

Further Reading

Krings T, Mull M, Gilsbach JM, Thron A. Spinal vascular malformations. Eur Radiol 2005;15(2):267–278

Krings T, Ozanne A, Chng SM, Alvarez H, Rodesch G, Lasjaunias PL. Neurovascular phenotypes in hereditary haemorrhagic telangiectasia patients according to age. Review of 50 consecutive patients aged 1 day-60 years. Neuroradiology 2005;47(10):711–720

Mandzia JL, terBrugge KG, Faughnan ME, Hyland RH. Spinal cord arteriovenous malformations in two patients with hereditary hemorrhagic telangiectasia. Childs Nerv Syst 1999;15(2-3):80–83

Prestigiacomo CJ, Niimi Y, Setton A, Berenstein A. Three-dimensional rotational spinal angiography in the evaluation and treatment of vascular malformations. AJNR Am J Neuroradiol 2003;24(7):1429–1435

Rodesch G, Hurth M, Alvarez H, Ducot B, Tadie M, Lasjaunias PL. Angio-architecture of spinal cord arteriovenous shunts at presentation. Clinical correlations in adults and children. The Bicêtre experience on 155 consecutive patients seen between 1981-1999. Acta Neurochir (Wien) 2004;146(3):217–226, discussion 226–227

CASE 64

Case Description

Clinical Presentation

A 20-year-old woman presents with the sudden onset of back pain that is located between the scapulae and spreads to the neck area. She also has bilateral upper and lower limb paresis that is more pronounced on the right side. Spinal MRI is performed.

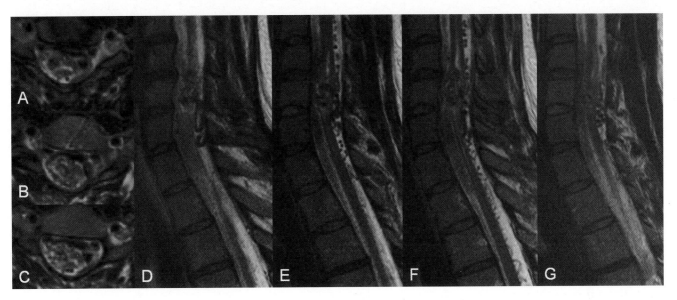

Fig. 64.1 (A–C) Axial and **(D–G)** sagittal T2-weighted MR images before treatment demonstrate hematomyelia as well as prominent intramedullary and perimedullary flow voids.

Radiologic Studies

MRI

MRI demonstrated hematomyelia with associated slight T2 hyperintensity and dilated perimedullary and intramedullary vessels. An intramedullary vessel outpouching was visualized on the anterior right aspect of the cord (**Fig. 64.1**).

DSA

After injection in the right ascending cervical artery, a dilated anterior spinal artery (ASA) was detected that fed a diffuse glomerular arteriovenous malformation (AVM) with a large intramedullary component and dilated perimedullary veins. On 3D angiography of the nidus, a focal outpouching was visualized within the nidus that coincided with the outpouching seen on MRI. Because the patient had presented with spinal hemorrhage, this area was considered to be the main target of therapy (**Fig. 64.2**).

Diagnosis

Spinal pial AVM of the glomerular type with an intranidal aneurysm and hematomyelia

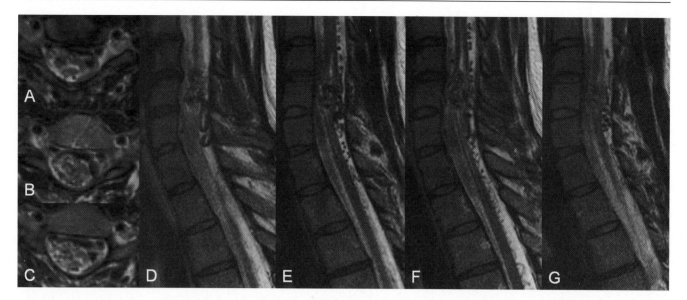

Fig. 64.2 DSA. Right ascending cervical artery angiograms in **(A)** AP view and **(B,C)** 3D reconstructions reveal a dilated ASA supplying a diffuse glomerular AVM that drains into dilated perimedullary veins. **(C)** A small focal outpouching within the nidus is noted, representing an intranidal (pseudo)aneurysm.

Treatment

EQUIPMENT

- Standard 5F access (puncture needle, 5F vascular sheath)
- 5F multipurpose catheter with continuous flush and a 0.035-in hydrophilic guidewire
- A 3 × 0.012-in flow-directed microcatheter (Magic; Balt International, Montmorency, France) with a 0.008-in guidewire (Mirage; ev3, Plymouth, MN)
- A 10% glucose solution
- Histoacryl/Lipiodol (1 mL/1.2 mL)
- Contrast material

DESCRIPTION

The 5F multipurpose catheter was placed distally into the ascending cervical artery. Flow-directed microcatheters, following steam shaping with 60- to 90-degree curves, were advanced via the ASA. The distal and inferior parts of the AVM harboring the aneurysm were catheterized via the sulco-commissural and vasa corona branches. A stable position of the catheter tip was confirmed with microcatheter injections before the injection of liquid embolic material. After the catheters had been flushed with glucose solution, a mixture of Histoacryl and Lipiodol (1:1.2) was injected into the AVM, with care taken to avoid any reflux along the catheter (**Fig. 64.3**). The follow-up control demonstrated significantly reduced flow through the AVM (the ascending branch of the ASA was now visible) and complete occlusion of the inferolateral compartment that harbored the aneurysm (**Fig. 64.4**). The patient had no new neurologic deficits following embolization. At clinical follow-up after 6 months, she had recovered significantly from the hematomyelia. She had a mild residual paresis of her right upper and lower extremity but was able to walk. Angiography demonstrated stable occlusion of the previously embolized branches and no new angioarchitectonic risk factors. There was still a significant amount of shunting; however, because the patient had no symptoms or signs suggesting venous congestion (presumably because of good outflow via radicular veins into the epidural venous plexus), no further therapy was undertaken. We continue to follow this patient clinically and with noninvasive imaging, and further therapy will be considered if changes in her neurologic symptoms or on follow-up MRI are detected.

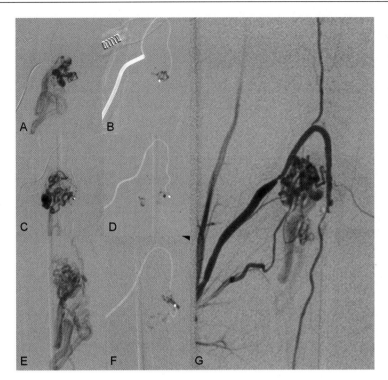

Fig. 64.3 (A,C,E) Superselective catheterizations and **(B,D,F)** corresponding glue casts targeting the compartment with the intranidal aneurysm. **(G)** Right ascending cervical angiogram following embolization demonstrates occlusion of the inferolateral compartment of the AVM.

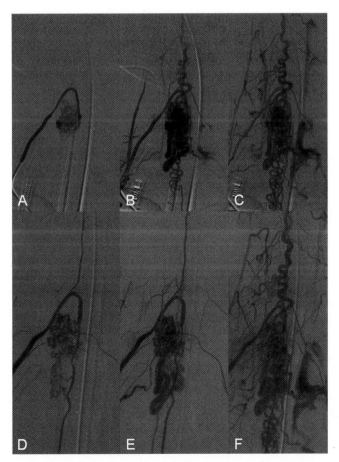

Fig. 64.4 (A–C) Comparison of initial angiography and **(D–F)** follow-up angiography shows reduced size of the AVM, no evident angioarchitectonic risk factors, and decreased flow through the AVM. Because the patient is asymptomatic, no further therapy is contemplated at this time.

Discussion

Background

Glomerular AVMs (also called plexiform or nidus-type AVMs) are the most frequently encountered spinal cord AVMs. The nidus resembles closely that of a brain AVM. This type of malformation usually has an intramedullary location, but superficial nidus compartments may reach the subarachnoid space. Because of the many anastomoses between the anterior and posterior arterial feeding systems of the spine, these AVMs typically have a multiple arterial supply from both the posterior and anterior spinal systems. Drainage is into dilated spinal cord veins. Therapy of spinal AVMs improves the prognosis in symptomatic patients, whereas in asymptomatic patients, its use has not been proven. Endovascular therapies are definitely the first line of treatment and should be tailored to the specific individual pathologic mechanisms and angioarchitectonics, as detailed below.

Noninvasive Imaging Workup

PHYSICAL EXAMINATION

- In patients with a suspected spinal cord AVM, especially those of the nidus type, the physical examination should include an inspection of the skin to rule out a spinal AV metameric syndrome (SAMS, or Cobb syndrome), which demonstrates skin, bone, and spinal cord involvement.
- Given their intramedullary location, nidus-type or glomerular AVMs are more prone to become symptomatic with intramedullary than with subarachnoid hemorrhage; venous congestion can occur in lesions that have a large shunting volume. Space-occupying effects and arterial steal have also been described as potential pathologic mechanisms. The combination of clinical findings, cross-sectional imaging features, and angioarchitectonics is of importance to define the target of treatment.

CT/CTA

- CT may play a role in demonstrating bone involvement in metameric syndromes; otherwise, CT and CTA play no significant role in the evaluation of nidus-type or glomerular AVMs.

MRI/MRA

- The typical appearance of a spinal cord AVM is a conglomerate of perimedullary and intramedullary dilated vessels that are demonstrated on T2-weighted sequences as flow voids. On T1-weighted sequences, depending on their flow velocity and direction, they appear as mixed hyperintense and hypointense tubular structures. Contrast enhancement may vary.
- Venous congestive edema may be present and appears as intramedullary hyperintensity on T2-weighted images with concomitant swelling of the cord.
- Intraparenchymal hemorrhages may be present that demonstrate varying signal intensities, depending on the time elapsed between bleeding and imaging. A subarachnoid hemorrhage may be present.
- MRI should be able to identify the location of an AVM in relation to the cord (intramedullary vs. perimedullary, anterior aspect vs. central vs. posterior aspect, number of longitudinal segments involved).
- Involvement of the bone, muscles, or skin must be ruled out (to differentiate metameric syndromes from cord AVMs).
- MRA can detect the main feeder of an AVM; however, given its low spatial resolution, complete catheter angiography is still necessary.

Invasive Imaging Workup

- As in fistulous AVMs, the first step is to perform complete angiography to determine the collaterals, main feeders, and number of different and/or overlapping compartments.
- To demonstrate focal weak points within the nidus (focal outpouchings, false aneurysms), 3D reconstructions will be helpful.
- Conventional series must include the venous phase because the appearance of contrast stagnation in intranidal outpouchings (pseudoaneurysms) is a classic sign of the point of rupture.
- Most "glomerular" AVMs have additional fistulous compartments. If a patient presents with venous congestion, these compartments must be identified so that they can be targeted first during embolization to reduce the AV shunt.
- If in addition to an intramedullary AVM a radicular AVM shunt is present in the metameric muscle or bone, a spinal metameric syndrome (Cobb syndrome) can be diagnosed.

Differential Diagnosis

- Nidus-type or glomerular AVMs have both intramedullary and perimedullary dilated vessels and can thereby be differentiated from other vascular shunting malformations.
- Hemangioblastomas may demonstrate dilated perimedullary vessels and an intramedullary mass lesion that enhances with contrast; however, dense, well-defined contrast enhancement and possibly cystic components are typical of these lesions and are not seen in AVMs.
- If involvement of the muscle, bone, or nerve roots is identified, a metameric syndrome (Cobb syndrome) is present.

Treatment Options

CONSERVATIVE OR MEDICAL MANAGEMENT

- A conservative approach should be considered in asymptomatic patients with no evidence of cord edema and no angioarchitectonic weak points.
- Following partial embolization, if symptoms become stable, further conservative management may be adopted if treatment-related risks are expected to be high.

SURGICAL TREATMENT

- Depending on the location of the AVM and its supply, surgical excision of a spinal cord AVM can be challenging. A staged approach may not be possible. Transmedullary feeders as well as compartments of the AVM fed by the ASA are difficult to reach. Therefore, endovascular therapies are the first line of treatment in most centers.

ENDOVASCULAR TREATMENT

- In our practice, embolization with liquid material (diluted glue) is the therapy of choice after a specific target has been defined.
- Partial treatment has been shown to improve the natural history of these lesions, whereas complete eradication of an AVM may result in greater treatment-related morbidity.
- Given the lower flow rates in these lesions compared with those in brain AVMs or fistulous spinal AVMs, particle embolization that results in venous stagnation may in selected patients lead to venous thrombosis and subsequent occlusion of the AVM.
- Postprocedural heparin may be recommended if passage of the liquid embolic agent has been significant to prevent excessive venous thrombosis.

Possible Complications

- Failure to penetrate the proximal vein with embolic material may lead to delayed reopening of the AVM.
- Aggressive embolization may lead to angiographically "nice" pictures but can be associated with significant morbidity.
- Endovascular therapy is contraindicated if a safe catheter position cannot be reached. The term safe, however, implies a profound understanding of the angioarchitecture of the spinal cord.

Published Literature on Treatment Options

The therapeutic approach to asymptomatic AVMs is difficult because data on the prognosis without treatment are not available; however, in patients with symptomatic AVMs, therapy improves the prognosis. In comparison with brain AVMs, spinal AVMs exhibit some fundamental differences. First, hyperacute treatment is rarely indicated because in our experience acute rebleeding is exceptional. Instead, after bleeding from a spinal AVM has occurred, we typically wait for 2 to 6 weeks for potential vasospasm to resolve and the hemorrhage to be absorbed. Second, whereas brain AVMs must be completely treated to avoid the risk for rebleeding, this seems not to be the case with spinal AVMs, in which partial treatment appears to be sufficient to dramatically improve the prognosis, especially for patients in whom a complete eradication of the AVM is likely to produce neurologic deficits. Especially in unruptured spinal AVMs that have become symptomatic because of venous congestion rather than hemorrhage, the goal must be to reduce the shunting volume rather than to produce an angiographically "nice" picture that carries a high risk for treatment-related morbidity. Third, because of the low flow rate in some glomerular AVMs, endovascular therapies with particles seem to yield a better and more stable result if venous stagnation (with subsequent venous thrombosis of the outlet) occurs (**Fig. 64.5**). Fourth, in the authors' opinion, there is currently no role for radiosurgery in the treatment of symptomatic spinal AVMs, given the longer latency period until the effects of the radiation take place and given the "eloquence" of the surrounding tissue. Target definition will play a major role in limiting treatment with radiosurgery because there is a considerable amount of movement in the spinal cord due to cerebrospinal fluid pulsation. Surgery remains an option in selected cases, especially when the endovascular route is too long (e.g., when an AV fistula is located

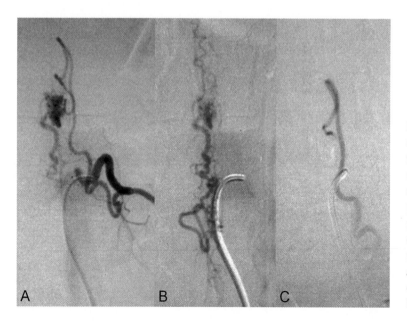

Fig. 64.5 (A) Left T9 segmental artery angiogram and **(B)** superselective microcatheter injection in AP view demonstrate a small glomerular AVM supplied by a radiculopial artery. This patient underwent embolization with particles. **(C)** Superselective microcatheter injection after embolization reveals complete obliteration of the AVM. There were no new neurologic deficits. The results were stable at follow-up after 6 months.

at the filum terminale). However, it is generally accepted that the endovascular route should be the modality of choice in most instances.

In most glomerular AVMs, the pathologic mechanism can be identified before the procedure, so that an individually tailored therapeutic strategy is possible. AVMs that have become symptomatic with hemorrhage may demonstrate a focal weakness that can be targeted with embolization. In cases in which the symptoms can be attributed to venous congestion, the aim will be to reduce the amount of shunting as much as possible. Taking into consideration the anatomic characteristics of the spinal cord vessels, the safest vessels through which embolization can be performed are the posterior spinal ones. Because of the vast anastomotic network, compartments belonging to the ASA axis can often be reached via the posterior spinal system as well. If treatment with particles is to be performed, then they must be very well diluted and injected slowly until venous stagnation occurs. Liquid embolic agents have the major advantage of being stable; however, the reported complication rates are higher (in the large series, ~10%), and only rarely will a complete obliteration be possible. In diffuse angiomas (SAMS or Cobb syndrome), a complete obliteration or resection is almost never possible. In these cases, we again adopt the strategy of a partially targeted embolization to reduce shunting zones and obliterate potential focal weak points.

PEARLS AND PITFALLS

- An assessment of the clinical symptoms and MR findings and a complete angiographic workup are essential in determining the treatment of spinal glomerular AVMs.
- Partial treatment tailored to the individual pathologic mechanism may be sufficient to relieve the patient's symptoms.
- Understanding the anatomy is key for a safe approach to this rare disease.

Further Reading

Boström A, Krings T, Hans FJ, Schramm J, Thron AK, Gilsbach JM. Spinal glomus-type arteriovenous malformations: microsurgical treatment in 20 cases. J Neurosurg Spine 2009;10(5):423–429

Krings T, Geibprasert S, Luo CB, Bhattacharya JJ, Alvarez H, Lasjaunias P. Segmental neurovascular syndromes in children. Neuroimaging Clin N Am 2007;17(2):245–258

Rodesch G, Hurth M, Alvarez H, David P, Tadie M, Lasjaunias PL. Embolization of spinal cord arteriovenous shunts: morphological and clinical follow-up and results—review of 69 consecutive cases. Neurosurgery 2003;53(1):40–49, discussion 49–50

Thron A. Vascular Anatomy of the Spinal Cord: Neuroradiological Investigations and Clinical Syndromes. New York, NY: Springer; 1988

CASE 65

Case Description

Clinical Presentation

A 32-year-old man presents with a bruit following a history of minor blunt trauma to the neck. Physical examination reveals a pulsatile bruit at the left side of the neck; his neurologic examination is normal. Angiography is performed.

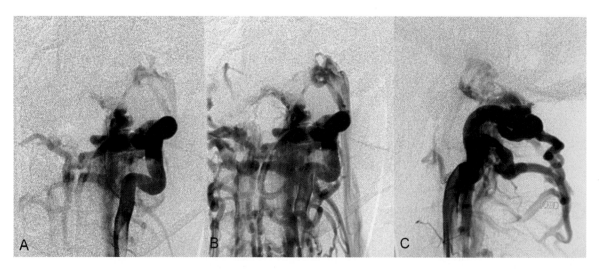

Fig. 65.1 DSA. Left vertebral angiogram in AP view of the **(A)** arterial and **(B)** venous phase and **(C)** in lateral view of the arterial phase.

Radiologic Studies

DSA

The left vertebral angiogram showed a direct arteriovenous (AV) shunt at the C2-C3 segment of the left vertebral artery (VA) that drained into the vertebral plexus before further draining into the internal jugular vein (**Fig. 65.1**). The right vertebral angiogram (not shown) also demonstrated retrograde filling of the fistula, with additional supply through collaterals from enlarged muscular branches of the left occipital artery.

Diagnosis

Left traumatic vertebrovertebral fistula (VVF)

Treatment

EQUIPMENT

- Standard 7F access (puncture needle, 7F vascular sheath)
- Standard 7F guiding catheter with continuous flush and a 0.038-in hydrophilic guidewire

- GOLDBAL3 gold valve detachable balloon (Balt International, Montmorency, France)
- Magic BD PE 1.8F catheter for detachable balloon (Balt)
- Isotonic contrast solution for balloon inflation
- Contrast material
- Heparin 3000 units

DESCRIPTION

After diagnostic angiography, 3000 units of heparin was given intravenously. The 7F guiding catheter was advanced carefully into the proximal left VA. The detachable balloon was prepared and mounted onto the detachable catheter system. A roadmap was done, followed by introduction of the balloon and detachable system into the guiding catheter. After the balloon was within the left VA, it was slightly inflated with 0.1 mL of isotonic saline solution to facilitate navigation into the fistula. After the balloon entered the vertebral plexus, it was inflated, with several hand injection angiograms through the guiding catheter to check its position. When the balloon was correctly placed within the first venous pouch, the one closest to the site of the fistula, it was fully inflated and detached. The detachable catheter system was then removed, and a final control run showed complete obliteration of the fistula (**Fig. 65.2**).

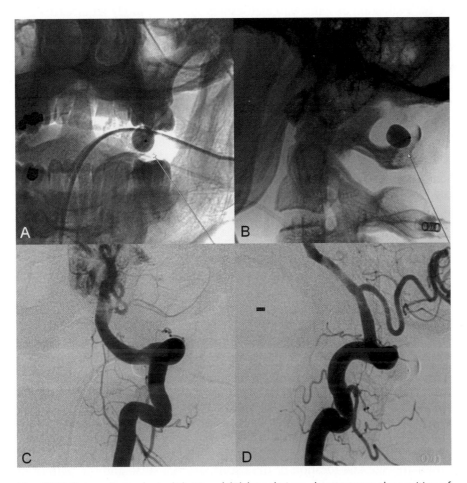

Fig. 65.2 Plain radiography in **(A)** AP and **(B)** lateral views demonstrates the position of the balloon within the first venous pouch. DSA. Left vertebral angiogram in **(C)** AP and **(D)** lateral views shows complete obliteration of the fistula after embolization.

Discussion

Background

VVFs are abnormal connections between the VA or its branches and the adjacent veins. They are rare and can be either traumatic or spontaneous in origin. Penetrating neck injury is a common traumatic cause; other, less frequent causes include placement of a central line, neck surgery, and fractures of the cervical spine. Spontaneous fistulae are known to be associated with vessel wall disorders, such as neurofibromatosis type 1, fibromuscular dysplasia, and Ehlers-Danlos syndrome type 4. Lesions may be asymptomatic, with only a neck bruit, or they may cause vertigo, cervical radiculopathy, or even more severe symptoms of vertebrobasilar insufficiency related to arterial steal and cervical myelopathy resulting from cervical cord compression by dilated epidural venous pouches. Although symptoms related to venous hypertension have been reported in the literature, actual reflux into the perimedullary or posterior fossa veins is extremely rare. Common locations are above the C2 level for spontaneous fistulae and below C5 for traumatic fistulae.

Noninvasive Imaging Workup

CT/MRI

- MRI is the standard for the evaluation of spinal vascular lesions, and CT is rarely required. CT can be used to evaluate calcifications and bone involvement (bone erosion in long-standing lesions, associated bone fractures in traumatic fistulae).
- The presence of flow-void structures on both T1- and T2-weighted sequences within the spinal canal and neural foramina suggests the diagnosis. Occasionally, heterogeneously increased signal may be seen within the venous pouches on both T1 and T2, caused by turbulence. These changes may mimic those of a tumor.
- The dilated epidural pouches can compress the nerve roots within the neural foramen or the spinal cord in the spinal canal.
- Focally increased T2 signal intensity within the cord is usually related to compressive myelopathy; however, if the increased signal is more extensive or there is no evidence of cord compression, the myelopathy may be related to venous hypertension resulting from retrograde perimedullary venous reflux.
- The site/level of the fistula is suggested by visualization of a connection between the VA and venous pouch.

CTA/MRA

- CTA has a major role in the evaluation of traumatic neck lesions.
- Early filling of the vertebral plexus and enlargement of the involved proximal VA can be seen on both CTA and MRA.
- Dynamic CTA and MRA may be required to identify the exact site of a fistula.

Invasive Imaging Workup

- Angiography is not required for the diagnosis of VVFs but is needed for pre-treatment evaluation.
- Both VAs are evaluated for the site and location of the fistula, arterial steal, and the pattern of venous drainage. Additional evaluation of the ipsilateral occipital artery and ascending and deep cervical arteries may be required to better delineate the exact location of the shunt and the first venous pouch.

- In patients with nontraumatic lesions, an evaluation of other vascular territories may be helpful to identify an underlying vasculopathy. Catheterization must be done very carefully in these circumstances.

Treatment Options

SURGICAL TREATMENT

- Proximal surgical ligation of the parent artery is no longer performed.
- Surgical procedures are rarely warranted in most circumstances and include direct surgical ligation of the fistula with packing of the venous pouches and surgical trapping of the VA. A bypass venous graft from the subclavian to the distal VA combined with endovascular occlusion of the remaining, proximal VA is used for large, complex fistulae.

ENDOVASCULAR TREATMENT

- The aim in the treatment of VVFs is to close the fistula and preserve the parent VA. This can be achieved with endovascular treatment and rarely with surgery.
- Balloons, coils, and liquid embolic agents can all be used to occlude a fistula, with the first venous pouch the main target of embolization. Balloons are in many centers the first line of treatment because they can rapidly occlude a fistula and are more easily controlled than coils and liquid embolic agents. If more than one balloon is required, then the first balloons are navigated further into the vertebral plexus, and the last balloon is placed at the first venous pouch closest to the fistula site.
- The use of other materials such as stents and Amplatzer vascular plugs has been reported, but these are not routinely used in our practice.
- Occasionally, the VA cannot be preserved, and sacrifice is required. The VA must be closed both distally and proximally, as close as possible to the fistula, to prevent recanalization by collateral segmental arteries.
- Heparin is routinely given to all patients.
- In our institution, all patients are prescribed absolute bed rest for at least 72 hours following the procedure to avoid balloon migration. Aggressive medication for nausea, vomiting, hiccups, and coughing may be needed.
- If early deflation of the balloon occurs within this period, then the bed rest is cancelled and the patient is rescheduled for another embolization after 1 month. This waiting period is often necessary for the first balloon to deflate sufficiently that placement of the second or third balloon is not obstructed.
- If the VVF recurs after the second embolization, the period of bed rest may be extended up to 5 days, or the use of other embolic materials, such as coils and/or liquid agents, is considered.

Possible Complications

- Migration or early deflation of the balloon
- Worsening of cervical radiculopathy as a consequence of nerve root compression by the balloon or embolic material
- Delayed occlusion of the involved VA, in particular in patients with underlying vascular wall disorders, such as neurofibromatosis type 1

Published Literature on Treatment Options

In the large VVFs series, endovascular treatment was considered the treatment of choice, performed in 67 to 75% of cases. Immediate occlusion of the fistula was achieved in up to 91 to 93% of cases, and the VA was preserved in 78 to 91% of cases. In these series, a transarterial route with either balloon or coils was used. In cases of VVFs that occur after penetrating injuries, with subsequent, more extensive damage to the VA, preservation of the parent artery is less likely, and occlusion of the parent vessel may be necessary. As for a transvenous approach to the treatment of VVFs, it is often more difficult to reach the vertebral plexus and thus the site of a fistula with a transvenous route than with a transarterial route. This technique is therefore reserved for cases in which transarterial embolization has failed. Several cases in which covered stents or stent-grafts were used have been reported by various authors; however, long-term follow-up is not available for these cases.

PEARLS AND PITFALLS_____

- VVFs can be traumatic or spontaneous in origin.
- Endovascular management is the treatment of choice. The aim is to close the fistula and preserve the parent artery. A transarterial route is the first line of treatment; however, if the fistula hole is too small, then a transvenous route may be used.

Further Reading

Beaujeux RL, Reizine DC, Casasco A, et al. Endovascular treatment of vertebral arteriovenous fistula. Radiology 1992;183(2):361–367

Gobin YP, Duckwiler GR, Viñuela F. Direct arteriovenous fistulas (carotid-cavernous and vertebral-venous). Diagnosis and intervention. Neuroimaging Clin N Am 1998;8(2):425–443

Goyal M, Willinsky R, Montanera W, terBrugge KG. Spontaneous vertebrovertebral arteriovenous fistulae. Clinical features, angioarchitecture and management of twelve patients. Interv Neuroradiol 1999;5:219–224

Kai Y, Hamada JI, Mizuno T, Kochi M, Ushio Y, Kitano I. Transvenous embolization for vertebral arteriovenous fistula: report of two cases and technical notes. Acta Neurochir (Wien) 2001;143(2):125–128

CASE 66

Case Description

Clinical Presentation

A 56-year-old man presents with paresthesia in the left lower limb in the L5 distribution. He was successfully treated for prostate carcinoma several years ago. CT is requested to evaluate the possible compression of neural elements in the lumbar spine.

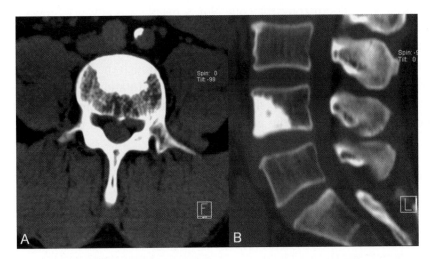

Fig. 66.1 (A,B) CT of the lumbar spine.

Radiologic Studies

CT

CT of the lumbar spine demonstrated a left-sided paramedian disk herniation at the L4-L5 level with compression of the left L5 nerve root. As an incidental finding, a large osteodense lesion with irregular spicular margins was noted in the L4 vertebral body (**Fig. 66.1**). Given the absence of this lesion on CT scans 4 years previously, together with the patient's history, an osteoblastic malignant lesion was suspected. Comparable lesions in other locations were not detected on extensive CT imaging of the thorax and abdomen or on bone scintigraphy. Therefore, a percutaneous biopsy of the lesion in the L4 vertebral body was planned.

Biopsy

EQUIPMENT

- Lidocaine (Linisol 2%; B Braun, Melsungen, Germany)
- Cutter (surgical blade)
- An 11-gauge, 10-cm M1M Cook bone biopsy needle with a beveled edge
- Kocher clamp (used to hold the biopsy needle)

- Orthopedic hammer
- A 20-mL syringe
- Closed recipient partially filled with 10% formalin

DESCRIPTION

The patient was placed prone on the table of the angiography suite and instructed to breathe slowly and not move. Strictly PA and lateral views of the L4 vertebral body were used. To reach the antero-inferior lesion in the vertebral body, a steep craniocaudal trajectory was needed from the pedicle toward the lesion. Therefore, the entry point in L4 was planned to be high in the pedicle or just above the pedicle. Because the lesion was located in the midline of the vertebral body, the biopsy needle had to be directed from the pedicle toward the midline. With the use of fluoroscopy, a skin entry point was chosen accordingly, superolateral to the right pedicle of L4.

After disinfection and local anesthesia, a 4- to 5-mm-wide incision was made in the skin, and the bone biopsy needle was introduced. With fluoroscopy, the bone biopsy needle was advanced toward the superolateral aspect of the right pedicle until bone contact was felt.

With the tip of the needle in contact with the bone, its position was determined on fluoroscopy to be just superior to the pedicle. Additional local anesthetic was injected through the biopsy needle to anesthetize the periosteum. Firm but controlled pressure, if necessary with rotation of the needle, was used to penetrate the cortical bone. (The needle tip should never pass beyond the inner margin of the pedicle on the AP view unless it has reached the posterior wall of the vertebral body on the lateral view.)

With lateral fluoroscopy, the needle tip position was determined to be superolateral within the vertebral body. The beveled edge was turned cranially and slightly laterally to help the needle tip slide caudally and medially toward the lesion (**Fig. 66.2**).

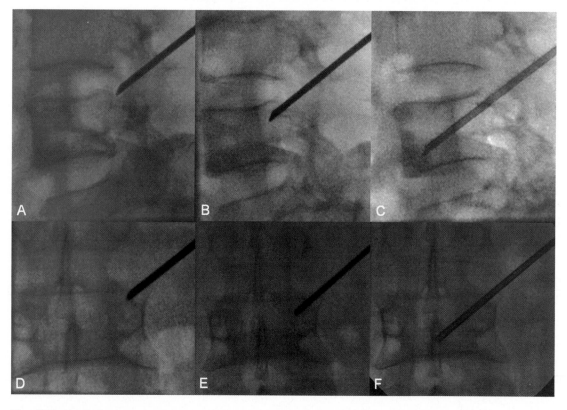

Fig. 66.2 (A–F) Fluoroscopy guidance in lateral and PA views with the use of a low dose of radiation.

Before the lesion was reached, the inner needle was removed. (The inner needle is necessary to penetrate cortical bone, but not trabecular bone. When the biopsy needle is advanced toward and into the lesion, normal trabecular bone and eventually abnormal bone tissue will enter the hollow shaft of the needle. It is often helpful for the interpreting pathologist if the transition zone between normal and abnormal bone is included in the biopsy sample.)

In this patient, it was necessary to tap the needle with a small orthopedic hammer to penetrate the osteodense lesion. After the lesion had been entered for a distance of more than 5 mm, the biopsy needle was rotated under pressure and retracted while negative pressure was maintained with a 20-mL syringe mounted on the hollow biopsy needle. (In the authors' experience, this may help to keep the biopsy sample within the biopsy needle.) The inner needle was used to push the biopsy sample from the biopsy needle into the recipient. The biopsy sample was visually inspected; the transition zone from normal bone marrow (red color) to abnormal bone marrow (white color) was seen, and the size of the sample of abnormal bone marrow was considered sufficient for pathologic examination. No second biopsy sample was taken. Pathology revealed infiltration by an osteoblastic tumor that was a prostate cancer metastasis.

Discussion

Background

Vertebral biopsy is often indicated in cases of suspected neoplastic lesions or infectious spondylitis. Historically, open surgical biopsy of the spine was the only option for a definitive diagnosis. In recent decades, percutaneous, image-guided vertebral biopsy procedures have been developed and are routinely used; these procedures are faster and more cost-effective, with an overall lower risk for complications. Fluoroscopy and CT are most commonly used for image guidance. The reported accuracy of core biopsy ranges from 77 to 97%.

Noninvasive Imaging Workup

Direct communication between the radiologist and referring physician, with a review of previous imaging and laboratory examinations, is needed to establish an indication for percutaneous vertebral biopsy; the benefits of a definitive diagnosis of a suspected vertebral lesion by biopsy must outweigh the risks of the biopsy procedure.

PHYSICAL EXAMINATION/LABORATORY RESULTS

- Exclude skin lesions (e.g., infection, wound, hemangioma) at the expected skin entry site.
- Laboratory parameters to be determined prior to the procedure are as follows: hematocrit, hemoglobin, platelet count, prothrombin time (PT), partial thromboplastin time (PTT), international normalized ratio (INR), blood urea nitrogen (BUN), and creatinine.
- Interrogate the patient regarding allergies and the use of anticoagulants.

CT/MRI

- Find other, similar lesions at locations that are more easily reached (with a lower risk for complications) for biopsy.
- Evaluate the location and size of the lesion to determine the biopsy trajectory, size of the needle, and type of imaging guidance.
- Evaluate for any associated soft-tissue mass effect of the lesion; sometimes, such tissue can more easily be reached for biopsy.
- Evaluate for intraspinal and foraminal tumoral extension. Be aware that mass effect on the thecal sac or nerve roots may increase in case of hemorrhage during or after the procedure.

PLAIN FILM

- Evaluate if the lesion is sufficiently visible on plain film.
- In case of bone destruction, evaluate if the vertebral outlines necessary for visual navigation of the biopsy needle are sufficiently visible or can be inferred adequately from adjacent vertebral structures. For example, enlargement and bone destruction may cause a pedicle to be invisible on plain film; however, a biopsy can be performed confidently in such a pedicle by using other landmarks of the vertebral body or adjacent vertebrae.

Differential Diagnosis

- Primary bone lesions and tumors
- Secondary bone tumors
- Infectious spondylitis/spondylodiscitis

Procedure Options

SURGICAL PROCEDURE

- Open surgical biopsy may make it possible to obtain larger samples and multiple samples.
- Open surgical biopsy is preferred if the patient is undergoing spinal decompression or stabilization at the same time.

PERCUTANEOUS PROCEDURE

- In our practice, we most often use local anesthesia of the skin and periosteum and reassure the patient verbally. General anesthesia is rarely needed and should be reserved for surgical open biopsy.
- A large array of percutaneous biopsy needles and systems is available. Stylet-bearing 20- or 22-gauge needles can be used for aspiration biopsy. Trephine or beveled-tip 10- to 14-gauge needles are available for core biopsy.
- A core biopsy can be obtained with a coaxial or a tandem technique. In the tandem technique, the needle used for local anesthesia is directed toward the lesion and serves as a visual guide for placing the biopsy needle alongside it. In the coaxial technique, the biopsy needle is placed over the guiding needle (removable hub), and multiple needle passes for biopsy can be performed through the guiding cannula, which remains in place.
- Beveled-tip needles have two intrinsic advantages. Inside the pedicle, the beveled side is turned toward the medial margin of the pedicle to avoid cortical penetration and injury to structures within the spinal canal; inside the vertebral body, the bevel can be used to push against bone, and the needle tip may be redirected slightly away from the beveled side.
- Several approaches to the vertebral body are possible. At lumbar levels, a trans-pedicular or posterolateral approach is used. Thoracic vertebral bodies are entered via a trans-pedicular or trans-costovertebral approach. Cervical levels are most frequently biopsied via an anterolateral approach, with displacement of the carotid vessels.

Possible Complications

- Hematoma and active bleeding: When a trans-pedicular approach is used, hematoma can be avoided by applying pressure to the soft tissues manually after the biopsy needle has been withdrawn. However, when a posterolateral approach is used, retroperitoneal bleeding may occur (which cannot be compressed manually).

- Vascular injury may be the result of direct puncture of arteries or veins, most notably the aorta and inferior vena cava adjacent to the vertebral bodies.
- Neural injury may result from direct puncture of spinal cord or nerves or from an indirect mechanism through vascular injury (anterior spinal artery).
- Pneumothorax may occur.
- Rib fracture: Forceful pressure on the patient's back may cause a rib fracture (e.g., in a patient with osteoporosis).
- Infection may develop, and possibly intraspinal abscess or meningitis.

Published Literature on Treatment Options

Percutaneous spine biopsy has widely replaced open biopsy. The adequacy, accuracy, and complication rates of percutaneous spine biopsy increase with the inner diameter of the biopsy needles used. CT guidance and fluoroscopy guidance do not differ significantly in adequacy and accuracy of tissue sampling. The complication rate of 5.3% for fluoroscopy is higher than the rate of 3.3% for CT guidance. The type, level, and vertebral location of the lesion, together with the expertise of the physician, may determine the choice between fluoroscopy or CT guidance.

Percutaneous spine biopsy has a specific role in reaching the definitive diagnosis of suspected vertebral lesions; a combined clinical, radiologic, and pathologic approach to these lesions provides an excellent diagnostic yield.

PEARLS AND PITFALLS_____

- Review the indication for biopsy with the referring physician, and review the patient's chart (coagulation, allergy).
- Anesthetize the skin, and also the periosteum.
- A Kocher clamp is used to hold the needle during intermittent fluoroscopy, so that the hands of the performing physician are not exposed to radiation. Pulsed fluoroscopy, a low tube current, and a small field of view are key to minimizing the physician's and patient's exposure to radiation while providing sufficient image quality. Some physicians prefer to use leaded gloves.
- Always know the exact position of the needle tip by using both lateral and PA fluoroscopy
- If the lesions are too small or the vertebral landmarks are not easy to locate at fluoroscopy, use CT guidance.

Further Reading

Geremia G, Joglekar S. Percutaneous needle biopsy of the spine. Neuroimaging Clin N Am 2000;10(3):503–533

Nourbakhsh A, Grady JJ, Garges KJ. Percutaneous spine biopsy: a meta-analysis. J Bone Joint Surg Am 2008;90(8):1722–1725

Stoker DJ, Kissin CM. Percutaneous vertebral biopsy: a review of 135 cases. Clin Radiol 1985;36(6):569–577

Tehranzadeh J, Tao C, Browning CA. Percutaneous needle biopsy of the spine. Acta Radiol 2007;48 (8):860–868

CASE 67

Case Description

Clinical Presentation

A 72-year-old woman living in a coastal city enjoyed her daily long walks on the beach. She has no previous medical history. One morning, she wakes up with a severely painful back, which leaves her immobilized in bed. Rest and pain medication are not helpful in alleviating the pain, and with great difficulty she manages to get to the local hospital a few days later. Laboratory findings are normal. Clinical examination and plain films of the lumbar spine are not considered suggestive of painful vertebral compression fracture (VCF). The patient is sent back home with a presumed diagnosis of fecal impaction but is bedridden with persistent pain. Her nephew, a nurse at the radiology department of our hospital, 100 miles inland, arranges to transfer the patient to our unit for MRI.

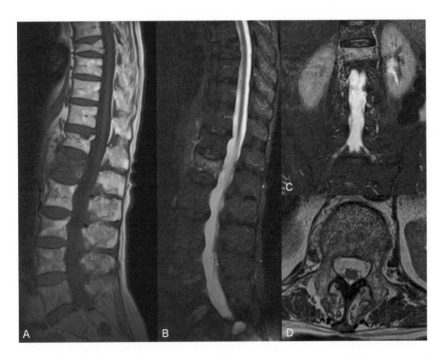

Fig. 67.1 (A–D) Sagittal T1-weighted and STIR MR images, coronal STIR image, and transverse T2-weighted MR image.

Radiologic Studies

MRI

MRI of the lumbar spine revealed multiple VCFs. The VCFs at levels L3, T12, and T8 demonstrated normal bone marrow signal on STIR (short T1 inversion recovery) and T1-weighted images and were considered healed fractures. The VCF at level L1 showed diffusely increased signal on STIR images and decreased signal on T1-weighted images, strongly suggestive of an acute VCF. Coronal STIR images with a large field of view excluded the presence of acute VCFs at other levels and demonstrated no sacral insufficiency fracture. Transverse T2-weighted images excluded displacement of the posterior wall of the vertebral body and medullary compression. The latter images were useful to plan the trans-pedicular bone needle trajectory for vertebroplasty by demonstrating the size and direction of the pedicles (**Fig. 67.1**).

Diagnosis

Acute VCF of L1

Treatment

EQUIPMENT

- Kocher clamp
- Cutter
- Two 11-gauge, 10-cm Cook M1M bone needles with beveled tips
- Cement (liquid monomer and powder)
- One 20-mL Janet-type syringe
- Seven 1-mL syringes with reinforced plungers (Medallion)
- Steri-Strips

DESCRIPTION

The patient underwent general anesthesia and was gently turned into a prone position on the table in the angiography suite. Supporting cushions at the upper thorax and pelvis helped to bring the spine into a hyperlordotic position (sometimes helpful for restoring height) and to prevent rib fractures. Sterile draping and sterile cleansing of the skin were done. On the left, a trans-pedicular approach toward vertebral body L1 was chosen. The skin entry site was determined with PA fluoroscopy, and a 5-mm-wide skin incision was performed. The skin entry site was 2 cm lateral to the pedicle, and the needle was pushed through the soft tissues toward the outer margin of the pedicle until bone contact was felt. With the tip of the needle between the mammillary process and accessory process of the pedicle and with the bevel turned laterally, the cortical bone could be penetrated by using short rotating movements. Once the needle tip was inside the pedicle, its position was checked on lateral fluoroscopy. On PA view, the needle was advanced deeper into the pedicle. Care was taken not to pass beyond the inner or lower margin of the pedicle to avoid intraspinal or nerve root damage; therefore, the bevel was turned medially or inferiorly if the needle tip approached the margins on the PA view. Once the needle tip was inside the vertebral body on the lateral view, the bevel could be turned laterally again to help slide the needle tip toward the midline of the vertebral body. On the right, an extrapedicular approach with a more craniocaudal trajectory was chosen, and therefore the skin entry site was 2 cm lateral and 2 cm superior to the pedicle. The needle was advanced in a craniocaudal direction through the soft tissues and aimed at the superolateral side of the pedicle until bone contact was felt. Cortical bone on the superior side of the pedicle base or on the postero-superior side of the vertebral body was penetrated with the bevel turned cranially. Once inside the trabecular bone of the vertebral body, the needle was advanced toward the midline of the vertebral body with the bevel directed cranially and/or laterally (**Fig. 67.2**).

After both needle tips were positioned in the anterior one-third of the vertebral body, cement was prepared. A 20-mL Janet-type syringe was filled with the liquid cement and used to fill the 1-mL syringes. The syringe filled first was used to intermittently test the liquidity of the cement. While the plunger is pushed gently, the liquid cement initially drips out of the syringe, and as the cement

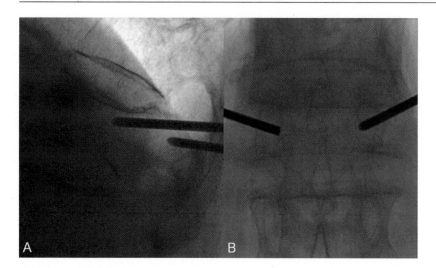

Fig. 67.2 (A,B) Lateral and PA fluoroscopy view. The left bone needle has a transpedicular trajectory, and the bevel is turned medially (toward the inner margin of the pedicle) to avoid cortical penetration toward the spinal canal. The right bone needle has an extrapedicular trajectory; because the needle tip has already passed the posterior wall of the vertebral body, the bevel is turned laterally to help slide the needle tip toward the midline of the vertebral body.

slowly becomes more viscous, the drip rate slows. When the cement curls like tooth paste at the tip of the syringe and does not drip any longer, it is ready to be injected.

Cement was injected very slowly under continuous fluoroscopic control in the lateral view as careful attention was paid to the spread of cement inside the vertebral body and eventually to stop the cement injection in case of leakage outside the vertebral body. A trabecular spread of cement (honeycomb or spicular pattern) is indicative of the interdigitation of cement with trabecular bone (**Fig. 67.3**). After the inner needles were repositioned within the bone needles (pushing the cement out of the bone needles), the bone needles were retracted without causing a cement antenna in the soft tissues. The skin incisions were cleansed and closed with Steri-Strips. After 10 minutes of cement hardening, the patient was turned to a supine position and awakened. She had to remain in

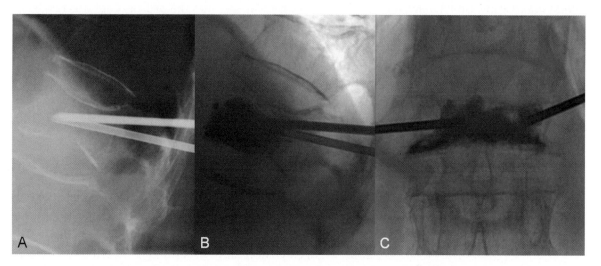

Fig. 67.3 (A–C) Lateral and PA views. With the needle tips in the anterior one-third of the vertebral body, cement is slowly injected with the use of continuous lateral fluoroscopy. Note the trabecular spread of cement.

bed (supine position on a flat mattress) for 4 hours to allow the cement to harden completely. The patient was discharged the next day and returned within a week to her normal level of daily activity with strongly reduced pain scores. The patient has now resumed her long walks on the beach and invites her nephew to come along.

Discussion

Background

Osteoporosis is a skeletal condition characterized by low bone mass and abnormal bony microarchitecture, which lead to an increased risk for fracture with minimal trauma. Aging, menopause, and other factors, such as alcohol and smoking, can result in bone loss and eventually low bone mass. Vertebral fractures account for almost half of all symptomatic osteoporotic fractures, and patients with these fractures have an increased mortality (up to 25–30%) compared with age-matched controls. In the Unites States, 700,000 to 1,200,000 new VCFs result from osteoporosis each year, with direct costs exceeding $15 billion. The risk for subsequent vertebral fracture is sevenfold to 10-fold higher in individuals who sustained a previous vertebral fracture, and the incidence of a new vertebral fracture within a year after a vertebral fracture approaches 20%.

Deramond and Galibert in France performed the first percutaneous vertebroplasty in 1984 when they injected bone cement into a C2 vertebral body weakened by an aggressive hemangioma. The extensive French experience with this technique was presented in 1993 at the second World Federation of Interventional and Therapeutic Neuroradiology Congress in Vancouver, BC, Canada, after which several North American teams became interested in the technique. In the United States, it began to be applied widely after investigators at the University of Virginia reported an 85 to 90% rate of significant pain relief in patients with osteoporotic compression fractures. During the following decade, percutaneous vertebroplasty developed into a routine clinical technique that is indicated for patients with pain resulting from osteoporotic VCFs that are not effectively treated by medical or conservative therapy. Additional indications were established for patients with painful destruction of vertebral bodies resulting from multiple myeloma, aggressive hemangioma, or metastasis.

Noninvasive Imaging Workup

PHYSICAL EXAMINATION AND LABORATORY ANALYSIS

- It is important to correlate the symptoms and location of pain with the findings on imaging (MRI); do not base a treatment decision on the imaging findings alone. Tapping the spinal processes and an axial compression test of the spine are useful to locate the source of back pain. Pain radiating into the lower limbs may be present but should not be the primary indication for cement augmentation
- Use pain scores (Visual Analogue Scale) and scores of daily life activity (e.g., Roland-Morris Disability Index) to evaluate patients before and after treatment.
- A routine blood analysis, including coagulation parameters, is necessary before the procedure

RADIOGRAPHY

- Strictly lateral and AP radiographs are used.
- Apply the Genant classification: semiquantitative visual grading of vertebral fractures regarding height loss (grade 0: normal height; grade 1 or mild fracture: 20–25% height loss; grade 2 or moderate fracture: 25–40% height loss; grade 3 or severe fracture: ≥ 40% height loss) and shape (wedge, biconcave, or crush fracture).

CT

- CT can be useful to evaluate displacement of the posterior wall, cortical breaches, and the direction of trabecular fracture lines (predicting cement distribution or leakage).
- CT can be used to search for signs of pathologic fracture, such as osteolytic areas or soft-tissue and epidural mass.

MRI

- Use inversion recovery (STIR or TIR [turbo inversion recovery]) sequences to detect bone marrow edema; T2-weighted sequences with fat saturation may be used as an alternative. Confirm areas of bone marrow edema on T1-weighted images.
- Add a coronal STIR sequence with a large field of view to detect other recent VCFs or paravertebral rib fractures, and to exclude (insufficiency) fractures of the sacrum (sacral wings).
- Evaluate bone marrow edema to confirm acute fracture or incompletely healed fracture. Differentiate bone marrow edema due to fracture from Modic type 1 changes, tumor, inflammatory spondylitis, and infectious spondylodiscitis.
- Search for signs of pathologic fracture, tumoral bone marrow involvement, or soft-tissue mass.
- In case of posterior wall displacement, evaluate possible compression of the cord or the cauda equina.
- Detect bone marrow edema in posterior elements of the vertebrae, such as the lamina and spinous process, and soft-tissue edema in interspinous or supraspinous ligaments; these findings in association with a (wedge) fracture of the vertebral body may indicate an increased risk for delayed healing or further compression if conservative treatment is chosen.
- Detect bone marrow edema in the pedicles; if a fracture in the pedicles is present, one may leave a cement antenna within the pedicle at the end of the cement injection when retracting the working cannula that is positioned following a trans-pedicular trajectory.
- Assess the size and direction of the pedicles of the fractured vertebra.

BONE MINERAL DENSITOMETRY

- Bone mineral densitometry is useful to establish the diagnosis of (postmenopausal) osteoporosis and to predict fracture risk. In Caucasian American women older than 64 years of age, for each decrease of one standard deviation in bone mineral density at the hip (Z-score), the relative risk for hip fracture increases 2.6-fold.
- Dual-energy x-ray absorptiometry (DEXA) is a 2D projection technique, and osteoporotic change may sometimes be obscured in the spine. Impacted, fractured bone is more compact and therefore may appear denser, and degenerative changes with osteophyte formation and subchondral sclerosis may also result in increased density. Therefore, an additional measurement of bone mineral density at the femoral neck is useful (except for patients with bilateral hip prostheses).

NUCLEAR MEDICINE STUDIES

- Imaging is performed 3 hours after the intravenous injection of technetium Tc 99m methylene diphosphonate (555–925 MBq).
- Increased tracer uptake reflects osteoblastic activity in bone; bandlike, intense tracer accumulation is seen in the vertebral bodies in osteoporotic or traumatic VCFs.
- In elderly patients, imaging should be delayed for 72 hours after trauma (or the onset of pain) because osteoblastic bone repair may be slower or weaker in them than in younger individuals.
- Tracer accumulation in vertebral fractures is very intense during the first months, then gradually diminishes to nearly normal after 18 to 24 months; therefore, the bone scan is able to distinguish between (sub)acute and older collapses.
- Nuclear medicine studies easily detect additional VCFs and paravertebral rib fractures.

Differential Diagnosis

- VCF caused by weakened bone associated with primary or secondary bone tumors or osteomalacia
- Rib fracture (with or without VCF)

Treatment Options

CONSERVATIVE OR MEDICAL MANAGEMENT

- Pain medication
- Relative bed rest
- External bracing
- Physiotherapy
- Peroral or intravenous biphosphonates

PERCUTANEOUS TREATMENT

- Percutaneous vertebroplasty
- Percutaneous kyphoplasty (performed with a balloon, a balloon and stent, or a radiofrequency technique)

SURGICAL TREATMENT

- Instrumented (posterior) vertebral fixation

Possible Complications

- During instrument positioning: Damage to intraspinal or paraspinal neural or vascular structures may occur.
- During cement injection: If the cement is too liquid during injection, it will not displace the bone marrow. Instead, it will enter the vascular channels and leak outside the vertebral body into paravertebral veins. This liquid cement may flow quickly toward the right atrium of the heart and form cement emboli in the pulmonary arteries. If a patent foramen ovale is present, cement emboli may even cause paradoxical infarctions. Cement leakage into vascular channels connecting to the central veins posteriorly in the vertebral body may cause cement to enter the anterior epidural venous plexus. Cement leakage in the paravertebral soft tissues is less important except when the upper side of the neural foramen is involved (injury to exiting nerve root by compression or thermal effect) or when the cement leaks into the spinal canal (compressing intraspinal neural structures). Cement leakage into the intervertebral disk space is clinically less important, but in some cases it may cause acute, painful Schmorl's nodes or even endplate fractures of adjacent vertebrae.
- When the bone needles are retracted after cement injection, cement antennas in the posterior soft tissues should be avoided. Therefore, all cement should be pushed out of the bone needles into the vertebral body, and the bone needles should be retracted with the use of lateral fluoroscopy. If cement is left in the bone needle, one should wait until the cement has hardened before retracting the needle (wiggling the bone needle may help to break the cement cylinder at the transition between bone and soft tissue). If, nevertheless, a cement cylinder forms in the soft tissues, one may often be able to retrieve it with the bone needle under fluoroscopy.
- After the procedure, additional VCFs may occur at other (adjacent or nonadjacent) levels.

Published Literature on Treatment Options

Conventional open surgery for vertebral fractures is associated with risks resulting from open reduction and internal fixation and is therefore usually reserved for fractures that cause neurologic impairment. Surgical fixation in osteoporotic bone has been unsuccessful because of loosening of the intraosseous screws.

Conservative treatment is effective (often only in the long run), but considerable morbidity and mortality are associated if prolonged relative immobilization of the patient is needed. Morbidity includes pneumonia, deep vein thrombosis and pulmonary emboli, gastrointestinal dysfunction, muscle wasting, and depression.

Percutaneous vertebroplasty, a minimally invasive procedure, has been shown to have substantial benefits for patients with osteoporotic VCFs, in particular during the first month after fracture. These include considerable and often immediate reduction of pain, improved ability to perform the activities of daily living, decreased use of pain medication, and shorter hospital stay.

Recently, two randomized studies published in *The New England Journal of Medicine* have questioned the benefits of percutaneous vertebroplasty; the results of these studies suggested that percutaneous vertebroplasty is no more effective than placebo treatment. This contradicts the personal experience of many radiologists and surgeons, as well as the results of most of the studies previously published. A commentary of the North American Spine Society suggested that potential confounding factors (e.g., patient selection) might have caused the described neutral results; patients were enrolled up to 1 year after the fracture occurred (instead of up to 6 weeks after fracture). Because patients were informed that they might be randomized into the placebo group, those with the most severe pain were less likely to enroll in the study. The upcoming results of another randomized, controlled multicenter study (VERTOS [Percutaneous Vertebroplasty Versus Conservative Therapy] II) will soon shed more light on the present contradiction in the literature.

PEARLS AND PITFALLS

- Strictly lateral and PA views are necessary to avoid inadvertently positioning the needle within or throughout the spinal canal.
- The beveled edge of the intrapedicular bone needle is turned toward the inner and/or lower margin of the pedicle to avoid passing beyond the cortical bone and damaging intraspinal structures or a nerve root sleeve. It is also useful to direct the tip of the needle within trabecular bone.
- The direction of the pedicle of L5 is often 45 degrees relative to the posterior wall of the vertebral body. With a straight PA trans-pedicular trajectory of the bone needle, the final position of the tip of the bone needle will be lateral to the vertebral body, and cement will be injected into the paravertebral soft tissues.
- The transverse shape of dorsal vertebral bodies may be triangular, and the final position of the tip of the bone needle may easily be lateral to the vertebral body if it is not directed toward the midline. Therefore, study the axial CT or MR images before the procedure.
- The viscosity of the cement is a crucial factor to avoid cement leakage or embolization. If the cement is more liquid than bone marrow, the cement (instead of the bone marrow) will be pushed into the vascular channels and prevertebral veins, and cement emboli may form.
- High-quality fluoroscopy is of paramount importance for a safe cement injection because it makes possible the early detection of cement leakage. If biplanar fluoroscopy is not available, use the lateral view during cement injection and intermittently check the PA view.

Further Reading

Alvarez L, Alcaraz M, Pérez-Higueras A, et al. Percutaneous vertebroplasty: functional improvement in patients with osteoporotic compression fractures. Spine (Phila Pa 1976) 2006;31(10):1113–1118

Anselmetti GC, Corrao G, Monica PD, et al. Pain relief following percutaneous vertebroplasty: results of a series of 283 consecutive patients treated in a single institution. Cardiovasc Intervent Radiol 2007;30(3):441–447

Buchbinder R, Osborne RH, Ebeling PR, et al. A randomized trial of vertebroplasty for painful osteoporotic vertebral fractures. N Engl J Med 2009;361(6):557–568

Evans AJ, Jensen ME, Kip KE, et al. Vertebral compression fractures: pain reduction and improvement in functional mobility after percutaneous polymethylmethacrylate vertebroplasty retrospective report of 245 cases. Radiology 2003;226(2):366–372

Galibert P, Deramond H, Rosat P, Le Gars D. [Preliminary note on the treatment of vertebral angioma by percutaneous acrylic vertebroplasty]. Neurochirurgie 1987;33(2):166–168

Genant HK, Wu CY, van Kuijk C, Nevitt MC. Vertebral fracture assessment using a semiquantitative technique. J Bone Miner Res 1993;8(9):1137–1148

Hasserius R, Karlsson MK, Jónsson B, Redlund-Johnell I, Johnell O. Long-term morbidity and mortality after a clinically diagnosed vertebral fracture in the elderly—a 12- and 22-year follow-up of 257 patients. Calcif Tissue Int 2005;76(4):235–242

Kallmes DF, Comstock BA, Heagerty PJ, et al. A randomized trial of vertebroplasty for osteoporotic spinal fractures. N Engl J Med 2009;361(6):569–579

Legroux-Gérot I, Lormeau C, Boutry N, Cotten A, Duquesnoy B, Cortet B. Long-term follow-up of vertebral osteoporotic fractures treated by percutaneous vertebroplasty. Clin Rheumatol 2004;23(4):310–317

McKiernan F, Faciszewski T, Jensen R. Quality of life following vertebroplasty. J Bone Joint Surg Am 2004;86-A(12):2600–2606

North American Spine Society. Newly Released Vertebroplasty RCTs: A Tale of Two Trials. http://www.spine.org/Documents/NASSComment_on_Vertebroplasty.pdf.

Voormolen MH, Lohle PN, Lampmann LE, et al. Prospective clinical follow-up after percutaneous vertebroplasty in patients with painful osteoporotic vertebral compression fractures. J Vasc Interv Radiol 2006;17(8):1313–1320

Voormolen MH, Mali WP, Lohle PN, et al. Percutaneous vertebroplasty compared with optimal pain medication treatment: short-term clinical outcome of patients with subacute or chronic painful osteoporotic vertebral compression fractures. The VERTOS study. AJNR Am J Neuroradiol 2007;28(3):555–560

CASE 68

Case Description

Clinical Presentation

A 74-year-old man first experienced severe dorsal back pain while shoveling in his garden. Persistent sharp pain in his back caused him to stop working, and he lay down for the rest of the day. The next morning, he felt an increasingly dull pain and had difficulty getting out of bed and dressing himself because of the pain. The patient's general practitioner decided to treat him with relative rest and pain medication.

Four weeks later, the patient presents to the emergency department with persistent dorsal back pain that is impairing his daily life activities. Coughing and sneezing are very painful, breathing is difficult because of pain, and turning to a lateral decubitus from a supine position is painful. His pain score on the Visual Analogue Scale (VAS) is 8/10. His Roland-Morris Disability Index score is 18/24. Manual tapping of all dorsolumbar spinous processes reveals a focal, severe pain reaction at the middorsal level. The axial compression test (the patient stands tiptoe, then falls back on his heels) result is positive (immediate provocation of focal, bandlike pain at the middorsal level). The patient also describes pain radiating along his ribs at this level, but compression of the ribs does not aggravate the pain (making rib fractures less likely). Manual compression on the lateral sides of the iliac wings elicits no pain reaction.

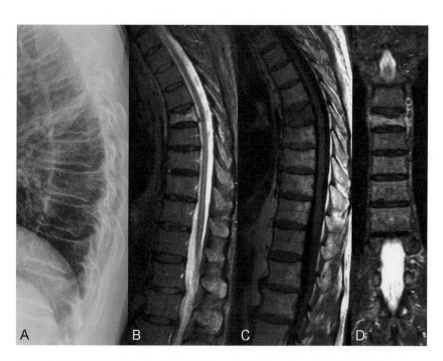

Fig. 68.1 (A–D) Plain film, sagittal STIR, sagittal T1, and coronal STIR MR images.

406

Radiologic Studies

PLAIN FILM

Radiographic examination demonstrated a single compression fracture of the dorsal spine at the level of T7. A wedge deformity with depression of the upper end plate and a height loss of 40% (Genant grade 2) were noted that resulted in a kyphotic angulation of the dorsal spine. Buckling of the anterior wall of the vertebral body was seen.

MRI

The T7 vertebral body demonstrated a diffuse change of signal intensity (i.e., decreased on T1-weighted images and increased on STIR [short T1 inversion recovery] images). Signal intensities in the adjacent vertebrae were normal.

Minor, focal displacement of the posterior wall at the lower half of the T7 vertebral body was noted, with impression on the thecal sac and possible contact with the cord. However, there was no sign of cord compression or myelomalacia. The intervertebral foramina were not narrowed because the height loss of the posterior wall of the vertebral body was minimal. On axial T2-weighted images, normally sized pedicles were seen, and a rounded anterolateral shape of this dorsal vertebral body was appreciated. On the coronal STIR images, there was no evidence of paravertebral rib fractures. Signs of edema were noted in the paravertebral soft tissues of T7 (**Fig. 68.1**).

NUCLEAR MEDICINE

At whole-body scintigraphy with technetium 99m, increased tracer uptake was seen in the body of the T7 vertebra.

DEXA

Bone densitometry with dual-energy x-ray absorption (DEXA) revealed normal bone density for the patient's age (according to the World Health Organization standards, based on a white female population), with mean bone mineral density values of 1.089 g/cm^3 at the lumbar spine and 0.922 g/cm^3 at both hips.

Diagnosis

Vertebral compression fracture (VCF) of T7 without radiologic signs of malignancy

Treatment

EQUIPMENT

- Kocher clamp
- Cutter
- KyphX HV-R Bone Cement (10 mL of liquid monomer and 20 g of powder polymer; Medtronic, Minneapolis, MN)
- Contrast medium
- Kyphon KyphoPak Express Tray and KyphX One-Step Osteo Introducer System (Medtronic) containing working cannulas with beveled tips and diamond tip stylets, bone drill, inflatable bone tamps (balloons), and bone fillers
- Steri-Strips

DESCRIPTION

Under general anesthesia, the patient was placed in the prone position with padding under the shoulders and pelvis in an attempt to reduce the dorsal kyphotic angle by using the patient's own body weight. A trans-costovertebral approach with both working cannulas was performed through a small skin incision (supero)lateral to the pedicle. Once the tips of the stylets in the working cannulas had reached bone lateral on, or superolateral in, the pedicle, the cannulas were aimed toward the middle third of the vertebral body on the PA view and the anterior third on the lateral view. (It is imperative not to pass beyond the inner or inferior cortical outline of the pedicles on the PA view until the tip of the working cannula has passed the posterior wall of the vertebral body on the lateral view. The trick of the beveled edge can be applied as described in Case 67. Working cannulas are in position when the tips have passed the posterior wall of the vertebral body.) A manual drill was advanced through each working cannula into the anterior third of the vertebral body to create a tunnel for positioning a balloon. A correct position of these tunnels was verified in PA and lateral views. By moving a bone filler back and forth, any rough edges in the walls of both tunnels were smoothed (to prevent balloon rupture). From markers on the drill, the length of the balloons needed was determined to be 15 mm. Biopsy was not performed before drilling in this case (**Fig. 68.2**).

Deflated balloons with markers indicating their tip and base were inserted through both working cannulas. Balloon position was locked by slight inflation up to 30 psi immediately after insertion.

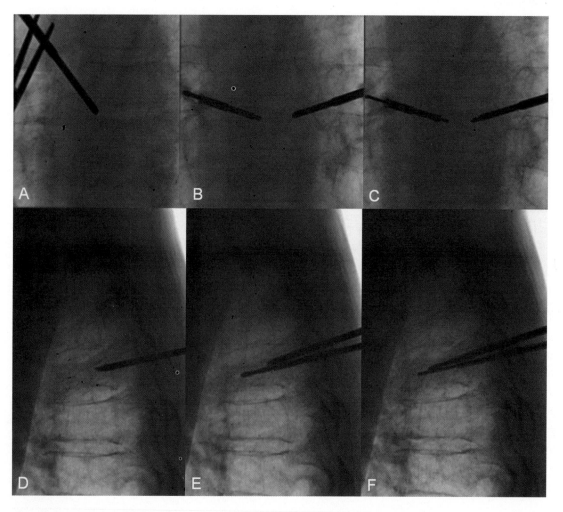

Fig. 68.2 (A–F) PA and lateral fluoroscopy views demonstrate needle insertion just beyond the posterior wall of the vertebral body, drilling of the vertebral body, and smoothing of the wall of the drilling channel with a bone filler.

(Balloons should be inflated only when both markers are outside the working cannula and inside the vertebral body.) Balloon inflation was stepwise and reached 150 psi. Inflating the balloons created a cavity in the vertebral body that was surrounded by a wall of compressed trabecular bone. As long as the balloon pressure dropped after each inflation, more cavity was being created (bone trabeculae were being compressed, and a slight elevation of the upper end plate was visible). When the end plate of the vertebral body was reached, the shape of the balloons was becoming flatter and pressure was no longer dropping as fast. This was considered the end point of the balloon insufflations (**Fig. 68.3**).

The volume of the insufflated balloons was 2 mL each, and therefore five bone fillers were prepared with cement. Once the cement had reached the correct viscosity (stopped dripping from the tip of the bone filler), the balloons were deflated and retracted. Cement was slowly injected with the tip of the bone filler positioned anteriorly in the created cavities. Injection was possible in the low-pressure bone cavities and was closely inspected with lateral fluoroscopy to detect possible cement leakage. At first, a rather homogeneous cement fill of the cavities was seen. This was followed by interdigitation of the cement with the surrounding trabecular bone. There was no cement leakage outside the vertebral body (**Fig. 68.4**).

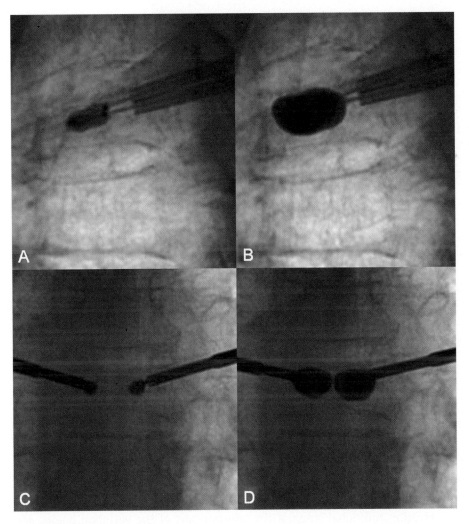

Fig. 68.3 (A–D) Lateral and PA views of balloon insufflations with contrast medium. Note flattening of the upper side of the balloon that is pushing against the upper end plate, resulting in some elevation of the upper end plate.

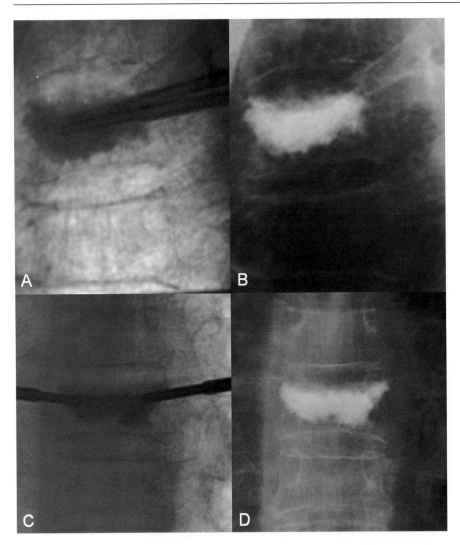

Fig. 68.4 (A–D) Lateral and PA views of cement injection with the bone fillers anteriorly in the cavities created by balloon insufflation.

After the working cannulas had been removed, the skin incisions were closed with Steri-Strips. After a 10-minute delay to allow the cement to harden, the patient was awakened and turned into a supine position. This position was maintained for 4 hours to allow the cement to harden completely. The next morning, the patient was discharged from the hospital with considerable pain relief (VAS score 2/10).

Discussion

Background

According to the International Osteoporosis Foundation, more than 40% of middle-aged women in Europe will sustain one or more osteoporotic fractures during their lifetime. The presence of one vertebral fracture increases the risk for a subsequent vertebral fracture fivefold. Of women with a recent osteoporotic vertebral fracture, 20% will sustain a new fracture within the next 12 months. Both symptomatic and asymptomatic vertebral fractures are associated with increased morbidity (e.g., decreased physical function and social isolation) and mortality. Kyphosis shifts the patient's center of gravity forward, creating additional stress at the anterior part of the vertebral bodies and increasing the risk for fracture. Kyphosis may also decrease the pulmonary vital capacity (adding to the restrictive lung disease of many elderly patients) and cause gastrointestinal difficulties.

Balloon-assisted kyphoplasty is a minimally invasive procedure used to treat VCF; the goals are to reduce pain, disability, and vertebral deformity by placing catheters with inflatable bone tamps inside the fractured vertebral body. Balloon inflation with contrast medium makes the surrounding cancellous bone more compact and creates a cavity inside the vertebral body. Furthermore, it may push the end plates apart, partly restore height, and correct angular deformity.

Indications for balloon-assisted kyphoplasty include osteoporotic, osteolytic (multiple myeloma, metastasis), and traumatic VCFs. Balloon-assisted kyphoplasty has been found particularly helpful when applied early after fracture (within 3 months), if the fracture deformity causes a kyphotic angle of more than 15 degrees, if there is an increased risk for cement leakage (large breaches in the cortical bone of the vertebral body), and if a good chance for height restoration is noted on the preoperative workup (wide horizontal cleft on CT/MRI, change in vertebral height on supine versus erect lateral radiography or during inspiration versus expiration in the supine position).

Instrumentation to perform kyphoplasty is constantly evolving. Current development strategies include the following: tools for creating cavities (bone scrapers or osteotomes to be used instead of the balloon); tools to maintain restored vertebral height when the balloon is deflated (balloon-with-stent technique); smaller tools to be used at higher dorsal levels; tools to inject cement from a distance (to decrease the physician's exposure to radiation); and restoration of height with pressurized (viscous) cement injection. The kyphoplasty instrumentation set used in this case consists of smaller tools and is found useful for the treatment of small vertebral bodies, vertebral bodies with narrow pedicles, and extremely compressed vertebral bodies.

Noninvasive Imaging Workup

PHYSICAL EXAMINATION

- Correlate the symptoms and location of pain with the imaging findings. Focal or bandlike back pain at the level of the fracture should be present. Radicular pain below the knees typically does not resolve after vertebral body augmentation.
- Use a pain-scoring scale (VAS) and instruments that measure quality of life and physical function (Roland-Morris Disability Index, SF-36 Physical Component Score [PCS], European Vertebral Osteoporosis Study [EVOS], EQ-5D).
- Routine blood analysis, including coagulation parameters, is required.

RADIOGRAPHY

- Strictly lateral and AP radiographs are used.
- Optionally, obtain lateral images with the patient in the prone and erect positions to detect changes in the height of the vertebral body and predict possible restoration of height with balloon kyphoplasty. In some cases, a change in vertebral height may also be seen with fluoroscopy during inspiration and expiration (lateral view, patient supine or prone).

CT

- CT is useful to evaluate fracture lines, cortical breaches, and displacement of bone fragments.
- Search for signs of pathologic fracture.

MRI

- Search for bone marrow edema to confirm acute fracture or incompletely healed fracture. Differentiate bone marrow edema due to fracture from Modic type 1 changes, tumor, inflammatory spondylitis, and infectious spondylodiscitis.
- In case of posterior wall displacement, evaluate for possible compression of neural elements.
- Assess the AP diameter of the fractured vertebra to choose the length of the balloon.

- Assess the shape of the vertebral body in the axial plane; the triangular or rounded shape of (dorsal) vertebral bodies may be invisible on fluoroscopy, so that the cortex may be breached at the anterolateral aspect of the vertebral body (often not appreciated by the performing physician), causing puncture of the aorta or leakage of a large volume of cement.

Differential Diagnosis

- Pathologic fracture: primary bone tumor, metastasis, multiple myeloma, vertebral hemangioma (aggressive type)
- Traumatic fracture versus insufficiency fracture
- Abnormal bone strength due to osteoporosis versus osteomalacia (e.g., Paget disease).
- Pain caused by paravertebral rib fracture, not (solely) by VCF
- Pain caused by other spinal disease (e.g., degenerative disk disease, facet degeneration, Baastrup disease, paraspinal hematoma); pain caused by nonspinal disease (e.g., pancreatic cancer)
- Bone marrow edema on MRI or increased tracer uptake on nuclear scan caused by degenerative changes (underlying active osteophyte formation), not directly by bone contusion or bone fracture. Degenerative changes may indirectly be the result of a previous compression fracture from several months or even more than a year earlier.

Treatment Options

- Percutaneous vertebral augmentation (vertebroplasty, kyphoplasty)
- Surgery with instrumented stabilization
- Preventive measures such as anti-osteoporosis medication (biphosphonates) and fall prevention programs

Possible Complications

- During instrument positioning: perforation of the inner wall of the pedicle and damage to structures in the spinal canal; perforation of the inferior wall of the pedicle and damage to the dural sleeve or exiting nerve root; perforation of the cortex of the vertebral body and damage to paravertebral structures (e.g., aorta, inferior vena cava, azygos vein), pneumothorax.
- During balloon inflation: breaching the cortex of the vertebral body instead of compressing trabecular bone toward the cortical bone; balloon rupture (the ruptured balloon can be replaced with another balloon after the ruptured one has been retracted).
- During cement injection: cement leakage if the cement is too liquid during injection. Cement leakage is reported to be less frequent with balloon kyphoplasty than with vertebroplasty, probably because a much lower injection pressure is needed to fill the created bone cavities in balloon-assisted kyphoplasty than is needed to fill the marrow spaces of trabecular bone in vertebroplasty

Published Literature on Treatment Options

The Fracture Reduction Evaluation (FREE) trial is a randomized, controlled multicenter trial comparing balloon kyphoplasty treatment with nonsurgical care in patients with VCFs less than 3 months old. Within the first month, kyphoplasty resulted in improvements in quality of life and disability measures and a reduction in back pain in patients with acute painful vertebral fractures. Although differences in improvement diminished by 1 year after treatment, a nonrandomized, controlled study performed by Grafe et al found that the addition of kyphoplasty to medical treatment persistently reduced pain, the occurrence of new vertebral fractures, and healthcare utilization for at least 12 months in patients with primary osteoporosis. In a case series with 2-year follow-up by Ledlie et al, kyphoplasty markedly improved clinical outcome and resulted in significant restoration of vertebral height.

PEARLS AND PITFALLS _____

- To know precisely the position of the tips of your instruments, strictly lateral and AP views should be available, and the performing physician should have studied the shape as well as the fracture lines of the vertebral body on preoperative transsectional imaging.
- Working cannulas should be positioned just beyond the posterior wall of the vertebral body before a drill or balloon is introduced.
- The primary goal of balloon insufflations is to create a cavity within the vertebral body that enables a low-pressure injection of cement. Pushing balloon insufflations to the limit to completely restore vertebral body height or correct a vertebral body deformity may result in complications.
- Slow and stepwise balloon insufflations from both sides are recommended to achieve symmetric height and reduce deformity. Check the drop in balloon pressure between insufflations, which is a measure of ongoing cavity creation.
- The cement injection should start in the anterior part of the created bone cavities to avoid cement leakage posteriorly (toward the spinal canal); use continuous fluoroscopic control in the lateral view to detect cement leakage early on.

Further Reading

Bouza C, López T, Magro A, Navalpotro L, Amate JM. Efficacy and safety of balloon kyphoplasty in the treatment of vertebral compression fractures: a systematic review. Eur Spine J 2006;15(7):1050–1067

Diel P, Reuss W, Aghayev E, Moulin P, Röder C; on behalf of the SWISSspine Registry Group. SWISSspine-a nationwide health technology assessment registry for balloon kyphoplasty: methodology and first results. Spine J 2009 October 8 (Epub ahead of print)

Grafe IA, Da Fonseca K, Hillmeier J, et al. Reduction of pain and fracture incidence after kyphoplasty: 1-year outcomes of a prospective controlled trial of patients with primary osteoporosis. Osteoporos Int 2005;16(12):2005–2012

Ledlie JT, Renfro MB. Kyphoplasty treatment of vertebral fractures: 2-year outcomes show sustained benefits. Spine (Phila Pa 1976) 2006;31(1):57–64

Taylor RS, Fritzell P, Taylor RJ. Balloon kyphoplasty in the management of vertebral compression fractures: an updated systematic review and meta-analysis. Eur Spine J 2007;16(8):1085–1100

Voggenreiter G. Balloon kyphoplasty is effective in deformity correction of osteoporotic vertebral compression fractures. Spine (Phila Pa 1976) 2005;30(24):2806–2812

Wardlaw D, Cummings SR, Van Meirhaeghe J, et al. Efficacy and safety of balloon kyphoplasty compared with non-surgical care for vertebral compression fracture (FREE): a randomised controlled trial. Lancet 2009;373(9668):1016–1024

Weisskopf M, Ohnsorge JA, Niethard FU. Intravertebral pressure during vertebroplasty and balloon kyphoplasty: an in vitro study. Spine (Phila Pa 1976) 2008;33(2):178–182

CASE 69

Case Description

Clinical Presentation

A 68-year-old man is referred by his oncologist for consideration of balloon kyphoplasty for vertebral compression fracture secondary to multiple myeloma (MM). Two months prior, he underwent surgical decompression and instrumented fusion for cord compression at T7 and T9 that left him with residual severe lower limb paraparesis and a Brown-Séquard syndrome. Now, acute, severe pain has developed in the lumbar spine, with a score of 8/10 to 9/10 on the Visual Analogue Scale (VAS). He is unable to bear weight or roll over in bed. Pain medications include oxycodone and gabapentin, which are titrated to his pain and activity levels. At the time of assessment, he has been unable to stand unassisted for 3 months, requires a wheelchair for mobility, and is struggling to manage the activities of daily living despite excellent support from his wife and daughter.

Physical examination demonstrates tenderness to palpation and percussion over the lumbar spine, with grade 4/5 power in the right lower limb and grade 3/5 power in the left quadriceps, knee extensors and flexors, and ankle flexors and extensors. There is no objective sensory abnormality. His knee and ankle reflexes are brisk on the left, normal on the right.

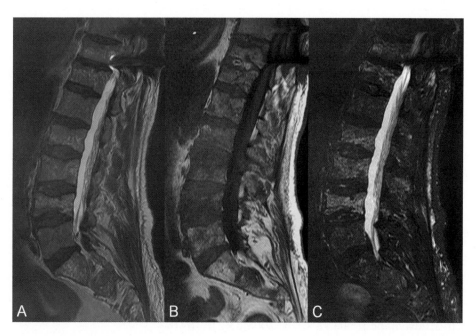

Fig. 69.1 (A–C) Sagittal T2-weighted, T1-weighted, and STIR MR images demonstrate superior and inferior end plate collapse, infiltration of the marrow with tumor, and compressed, edematous bone at multiple levels (T11, T12, L2, L3, and L4).

Radiologic Studies

On plain film, AP and lateral views of the lumbar spine demonstrated new vertebral compression fractures at L2, L3, and L4, which had not been present 3 months prior.

On MRI at 1.5 T, sagittal and axial T1, T2, and STIR (short T1 inversion recovery) sequences of the thoracic and lumbar spine demonstrated multifocal marrow signal abnormality: T1 hypointensity with STIR and T2 hyperintensity involving the T11, T12, L2, L3, and L4 levels. End plate compression fracture deformities were noted at L2 (inferior end plate), L3, and L4 (both the superior and inferior end plates). The loss of height was 20% (L2), 30% (L3), and 45% (L4). MM involved the sacrum, and anterior wedge compression fractures of the T7 and T9 vertebral bodies were noted, with an adequate thoracic surgical decompression and susceptibility artifact from the instrumentation (**Fig. 69.1**).

Diagnosis

Multilevel wedge and end plate compression fractures of the thoracic and lumbar spine, with new compression fractures at L2, L3, and L4 in a patient with known MM

Treatment

EQUIPMENT

- Scalpel with No. 11 blade
- A 10-mL syringe
- Straight, long-handled artery forceps (for holding needles)
- Small artery forceps
- Mallet
- KyphX Two-Step Osteo Introducer System (Medtronic, Minneapolis, MN)
- KyphX Xpander Inflatable Bone Tamp with 20/3 balloon
- KyphX Bone Filler Device
- KyphX HV-R (High-Viscosity Radiopaque) Bone Cement
- Kyphon Mixer
- Contrast

DESCRIPTION

The patient was offered a three-level balloon kyphoplasty at L2, L3, and L4. This was carried out as a day surgery procedure with conscious sedation, local anesthesia, and monitoring of the electrocardiogram, blood pressure, pulse, and oxygen saturation. The patient was placed in a prone position with bolsters and pillows supporting the pelvis and thorax to allow free diaphragmatic breathing. Treatment was performed with biplane fluoroscopy that was positioned over the pedicles in the AP plane with a craniocaudal angle parallel to the vertebral end plate. The AP tube was then angled 10 to 20 degrees in a right anterior oblique direction to view the right pedicle en face, with care taken to be able to visualize the medial cortex of the pedicle. The lateral fluoroscopy was centered on L2 perpendicular to the posterior cortex with the pedicles superimposed over each other.

Local anesthesia (50:50 mixture of 1% lidocaine and 0.5% bupivacaine) was deepened to the periosteum overlying the pedicle with a 22-gauge spinal needle. A 13-gauge Jamshidi (CareFusion, San Diego, CA) needle was introduced and positioned at the center of the right pedicle, at the junction of the upper and middle thirds, and then advanced under fluoroscopy into the posterior body without any breach of the medial cortex of the pedicle on the angled AP projection. A guidewire

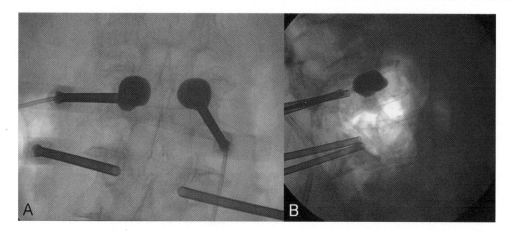

Fig. 69.2 (A,B) Balloon inflation at L2 in AP and lateral views with the cannula positioned anterior to the posterior cortex of the body.

was advanced to the anterior body before the Jamshidi needle was removed. The Osteo Introducer System was passed over the guidewire anterior to the posterior cortex. The hand drill was used to clear a track for the Bone Tamp device. This procedure was repeated to access the left pedicle at L2, then repeated at the L3 and L4 levels.

Six 20/3 KyphX Xpander Inflatable Bone Tamp devices were introduced through the cannulas and positioned adjacent to the compression fractures before inflation with 3 to 4 mL of contrast. (At this point, additional intravenous analgesia may be needed because the balloon expansion is painful. An option at this point is to use a KyphX Latitude Curette device to create a cavity in the body to facilitate balloon expansion.) The balloons were left inflated to provide hemostasis while the poly-methylmethacrylate (PMMA) cement was being mixed (**Fig. 69.2**).

The KyphX HV-R (High-Viscosity Radiopaque) Bone Cement was mixed, and the bone filler devices were filled with 1.5 mL of cement. When the cement had reached the appropriate viscosity,

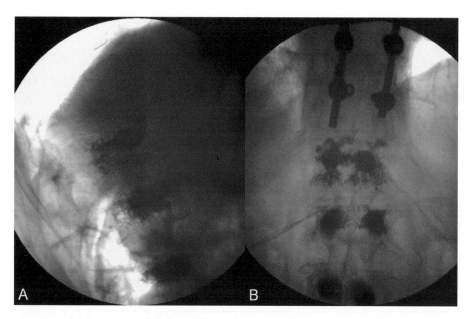

Fig. 69.3 (A,B) After PMMA injection in lateral and PA views. Infiltration into the matrix around the cavity demonstrates the severity of the osteopenia in MM.

the balloons were deflated and removed, the bone filler devices were introduced into the anterior part of the cavity, and the cement was injected without pressure under direct vision with monitoring for leakage beyond the cortical margins of the vertebra. There was no extravasation, with adequate filling of all the vertebral bodies (**Fig. 69.3**).

This stage of the procedure needs to be carefully timed to achieve satisfactory filling at three levels through six cannulas. If necessary, it can be done in two stages with a second batch of cement. Firm compression of the puncture sites to reduce bleeding into the tissues from the pedicle access points has been shown to reduce postprocedural pain and spasm. The patient was discharged approximately 3 hours after the procedure with a prescription for oral analgesia, instructions for postoperative wound care, and instructions about whom to contact regarding any potential complications or concerns. Appointments for clinical follow-up and follow-up imaging were arranged. Three days after the procedure, the patient was able to discontinue the opiate analgesia, taking acetaminophen as necessary for pain. He was able to bear weight free of pain during transfers and started mobilization with physiotherapy within the first week.

Discussion

Background

Metastatic disease in cancer is common, and 30 to 70% of the roughly 563,700 people who die annually of cancer in the United States have bone metastasis. Symptomatic epidural cord compression occurs in 5 to 14%. Despite advances in cancer therapy, the duration of patient survival following spinal cord compression with neurologic symptoms remains between 3 and 9 months. Multiple lesions at noncontiguous levels occur in 10 to 40% of patients in case series. Pain from vertebral body fracture, neurologic dysfunction, and cord compression are the most common clinical features at presentation.

The general criteria for predicting imminent spinal vertebral body collapse are the following: involvement of more than 50% of the vertebral body, tumor involvement of the pedicle, involvement of half of the body, and involvement of the anterior and posterior elements of the spine. In the thoracic spine specifically, the criteria for risk include involvement of 30% of the vertebral body with costovertebral joint destruction or involvement of 60% of the vertebral body with no destruction of other spinal components. The preservation of quality of life and function and the management of pain are the primary end points of therapy for these patients.

Noninvasive Imaging Workup

Plain films are very insensitive. A loss of bone mass of at least 50% must occur before a metastasis can be detected predictably; therefore, cross-sectional multiplanar imaging techniques are the standard of care.

CT is rapid and can quantitatively evaluate osteolytic and sclerotic lesions of bone and provide multiplanar reconstructions.

In neoplastic disease of the spine, MRI has become the modality of choice. The bone marrow signal changes as the marrow ages from hematopoietic (red) to fatty (yellow) marrow. Radiation accelerates this process. Metastases are seen directly as soft-tissue lesions replacing the marrow signal intensity and are visualized best on the T1-weighted sequence. The T2-weighted sequence is complementary, defining the canal. STIR or equivalent sequences are of critical importance to accurately detect fat infiltration, bone edema, and tumor within the marrow. STIR sequences can differentiate between an old, healed fracture and an edematous, active fracture. Pain relief after PMMA injection correlates significantly with this increased signal.

Treatment Options

CONSERVATIVE OR MEDICAL MANAGEMENT

- In the palliation of metastatic disease, pain control, preservation of function, and quality-of-life issues determine the choice of treatment.
- Bed rest, pain medication, and external bracing are conservative treatment options.

SURGICAL TREATMENT

- Surgical decompression with or without stabilization and instrumentation is an option.

PERCUTANEOUS APPROACHES

- Vertebroplasty
- Kyphoplasty (with a balloon, stents, or radiofrequency techniques)

Possible Complications

- Reported complications include cement leakage with pulmonary embolism, cord or nerve root compression, infection, retroperitoneal hematoma, and fractures of the adjacent segments.

Published Literature on Treatment Options

Of patients with acute cord compression, ~80% who are able to walk at the time of surgery remain ambulatory after treatment. Of patients who are paraplegic before intervention, only 6% regain ambulatory status. With radiotherapy alone, the ambulatory rate after treatment is ~45%. Mortality rates at 1 and 3 months are 9% and 29%, respectively. Postoperative complication rates are reported to be between 27% and 40%, the majority related to wound infection.

The benefits of vertebral stabilization and pain relief are offset by the complications, as previously stated. The incidence of pulmonary embolism is reported to be 0.6% with vertebroplasty and 0.01% with kyphoplasty; the incidence of neurologic complications with vertebroplasty is 0.6% and with kyphoplasty 0.03%. The overall rates of cement extravasation after vertebral augmentation are reported to be as high as 41% for vertebroplasty and 9% for kyphoplasty. Total complication rates are reported to be between 2 and 10%, with higher percentages in cancer patients. The safety profile supports kyphoplasty in the treatment of metastatic vertebral compression fractures.

The primary indication for vertebral augmentation is severe pain (score > 7/10 on the VAS) with the collapse of one or more vertebrae or bone destruction and a high risk for the collapse of one or more vertebrae. The secondary indication is a lower level of pain (score < 7/10 on the VAS) with significant loss of height, structural integrity, or stability.

There are significant contraindications to vertebral augmentation; however, in a palliative role, several "absolute" contraindications may be reconsidered as "relative" contraindications in the management of the patient as a whole. Absolute contraindications to this procedure are the following: contraindications to general or local anesthesia, pregnancy, bleeding disorders, infections (skin, systemic, urinary tract), pain unrelated to vertebral compression fracture, overt instability, severe cardiopulmonary insufficiency, and allergy to procedure-related drugs (PMMA). Relative contraindications are cord compression, lesions above T3, osteoblastic metastases, patient age younger than 40 years, technical difficulties (vertebra plana), and fractures with retropulsed bone.

Recent papers have suggested that vertebroplasty for painful osteoporotic fractures does not confer any benefit compared with a sham or placebo procedure. Careful patient selection, a clearly defined management strategy, and realistic therapeutic goals are important when this type of intervention is offered to a patient with metastatic spine disease. Prevention of a vertebral fracture may prevent a significant deterioration in the patient's quality of life. Vertebral augmentation is considered a relatively low-risk procedure compared with surgery when performed appropriately in carefully selected patients.

PEARLS AND PITFALLS

- If a diagnosis has not yet been made, bone biopsies can be performed during the same procedure with dedicated bone biopsy devices.
- Depending on which end plate has collapsed, the superior or inferior end plate can be selected to allow placement of the needle parallel to the uninjured cortex.
- Kyphoplasty is considered safer than vertebroplasty for patients with tumor.

Further Reading

Hussein MA, Vrionis FD, Allison R, et al; International Myeloma Working Group. The role of vertebral augmentation in multiple myeloma: International Myeloma Working Group Consensus Statement. Leukemia 2008;22(8):1479–1484

Kallmes DF, Comstock BA, Heagerty PJ, et al. A randomized trial of vertebroplasty for osteoporotic spinal fractures. N Engl J Med 2009;361(6):569–579

Lieberman I, Reinhardt MK. Vertebroplasty and kyphoplasty for osteolytic vertebral collapse. Clin Orthop Relat Res 2003; (415 Suppl)S176–S186

Mathis JM. Percutaneous vertebroplasty: complication avoidance and technique optimization. AJNR Am J Neuroradiol 2003;24(8):1697–1706

Taneichi H, Kaneda K, Takeda N, Abumi K, Satoh S. Risk factors and probability of vertebral body collapse in metastases of the thoracic and lumbar spine. Spine (Phila Pa 1976) 1997;22(3):239–245

Wardlaw D, Cummings SR, Van Meirhaeghe J, et al. Efficacy and safety of balloon kyphoplasty compared with non-surgical care for vertebral compression fracture (FREE): a randomised controlled trial. Lancet 2009;373(9668):1016–1024

CASE 70

Case Description

Clinical Presentation

An 84-year-old woman is referred to our institution from a geriatric rehabilitation center with a painful vertebral compression fracture (VCF). The patient has a history of low back pain that worsened significantly 3 months earlier after a fall that caused an L1 VCF. Initially, the patient responded to medical management, but now, after 3 months of conservative therapy, the intensity of her pain has increased to 7/10 on the Visual Analogue Scale (VAS). A physical examination reveals no focal neurologic deficit or radicular symptoms. For treatment planning, MRI and CT of the thoracolumbar spine are performed.

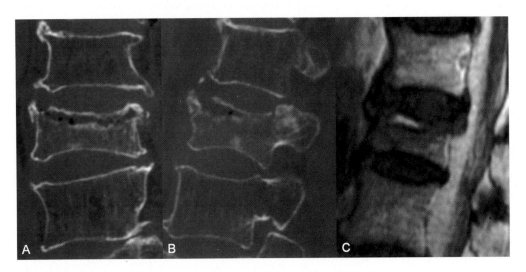

Fig. 70.1 (A–C) Plain CT (coronal, sagittal) and MRI (sagittal T2-weighted).

Radiologic Studies

CT

Plain CT of the spine demonstrated an L1 VCF. The fracture line extended from the anterior to the posterior margin (type A), but not into the posterior column. Osseous impaction of ~20% of the original height (grade 2) was noted (**Fig. 70.1 A,B**). The margins of the fracture were partially impacted and sclerotic, and the cleft was open when the patient was in the supine position, indicating a mobile fracture. Neighboring levels demonstrated reduced bone density, suggesting generalized osteoporosis.

MRI

No further fracture levels, no compression of neural elements, and no evidence of an epidural hemorrhage were detected on screening MRI. High signal on T2-weighted images demarcated fluid in the fracture cleft (**Fig. 70.1C**).

Diagnosis

Single-level VCF, type A, grade 2, mobile in osteoporosis

Treatment

EQUIPMENT

StabiliT Vertebral Augmentation System (DFine, San Jose, CA)
- 10-Gauge Introducer Needle and Navigational Osteotome
- Activation Element for Radio-Frequency Energy Delivery
- StabiliT ER2 Bone Cement and Hydraulic Assembly
- Multiplex Controller and Hand Switch for remote control of cement delivery

DESCRIPTION

After the patient was placed in the prone position on the angiography table, sedation was initiated, followed by local anesthesia of the skin, soft tissue, and periosteum. The 10-gauge Introducer Needle was used in a trans-pedicular approach through the right pedicle. The StraightLine Osteotome was then used to obtain a biopsy specimen and create an initial cavity within the anterior aspect of the vertebral body. Next, the Midline Navigational Osteotome was advanced into the vertebral body and through a series of articulations advanced across the midline in the anterior aspect of the vertebral

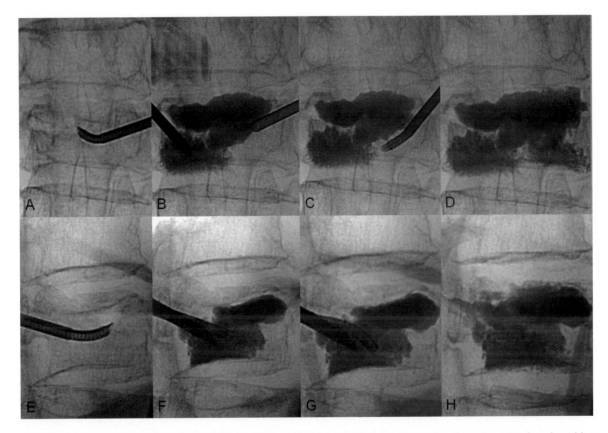

Fig. 70.2 (A–H) Radiofrequency kyphoplasty (AP/lateral, from left to right). Note that the navigational tool enables remote access and site- and size-specific cavity creation within the vertebral body. Preferential filling of these cavities as well as the interdigitation of cement with adjacent regions of compromised bone is then achieved.

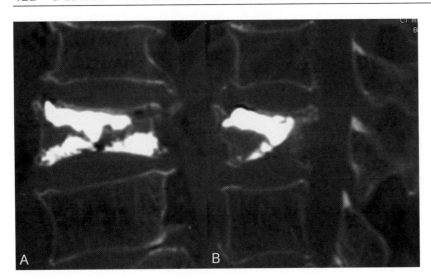

Fig. 70.3 (A,B) Plain CT after treatment (coronal, sagittal) demonstrates site-specific cement deposition.

body. The left side was accessed via a second trans-pedicular approach, and the same tool exchange was used to create cavities in and around the cleft of the fracture. High viscosity and slow application (hydraulic delivery system with remote control) facilitated excellent control, with an immediate effect on the intravertebral cement. Because of the high viscosity and surface tension of StabiliT ER2 Bone Cement after it passes through the Activation Element, it is not very susceptible to uncontrolled leakage. On the contrary, areas of cement deposition may expand and restore some of the height lost through impaction. Bilateral deposition with marked interdigitation was used to support the weakened bone and direct loading forces safely toward the lower end plate (**Fig. 70.2**). A total of ~6 mL of cement was injected. Following the procedure, the patient experienced immediate relief of her symptoms (**Fig. 70.3**).

Discussion

Background

Osteoporosis is a widespread and important disease of older patients. Untreated VCFs are associated with significant morbidity and mortality. Pain and reduced mobility are the main short-term effects, and kyphotic deformity the main longer-term effect. Most fractures are compression fractures without concomitant distraction or rotation injuries. Height loss can be graded to indicate the severity of the deformity according to the classifications of Genant and Magerl. Type A fractures can usually be treated successfully, with limitations arising depending on experience and equipment. Possible complications are spinal or foraminal stenosis due to compression or hemorrhage. Any neurologic deficit should raise suspicion and lead to a re-evaluation and possibly surgical treatment options.

Noninvasive Imaging Workup

PHYSICAL EXAMINATION

- Prior to kyphoplasty, a physical examination and neurologic examination should be performed. The typical presentation of a VCF before treatment should include the sudden onset of intense dorsal pain (VAS score > 7; minimum > 4) and the elicitation of pain by tapping or a mild axial load. Prone positioning of the patient should not be complicated by large hernias. Infection must be ruled out clinically and with laboratory tests.

RADIOGRAPHY

- In patients with typical clinical symptoms, radiography usually leads to the diagnosis of an osteoporotic VCF. The fracture grade is best appreciated when the patient is in an upright position (optimally in inclination).

CT

- Plain CT can further depict the extent of a vertebral fracture, especially involvement of the posterior wall in a burst fracture or an osseous distraction injury. Knowledge of the precise location of fracture clefts is advantageous to anticipate the effect of a cement injection and to avoid unexpected cement leakage. Trabecular impaction or fracture consolidation suggests that height restoration is less likely.

MRI

- Plain MRI should be performed if available and applicable. Ideally, T2-weighted, fat-saturated or other screening sequences will depict occult fractures and provide a full account of the symptomatic levels before treatment. MRI should exclude inflammation or previously unknown tumor and should evaluate potential cord involvement. Because kyphoplasty is not indicated in patients with old, settled fractures or osteochondrosis, the absence of bone edema or the presence of only Modic-type changes must be reported.

Invasive Workup

- Biopsy either is routinely performed or should be strongly considered before cement injection if the imaging findings cannot rule out infection or tumor.

Differential Diagnosis

- Osteoporosis is the most frequent cause of VCF. Osteolytic malignant neoplasm (myeloma, lymphoma, metastases), benign tumors (hemangioma), infection, or rarer entities (Paget disease) must be taken into account.

Treatment Options

CONSERVATIVE OR MEDICAL MANAGEMENT

- Conservative medical treatment and braces have long been the only and often sufficient treatment option for VCF.
- For patients who have an uncomplicated VCF with a low grade, conservative treatment should be the method of choice. Complications from unstable fractures and progressive deformity should be avoided, with the requirements of patient mobilization taken into account.
- When conservative treatment fails, interventional treatment is still an option.

INTERVENTIONAL MANAGEMENT

- Vertebroplasty and then kyphoplasty emerged in the mid- and late 1990s as minimally invasive treatment options for osteoporotic VCF. The indications for the two procedures do not differ and are primarily pain management and secondarily fracture stabilization. The term *kyphoplasty* was coined by manufacturers for procedures in which devices are used to create cavities and restore VCF height. Height restoration is, however, certainly not unique to these procedures and by itself not an indication to perform kyphoplasty. Developments in devices and procedures in recent years have broadened the clinical armamentarium for the interventional treatment of VCFs.

SURGICAL TREATMENT

- Surgery is the treatment of choice for complicated (not type A) VCFs with apparent or imminent neurologic compromise.

Possible Complications

- Spinal or foraminal bleeding or infection, radicular injury, dural leakage (seldom)
- Cement leakage (paravertebral, diskal, foraminal, spinal)
- Pulmonary cement embolism (not with high-viscosity cement)
- Pulmonary fat embolism

Published Literature on Treatment Options

"Radiofrequency" kyphoplasty is a minimally invasive procedure for the treatment of VCFs. It is performed with a dedicated vertebral augmentation system that has two main components designed to provide unique control of cement delivery and location: (1) a unique means of delivering an ultra–high-viscosity bone cement (gumlike) with an extended working time of ~30 minutes and (2) a proprietary Midline Osteotome, which is an articulating osteotome used to precisely create site- and size-specific cavities/channels throughout the vertebral body before cement application. Cement deposition is controlled with a hydraulic delivery system that can deliver the uniquely high-viscosity cement at a constant rate to fill the created cavities, as well as allow the cement to interdigitate with surrounding trabecular bone throughout the vertebral body. Cement in a cleft stabilizes or, if forced, drives a fracture. In simple cases, access via a single pedicle is often sufficient.

Two studies published in *The New England Journal of Medicine* in 2009 expressed doubts about the beneficial effects of percutaneous vertebroplasty in VCF. However, a recently published meta-analysis of more than 70 articles on vertebroplasty and kyphoplasty by McGirt et al suggests that physical disability is reduced and general health and pain relief are better following these procedures than after medical management within the first 3 months after intervention. Finally, the multicenter Fracture Reduction Evaluation (FREE) trial proved significant pain reduction in patients who had VCFs treated with cavity creation and adequate cement deposition.

PEARLS AND PITFALLS_____

- The uncontrolled application of cement causes rare but sometimes tragic complications. Always be sure to control the application of cement (i.e., the procedure).
- Even in complicated cases, a favorable balance between clinical benefit and technical risk must be maintained. If in doubt, re-evaluate and consider other treatment options. Always consider the patient's general physical and spine-specific status.
- Plan your treatment based on the imaging findings (consider that more is involved than just cement and two straight needles).

Further Reading

Buchbinder R, Osborne RH, Ebeling PR, et al. A randomized trial of vertebroplasty for painful osteoporotic vertebral fractures. N Engl J Med 2009;361(6):557–568

Genant HK, Wu CY, van Kuijk C, Nevitt MC. Vertebral fracture assessment using a semiquantitative technique. J Bone Miner Res 1993;8(9):1137–1148

Kallmes DF, Comstock BA, Heagerty PJ, et al. A randomized trial of vertebroplasty for osteoporotic spinal fractures. N Engl J Med 2009;361(6):569–579

Magerl F, Aebi M, Gertzbein SD, Harms J, Nazarian S. A comprehensive classification of thoracic and lumbar injuries. Eur Spine J 1994;3(4):184–201

McGirt MJ, Parker SL, Wolinsky JP, Witham TF, Bydon A, Gokaslan ZL. Vertebroplasty and kyphoplasty for the treatment of vertebral compression fractures: an evidenced-based review of the literature. Spine J 2009;9(6):501–508

Wardlaw D, Cummings SR, Van Meirhaeghe J, et al. Efficacy and safety of balloon kyphoplasty compared with non-surgical care for vertebral compression fracture (FREE): a randomised controlled trial. Lancet 2009;373(9668):1016–1024

CASE 71

Case Description

Clinical Presentation

A 44-year-old woman in whom multiple myeloma was diagnosed 10 months before the current presentation has undergone chemotherapy and radiation therapy of T11 and L2 osteolyses, but her thoracolumbar back pain has not significantly subsided during the course of treatment. The patient is referred to the oncology department of our institution for autologous stem cell transplantation. At the time of admittance, the pain level is 8/10 on the Visual Analogue Scale despite medical management with opioids. The physical examination does not reveal focal neurologic deficits or radicular symptoms. Routine MRI is not performed because of the patient's severe claustrophobia. Plain CT of the thoracic and lumbar spine is obtained.

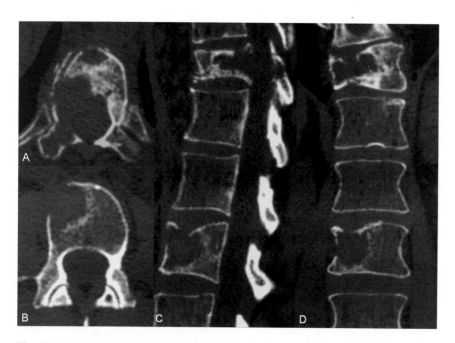

Fig. 71.1 (A–D) Plain CT (axial T11, axial L2, sagittal, coronal).

Radiologic Studies

CT

Plain CT of the thoracolumbar spine demonstrated two large osteolytic lesions (**Fig. 71.1**). At T11, a large, right-sided defect extended from the anterior to the posterior wall and involved the right pedicle. It was noted that the anterior wall provided a solid boundary, whereas the posterior wall did not show a calcified matrix. The pathologic right-sided compression fracture showed ~40% height loss and concomitant scoliosis. The L2 lesion led to an upper end plate fracture, with large defects in the upper end plate and the anterior and lateral walls. There was no noticeable spinal or foraminal tumor soft-tissue protrusion.

Diagnosis

Multiple myeloma (stage IIIA) with pathologic fractures at T11 and L2

Treatment

EQUIPMENT

StabiliT Vertebral Augmentation System (DFine, San Jose, CA)
- 10-Gauge Introducer Needle and Navigational Osteotome
- Activation Element for Radio-Frequency Energy Delivery
- StabiliT ER2 Bone Cement and Hydraulic Assembly
- Multiplex Controller and Hand Switch for remote control of cement delivery

DESCRIPTION

The patient was placed in the standard prone position under general anesthesia. A right extra-pedicular approach with the 10-gauge Introducer Needle was used for both levels. A biopsy was obtained with the StraightLine Osteotome. Carefully controlled cement delivery over an extended period of time was performed in each level until the cavities were optimally filled. Given the variable morphology of these lytic lesions, different strategies for cement application were employed at each level. In the T11 vertebra, a central deposition was made first. Afterward, a very slow delivery of cement from far anteriorly was performed to slowly drive a fairly solid front of cement posterolaterally. In the L2 vertebra, a slow injection was performed that started centrally (**Fig. 71.2**). In total, 6.0 mL of cement was administered in T11, and 2.0 mL in L2. Follow-up CT after the procedure demonstrated deposition of the cement within the previously seen osteolytic lesions (**Fig. 71.3**).

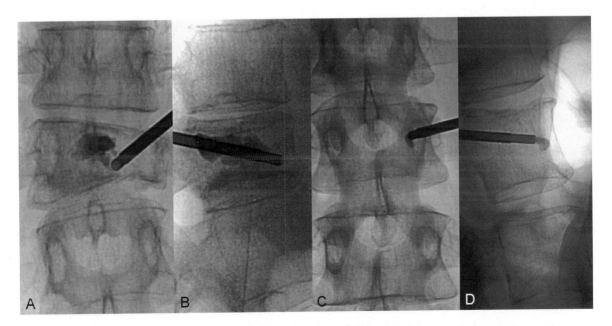

Fig. 71.2 (A–D) Radiofrequency kyphoplasty (AP/ lateral) of T11 and L2 with initial cement deposition.

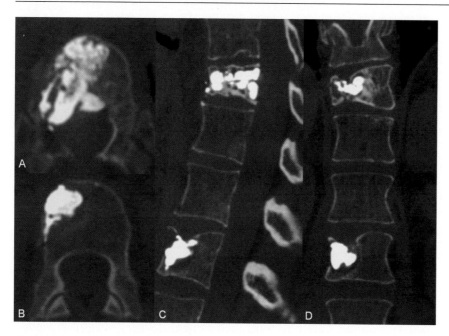

Fig. 71.3 (A–D) Plain CT after treatment (axial T11, axial L2, sagittal, coronal) demonstrates site-specific cement deposition.

Discussion

Background

Lytic tumors (i.e., multiple myeloma, metastases, and rarely hemangioma or other benign entities) are classically the lesions for which minimally invasive cement procedures such as vertebroplasty and kyphoplasty are indicated. Historically, the use of cement in non–spine-related cementoplasty with polymethylmethacrylate has been well documented. Pain may arise from hard tissue instability due to an unconsolidated pathologic vertebral compression fracture (VCF; simple end plate fracture or vertebral collapse), or the pain may be tumor-specific. Spinal or foraminal stenosis with radicular symptoms may be caused by tumor mass effect, fracture, or a combination of both. The principal purpose of minimally invasive cement injection is to alleviate pain. It is important not to consider vertebroplasty as antitumoral therapy. In nonpalliative care, it should be complementary to chemotherapy and radiotherapy, with the sequence determined in each case by the symptoms and treatment concept. Practice guidelines for each tumor entity should be followed. Technical limitations due to tumor bleeding or imminent neurologic deficit must be considered.

Noninvasive Imaging Workup

RADIOGRAPHY

- Most VCFs in patients with back pain are osteoporotic fractures with typical imaging findings. However, a pathologic vertebral fracture can lead to a cancer diagnosis, or a fracture may occur during the course of known cancer. Regardless, radiography is usually the first-line imaging modality. Generally, atypical radiographic findings without evidence of osteopenia or trauma should raise the index of suspicion for malignancy and lead to further imaging and clinical workup.

CT

- CT can be obtained for further diagnosis or for planning treatment. In our institution, a plain spine scan is performed routinely. In patients with symptomatic tumors, multiplanar reformats of scheduled contrast-enhanced thoracic or abdominal scans may also reveal compression fractures (either osteoporotic or tumoral). For the purpose of staging many entities, including multiple myeloma, CT can replace plain radiography. For planning treatment, a careful evaluation of the fractured vertebrae is mandatory. In planning the site of cement delivery and the amount to be delivered, knowledge of the fracture lines and especially the location of larger lytic defects is a prerequisite for a successful intervention. Purely osteoblastic lesions are not an indication for vertebroplasty or kyphoplasty.

MRI

- Plain MRI should be performed if available and applicable. Ideally, T2-weighted, fat-saturated or other screening sequences will depict tumoral lesions and occult fractures, providing a complete preoperative morphologic assessment. Contrast-enhanced imaging (T1-weighted, fat-saturated) further increases sensitivity and specificity. Inflammation or cord involvement must be evaluated.

Treatment Options

CONSERVATIVE OR MEDICAL MANAGEMENT

- Conservative medical treatment can be sufficient for many patients with tumor-associated VCF if adequate pain control can be achieved.
- In patients with uncomplicated pathologic fractures, conservative treatment should be the method of choice. Complications from unstable fractures and progressive deformity should be avoided, with the requirements of patient mobilization taken into account.
- When conservative treatment fails, interventional treatment is still an option.

RADIATION THERAPY

- Radiation therapy is effective for several radiation-sensitive entities, including myeloma.
- Tumor growth is controlled reliably in these entities. Symptoms (also neurologic) may lessen after radiation therapy or chemotherapy if the tumor size decreases.
- Pain relief is usually achieved in the course of therapy. The time interval depends on the dose concept and fractionation scheme. Pain from unstable fractures is less likely to decrease permanently.
- Stability is not significantly improved in the short term. In the long term, remineralization and sclerotic encasement may occur.

INTERVENTIONAL MANAGEMENT

- Vertebroplasty was first performed for a symptomatic hemangioma in 1984. Since then, vertebroplasty and later kyphoplasty have been performed frequently in patients with tumors.
- Indications for both procedures are primarily pain management and secondarily fracture stabilization. The pain usually decreases significantly during the days following the intervention. Stability is provided immediately after the intervention.
- To date, many systems are available for the treatment of pathologic VCF.
- In the case presented, radiofrequency kyphoplasty accomplished the following:
  - It provided unique control in the larger lytic defects adjacent to a structure at risk, such as the spinal cord or a nerve root.
  - It reduced the potential for the symptomatic extravasation of cement associated with the use of lower-viscosity cements and for balloon-related injuries associated with the use of inflatable balloons in severely lytic vertebrae with compromised posterior walls.

SURGICAL TREATMENT

- Surgery is the treatment of choice for patients with apparent or imminent severe neurologic compromise.

Possible Complications

- Spinal or foraminal bleeding or infection, radicular injury, dural leakage (rare)
- Cement leakage (paravertebral, diskal, foraminal, spinal) and pulmonary cement or fat embolism

Published Literature on Treatment Options

Published studies have proven that pain is reduced after vertebroplasty in patients with tumor-associated VCFs, although further studies should raise the level of evidence. In oncology patients, it is of special importance to establish an interdisciplinary approach to treatment and to respect tumor-specific practice guidelines. Given the careful administration of cement required in severely lytic vertebrae, an ultra–high-viscosity cement with an extended working time of more than 30 minutes facilitates a thoughtful and controlled procedure. The ability to deliver cement with a remotely controlled system, thereby reducing the operator's exposure to radiation, is attractive, given the length of time complicated procedures may require.

PEARLS AND PITFALLS_____

- As in the treatment of osteoporotic VCFs, biplanar (AP and lateral) fluoroscopy is ideal for this procedure. On occasion, CT guidance may be advantageous. In most cases, treatment planning based on preoperative cross-sectional imaging is advisable (CT/MRI). Critical cases may require both.
- The standard access is trans-pedicular for most lumbar VCFs and extrapedicular for most thoracic VCFs.

Further Reading

Boswell MV, Trescot AM, Datta S, et al; American Society of Interventional Pain Physicians. Interventional techniques: evidence-based practice guidelines in the management of chronic spinal pain. Pain Physician 2007;10(1):7–111

Galibert P, Deramond H, Rosat P, Le Gars D. [Preliminary note on the treatment of vertebral angioma by percutaneous acrylic vertebroplasty]. Neurochirurgie 1987;33(2):166–168

Hussein MA, Vrionis FD, Allison R, et al; International Myeloma Working Group. The role of vertebral augmentation in multiple myeloma: International Myeloma Working Group Consensus Statement. Leukemia 2008;22(8):1479–1484

McGirt MJ, Parker SL, Wolinsky JP, Witham TF, Bydon A, Gokaslan ZL. Vertebroplasty and kyphoplasty for the treatment of vertebral compression fractures: an evidenced-based review of the literature. Spine J 2009;9(6):501–508

Ofluoglu O. Minimally invasive management of spinal metastases. Orthop Clin North Am 2009;40(1):155–168, viii

CASE 72

Case Description

Clinical Presentation

A 56-year-old man has had left lateral lower back pain irradiating toward the left knee with local spinal tenderness for more than 3 months. The pain becomes worse with exertion and is worse in the mornings. Anti-inflammatory drugs give him only temporary pain relief.

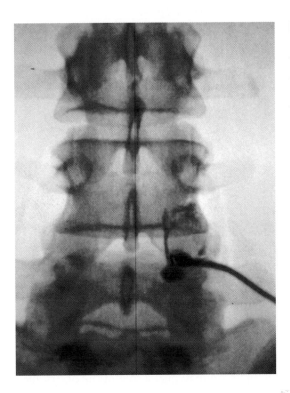

Fig. 72.1 Needle position in the left L4-5 facet joint before anesthetic injection, with the ring arthrogram verifying the intra-articular position of the needle tip.

Radiologic Studies

CT

Outside imaging with unenhanced CT of the lumbosacral spine demonstrated mild degenerative facet joint changes, most pronounced at the left L4-5 level, with osteophytic spurring. There was no evidence of a disk herniation or protrusion.

Diagnosis

Lumbar facet arthropathy left L4-5

Treatment

EQUIPMENT

- A 22-gauge spinal needle
- Contrast
- Local anesthetic (1 mL of 0.5% bupivacaine) with steroids (20 mg of triamcinolone)

DESCRIPTION

The patient was placed in the prone position on the angiography table. Following careful disinfection of the skin, the spinal needle was inserted over the inferomedial aspect of the joint and advanced until the tip touched the lamina. The correct position of the needle was confirmed on a lateral view. A small amount of contrast material was slowly injected to confirm the position of the needle within the facet joint and demonstrated a classic ring arthrogram (**Fig. 72.1**) outlining the borders of the joint without entering the superior synovial recess. As the mixture of local anesthetic and steroid was injected, the patient said that he felt his typical pain worsening. After completion of the injection, the needle was removed. The patient was observed for 1 hour in the recovery room and then sent home. He came back 1 week later, completely free of pain after the procedure.

Discussion

Background

Local spinal pain and radiculopathy are very common conditions that debilitate more than half of the population of the United States at some point during their lifetime. The prevalence of these conditions is at least 5% annually. The role of the facet joints as a source of low back pain has been well established. The facet joints are synovial joints, with a joint space, hyaline cartilage surfaces, a synovial membrane, and a fibrous capsule. Because of the presence of nociceptive fibers within the facet joints, pain may occur when the joints are subjected to increased loads. The facet joints are innervated by the medial branches of the dorsal rami of the spinal nerves, which means that pain may be referred to the buttocks, loins, groins, or legs. The exact pathologic mechanism and cause of the pain is unknown; microtrauma, osteoarthritis, distension or inflammatory changes of the synovium, meniscoid entrapment, synovial impingement, or joint subluxation may play a role in the occurrence of symptoms. The prevalence of lumbar facet arthropathy is higher in the elderly.

Noninvasive Imaging Workup

PHYSICAL EXAMINATION

- The classic symptom of facet joint arthropathy is low back pain radiating in a nonradicular pattern to the hip and buttock and to below or just above the knee. In addition, local spinal tenderness, the exacerbation of pain during exertion or rotation, and morning pain and stiffness may be present. Occasional relief may be obtained with anti-inflammatory drugs or the application of heat.

RADIOGRAPHY/CT/MRI/NUCLEAR MEDICINE FINDINGS

- Imaging abnormalities do not correlate with the symptoms in most cases.
- Abnormalities of the joints may be present, including hypertrophic facet joint arthropathy, osteophytic spurring, accumulation of fluid in the joint capsule, and synovial cysts.
- Mild enhancement may be seen in the affected joint.
- Bone scan may reveal locally increased bony turnover.

Invasive Imaging Workup

- Facet joint arthropathy is classically diagnosed on clinical grounds and confirmed by a facet joint block, which will eliminate the pain. The invasive procedure therefore has a dual role of diagnostic confirmation and symptomatic treatment.

Differential Diagnosis

- Lumbar degenerative disk disease, lumbar compression fracture
- Spondylolysis or spondylolisthesis
- Sacroiliac joint syndrome, piriformis syndrome
- Chronic pain syndrome, fibromyalgia, myofascial pain

Treatment Options

CONSERVATIVE OR MEDICAL MANAGEMENT

- Most cases of facet joint arthopathy are successfully treated conservatively with rest, physical therapy, and anti-inflammatory drugs.
- Chiropractic manipulations are commonly done, although physicians do not frequently recommend them to their patients.
- Local heat may relieve the symptoms.
- When conservative treatment fails, interventional treatment may be the next step in the escalation of therapy.

PERCUTANEOUS APPROACHES

- Intra-articular injections can be performed via either an oblique approach or a direct vertical posterior approach. The latter approach may be a better choice if the joint has a curved configuration or if excessive osteophytes are present.
- Occasionally, attempts to cannulate the joint fail, particularly in the presence of advanced degenerative changes. In this situation, a periarticular injection can be given, or a block of the medial branch of the posterior ramus of the spinal nerve attempted.
- Imaging can be performed under fluoroscopy or CT control; the latter is recommended in the presence of significant degenerative changes and offers advantages when difficult or small targets must be reached with a high accuracy rate.
- On fluoroscopy, the anterior aspect of the lumbar facet joint is best seen with a 30- to 45-degree angulation of the AP tube, whereas the posterior aspect is seen with a smaller degree of angulation. The target of the needle should be the posterior and inferior aspect of the joint; in the upper lumbar vertebrae, the approach will be more vertical, whereas in the lower lumbar vertebrae, the approach will be more oblique.

SURGICAL TREATMENT

- Surgical treatment is classically not indicated and may be reserved for the very small number of patients who fail all of the less invasive procedures. Very careful consideration of the risks versus the potential benefits of the intervention is mandatory before such a treatment plan is undertaken.

Possible Complications

- Cushing syndrome (especially if multiple levels are injected with steroids)
- Infection
- Allergic reactions to any of the injected fluids

- Nerve damage
- Hemorrhage

Published Literature on Treatment Options

Injection of the lumbar facet joints with local anesthetics and steroids is an established diagnostic and therapeutic procedure despite inconclusive evidence that it has a beneficial effect, according to a recent Cochrane Review by Nelemans et al. A randomized trial conducted by Lilius et al found no significant difference between intra-articular injection of steroid, periarticular injection of steroid, and intra-articular injection of saline; 64% of patients demonstrated an initially good response, but the proportion fell to 23% at 3 months. A study by Carette et al showed no statistical difference between corticosteroid and saline injection in patients with a previous positive response to local anesthetic, although the trend favored the corticosteroid group. The apparent beneficial effect of the saline injections may, however, not necessarily be due only to a placebo effect; it may also be related to some other factor, such as distension or rupture of the joint capsule. Despite the paucity of evidence, facet joint injections are still widely performed. In our opinion, the diagnostic component of the test is of major importance because the local anesthetic component of the injection can determine if the facet joints are the source of patient's pain. Patients with a good early response to the injection can be considered for a more permanent treatment, such as medial branch rhizotomy (neurotomy), radiofrequency ablation, or percutaneous cryodenervation of the facet joints.

PEARLS AND PITFALLS

- Because the procedure is easy and can be done quickly, prior disinfection of the skin may be neglected, which can lead to severe complications. The most important step of this procedure is, in our opinion, proper skin disinfection and absolutely sterile handling of the injection needle, contrast, and steroids/anesthetic to be injected. The smallest (22-gauge or smaller) needle possible should be used.
- A physician's preference for a given technique (CT/fluoroscopy) is largely related to training and experience and does not necessarily mean that the alternatives are inferior or more dangerous.
- Exacerbation of the patient's typical pain during injection of the anesthetic/steroids is a sign that the facet joints are indeed the culprit causing the pain (extension of the disk space), which typically regresses over the next 15 minutes.

Further Reading

Carette S, Marcoux S, Truchon R, et al. A controlled trial of corticosteroid injections into facet joints for chronic low back pain. N Engl J Med 1991;325(14):1002–1007

Gallucci M, Conchiglia A, Lanni G, Conti L, Limbucci N. Treatments for sciatica mimics: facets and sacroiliac joints. Neuroradiol J 2009;22:154–160

Lilius G, Laasonen EM, Myllynen P, Harilainen A, Grönlund G. Lumbar facet joint syndrome. A randomised clinical trial. J Bone Joint Surg Br 1989;71(4):681–684

Nelemans PJ, de Bie RA, de Vet HC, Sturmans F. Injection therapy for subacute and chronic benign low back pain. Cochrane Database Syst Rev 2000;(2):CD001824

Silbergleit R, Mehta BA, Sanders WP, Talati SJ. Imaging-guided injection techniques with fluoroscopy and CT for spinal pain management. Radiographics 2001;21(4):927–939, discussion 940–942

Index

Note: Page numbers followed by *f* and *t* indicate figures and tables, respectively.

435